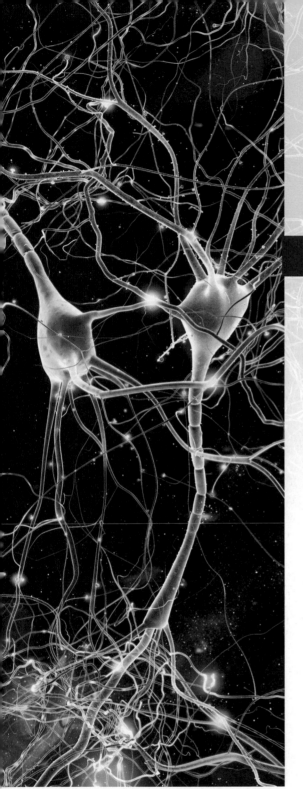

T0175210

The Only
NEUROLOGY
BOOK

You'll Ever Need

ALISON I. THALER, MD
MALCOLM S. THALER, MD

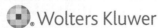
Wolters Kluwer

Philadelphia · Baltimore · New York · London
Buenos Aires · Hong Kong · Sydney · Tokyo

Acquisitions Editor: Joe Cho
Development Editor: Thomas Celona
Editorial Coordinator: Oliver Raj
Marketing Manager: Kirsten Watrud
Senior Production Project Manager: Alicia Jackson
Manager, Graphic Arts & Design: Stephen Druding
Art Director, Illustration: Jennifer Clements
Illustrator: TNQ Technologies
Senior Manufacturing Coordinator: Beth Welsh
Prepress Vendor: TNQ Technologies

Printed in Mexico

Library of Congress Cataloging-in-Publication Data

Names: Thaler, Alison I., author. | Thaler, Malcolm S., author.
Title: The only neurology book you'll ever need / Alison I. Thaler, Malcolm
  S. Thaler.
Description: Philadelphia : Wolters Kluwer, [2023] | Includes
  bibliographical references and index.
Identifiers: LCCN 2021053853 (print) | LCCN 2021053854 (ebook) | ISBN
  9781975158675 (paperback) | ISBN 9781975158712 (epub) | ISBN
  9781975158729 (epub)
Subjects: MESH: Nervous System Diseases | Case Reports | BISAC: MEDICAL /
  Neurology | MEDICAL / Test Preparation & Review
Classification: LCC RC346 (print) | LCC RC346 (ebook) | NLM WL 140 | DDC
  616.8--dc23/eng/20211209
LC record available at https://lccn.loc.gov/2021053853
LC ebook record available at https://lccn.loc.gov/2021053854

QUADM0822

Foreword

In this book, Drs. Alison I. Thaler and Malcolm S. Thaler have managed to complete an almost impossible task: to take a clinical discipline as complicated as neurology and break it down into its simple and digestible components. You will learn about stroke, seizures, aneurysms, neuropathies, migraines, and all manner of neurological disease. But you will also learn the *approach* to the neurological patient, told with the voices of those who have been there and seen it all. It is a companion that you want at your side.

In the early years of preclinical training, students are introduced to the endlessly complicated neuroanatomical pathways. Later, when they enter the wards and are confronted with patients suffering from neurological disease or injury, they can find it difficult to put those pathways into clinical practice. How should you approach a patient who presents with a neurological problem? When patients tell you that they haven't been able to move their right leg for the past two hours, what should you do? How worried should you be, and should you call for help? What might be going on, and what kinds of disease processes might leave the patient devastated if you don't react quickly and appropriately? This book provides you with the critical tools that you'll need to be able to think through questions like these in a clear and concise manner.

This is not a textbook in neurology. It is not an encyclopedic review of neuroanatomy or pathophysiology. Instead, it highlights *what you need to know*—as a third-year medical student studying for the shelf; a neurology resident preparing for night float; or a nurse, physician's assistant, or physician faced with evaluating and treating neurologic disease. The relevant neuroanatomy and pathophysiology are brought to life and given clinical context.

Look to this book for pearls about what to do in various clinical scenarios—how to triage, how to get a sense of which kinds of neurological presentations are emergencies and which can wait until the next day to try to figure out. You will learn how to diagnose and treat these patients in a straightforward and always evidence-based manner. And while learning about these neurological conditions, you will also be taken on a wonderful tour of the fundamentals of clinical neurology.

Michael Fara, MD, PhD
Assistant Professor of Neurology
Interim Director, Stroke Center at Mount Sinai Hospital
Icahn School of Medicine at Mount Sinai
New York, New York

Steven Galetta, MD
Chair of the Department of Neurology
Professor of Neurology and Neuro-Ophthalmology
NYU Grossman School of Medicine
New York, New York

Preface

Neurology has the reputation—well-deserved, if perhaps overstated—of being hard. Fascinating—yes. Intellectually stimulating—of course. Worth the investment in time and overworked neurons—without a doubt! But hard. So that's why we're here, and why we created this book. Not to make it easy—that would be a claim you could see through from a mile away—but to make it *easier*. To help you make sense of it all. To take all that anatomy and physiology, all those syndromes and categories and treatment protocols, and wrap them up into manageable bundles that are clear, concise, and practical. And while we're at it, we are going to make it fun. No, really. We promise you are going to enjoy mastering this material (OK, we admit that memorizing the brachial plexus may not be your ideal version of fun, but we will do our best!).

This book is different from other neurology books you may have encountered. The text is conversational. There are tons of illustrations and images. Clinical pearls—the kinds of things you won't find in other books—are sprinkled liberally throughout. Most importantly, we focus on those elements of neurology that matter most for patient care. Our goal is not to impress you with vast quantities of neuroanatomic esoterica; rather, we will stress over and over again the basic principles underlying neurologic diagnosis and management.

And there is something else that we believe makes this book special. It offers a dual perspective on neurology. One of us is a neurologist, the other an internist. Both of us devote a large portion of our time to academic clinical teaching. By combining the perspectives of our two specialties, we can share with you the most real-life and up-to-date details that only a neurologist would know, as well as the broader perspective and patient-oriented approach that is an internist's stock in trade. We dig deep when we have to and then pull back to make sure that everything we discuss is clinically relevant and patient centered.

This book can and should be used differently depending on who you are and what you want out of it. It covers everything you need for the medical student shelf examination but at times goes above and beyond, so if you want only streamlined and testable material, focus on the flashcards in the companion ebook and bolded topics in the text; use the rest of the book as a reference, to help clarify when something doesn't make sense, when you find yourself wanting to know more about a particular topic, or when you need to prepare a presentation for rounds. For preliminary interns and junior neurology residents, read it cover-to-cover. We have done our best to make sure it reads lightly and quickly (at least as far as medical textbooks go!), and it contains everything we wish we'd known at the start of our careers. You will be as well prepared for neurology residency as is possible, we promise. And for non-neurology trained physicians, nurses, NPAs and PAs who treat patients with neurologic illness, keep this by your side as a companion—an easily digestible *what-you-really-need-to-know* guide to the diagnosis and management of neurologic disease.

We can't let you get started without first acknowledging all of the extraordinary clinicians and academicians who reviewed our chapters, offered their subspecialized wisdom, rolled their eyes at times but were always kind, supportive, and as excited about this book as we are. In particular, we want to thank Drs. Laura Stein, Michael Fara, Stephen Krieger, Rajeev Motiwala, Susan Shin, Joanna Jen, Allison Navis, Mark Green, Anna Pace, Anuradha Singh, Caroline Crooms, Noam Harel, Amy Chan, Praveen Raju, Joshua Friedman, Benjamin Brush, Kenneth Leung, Emily Schorr, and Steven Galetta. We couldn't have done this without you. We also want to thank the amazing folks at Wolters Kluwer who saw this book through from inception to reality: Sharon Zinner, Lindsay Ries, Oli Raj, Thomas Celona, Chris Teja, Joe Cho, and the incredibly talented artists at TNQ. And lastly, we want to express our gratitude to our students for making us better teachers, and our patients who every day make us better human beings.

We dedicate this book to our families. It is a tiresome cliche to state how they stood by us even as we drove them crazy with all the time and energy we devoted to this project, but cliches are cliches for a reason. So thank you Ben and Nancy and Jon and Tracey—we love you, couldn't live without you, and promise we will be back in touch as soon as we finish plotting out the next edition!

Alison I. Thaler
Malcolm S. Thaler

Contents

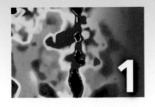

Let's Get Started: Your Neurologic Toolbox

1

In this chapter, you will learn:

1 | The basic anatomy of the nervous system in a streamlined and straightforward way that you can apply directly to clinical practice

2 | How to take a useful neurologic history

3 | The essentials of the neurologic examination, and what each test can tell you about the localization (*i.e.*, the anatomy) of the patient's problem

4 | The tools to help you in the diagnosis and management of neurologic issues; these include imaging (computed tomography [CT], magnetic resonance imaging [MRI] and some other tests you may not be as familiar with), lumbar puncture, electroencephalography (EEG), nerve conduction tests (NCS), and electromyography (EMG)

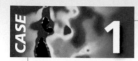

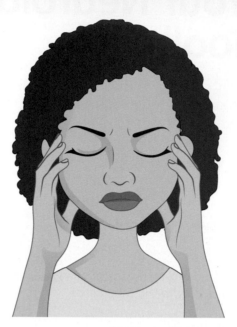

Your Patient: Hailey, a 30-year-old woman with no past medical history, comes to the emergency department complaining of a worsening headache. She has a long history of headaches but they typically resolve with ibuprofen and a good night's sleep. This headache, however, has persisted for more than 7 days and nothing seems to make it better. Her vitals are stable and her neurologic examination is normal. She is given metoclopramide and ketorolac and within an hour feels significantly better. Your attending asks you if you think she's ready for discharge. What's your answer—is Hailey ready to return home?

By the time you have finished this chapter, you will be exhausted (there are no two ways about it; there is a lot of material to learn) but ready to take on the world of neurologic disease!

In a broad sense, all disease is experienced through the nervous system. Physical pain, emotional pain—really, any kind of sensation, good or bad—is sensed, transmitted, and perceived by the neurologic system. Our thoughts, feelings, and memories are neurologic as well, and when they go awry you can point your finger at the brain as the responsible party.

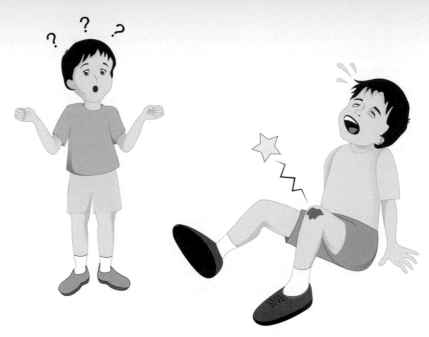

It's all in your head, whether it's mental confusion or a skinned knee.

However, what we mean when we speak of neurologic disease, and what you expected when you picked up this book, is any disorder where *the primary pathology resides in the brain, spinal cord, or peripheral nerves* (the *neuromuscular junction and muscles* are included in the domain of neurology as well, and we won't overlook them). And there are plenty of these conditions to keep us busy for the next several hundred pages!

Neuroanatomy: The Basics

Before we go any further, let's walk through the basic structure of the nervous system. The nervous system can be conceived of as being divided into three parts: the central, peripheral, and autonomic nervous systems.

1. The *central nervous system (CNS)* includes the brain, brainstem, and spinal cord. All are protected by bone and three thin membranes called the *meninges*: the *dura, arachnoid,* and *pia.* Most of the brain is also protected by the *blood-brain barrier,* a term that refers to a special property of the cerebral blood vessels that limits the passage of many potentially harmful substances, such as circulating hormones, toxins, and pathogens, from the blood into the extracellular fluid of the brain.

2. The *peripheral nervous system (PNS)* includes all the neurons and ganglia (*i.e.,* groups of nerve cell bodies) that lie outside of the brain and spinal cord. The cranial nerves, with the exception of the olfactory (CN1) and optic nerve (CN2), are part of the PNS. Unlike the CNS, the PNS is not protected by bone, meninges, or the blood-brain barrier and is therefore more vulnerable to injury. The PNS is divided into somatic and autonomic divisions.

a. The *somatic division* consists of sensory and motor neurons. Specifically, we speak of *sensory afferents* (afferent means conducting inward), which receive and pass on sensory information from the outside world, and *motor efferents* (efferent meaning conducting outward), which enable voluntary movement. These neurons are also responsible for deep tendon reflexes (see page 26).

b. The *autonomic division* is part of the overall autonomic nervous system (see below) and includes both the sympathetic and parasympathetic nerves. The sympathetic nerves use the neurotransmitters acetylcholine and norepinephrine to communicate, whereas the parasympathetic nerves use only acetylcholine. These two systems typically function in opposition to each other, triggering an event or response that is countered by the other system. The sympathetic nerves mediate the 'fight or flight' response (for example, pupillary dilation to allow more light to enter the eye; bronchodilation to promote oxygen exchange; and vasoconstriction to divert blood flow away from the GI tract and skin and redirect it to the skeletal muscles). The parasympathetic nerves mediate the 'rest and digest' response (for example, pupillary constriction; bronchoconstriction; and vasodilation to the GI tract and skin).

3. The *autonomic nervous system* regulates visceral functions such as digestion, temperature, heart rate, and blood pressure. It is made up of components of both the PNS (the autonomic division, as above) and CNS (including structures we haven't discussed yet—the insular cortex, brainstem, and hypothalamus, among others). The autonomic nervous system also contains the enteric nervous system, which integrates information about the gastrointestinal (GI) tract and provides output to control and coordinate GI tract functions and local blood flow.

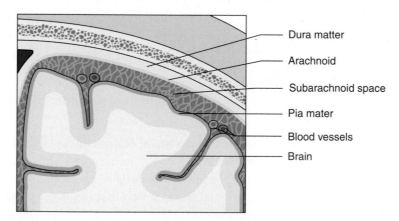

The meninges. The dura is the outermost and toughest layer that lies directly beneath the skull. The arachnoid, a thinner, spidery membrane, is separated from the dura by a potential space; in other words, under normal conditions, the dura and arachnoid are touching one another, but under pathologic conditions (a subdural bleed, for instance), they can become separated as the space fills with fluid. The pia is the innermost and most delicate layer; it clings to the gyri (the folds) of the brain. Cerebrospinal fluid (CSF) flows between the arachnoid and pia in the subarachnoid space. Together, the arachnoid and pia are known as the leptomeninges.

Box 1.1

The brain—even yours (even ours!)—is incontrovertibly amazing. The human brain weighs about 3 pounds and has the consistency and appearance of tofu. Estimates vary, but the average brain has around 100 billion neurons with trillions of connections among them. Our whole life is lived inside our brain. Everything we perceive about the world around us is nothing but a panoply of electrical signals whizzing from neuron to neuron. The sky, after all, isn't really "blue" in the way we might be tempted to think of blue—photons aren't intrinsically blue—rather, they have a wavelength that appears blue to us because of the way the brain interprets the electrical signals generated by our looking at the sky. Nor do sound waves intrinsically sound like Beyoncé or Beethoven. And what is a thought or a feeling or a memory other than a way of integrating and interpreting electrochemical currents racing through our cerebral cortex? It's pretty incredible when you stop to think about it.

There is a lot of complex anatomy that goes into each of these systems. But rather than burden you with all of it at once, we will give you the basics now and fill in many of the details later as we need them.

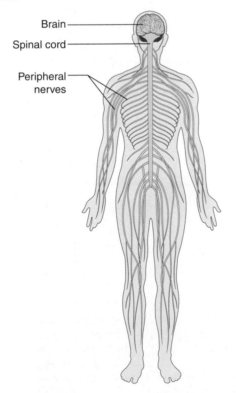

The nervous system.

Brain Anatomy 101. The brain consists of the *cerebrum*, the *brainstem*, and the *cerebellum*. The cerebrum is divided into two hemispheres (left and right), which communicate electrically across a band of nerve fibers called the *corpus callosum*. There are four lobes on each side: the frontal, parietal, temporal, and occipital lobes. The outermost layer of the cerebrum, the cerebral cortex, contains *gray matter*—the cell bodies of the neurons—and the interior consists of *white matter*—the nerve fibers, or axons. The structures that lie deep within the brain (including the thalamus and the basal ganglia) are also gray matter. The brainstem consists of the midbrain, pons, and medulla. The cerebellum lies posterior to the cerebrum and brainstem.

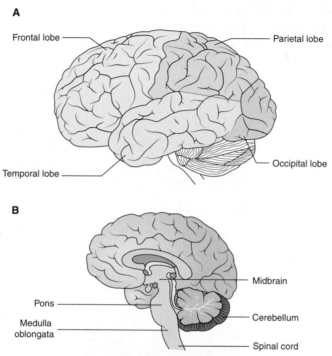

(*A*) The four lobes of the cerebrum. (*B*) The brainstem and cerebellum.

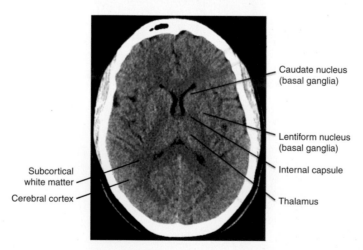

A CT of the head, showing the cerebral cortex, subcortical white matter, and deep gray matter structures, including the thalamus and basal ganglia (which includes the caudate and lentiform nucleus). As we will discuss later in this chapter, white matter (such as the internal capsule) actually appears dark on CT (owing to the high content of myelin, which is a fatty substance and therefore relatively low density compared with the cellular gray matter), and gray matter (such as the cortex, the basal ganglia and thalamus) appears bright. (Modified from Farrell TA. *Radiology 101*. 5th ed. Wolters Kluwer; 2019.)

The brain is protected by the skull and the three meninges. The blood supply to the brain can be divided into two sources: (1) the anterior (carotid) circulation and (2) the posterior (vertebrobasilar) circulation. They are linked by anastomoses at the base of the brain in a structure called the circle of Willis (see Chapter 2, page 50). Venous sinuses lie within the dura, and these drain both blood and CSF.

The brain is also home to four ventricles: two lateral ventricles, the third ventricle, and the fourth ventricle. The ventricles are hollow spaces within the brain and brainstem that contain the CSF. CSF is produced by modified ependymal cells known as the choroid plexus that are located within the ventricles. CSF flows from the lateral ventricles down through the third ventricle, fourth ventricle, the central canal of the spinal cord, and into the subarachnoid space, where it will ultimately be passively reabsorbed by arachnoid villi (also known as granulations; these are small protrusions of arachnoid into the dura) into the dural venous sinuses.

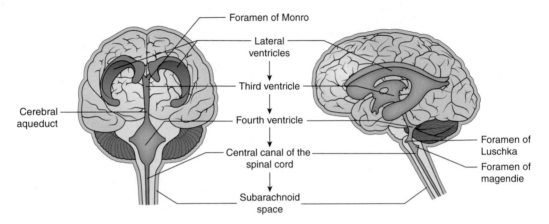

The pathway of the ventricular system. The CSF flows from the lateral ventricles into the third ventricle (via the foramen of Monro), into the fourth ventricle (via the cerebral aqueduct), into the central canal of the spinal cord (via the foramen of Magendie and Luschka), and finally into the subarachnoid space that surrounds the spinal cord and the brain.

Electrophysiology in Two Pages

The basic unit of the nervous system is the *neuron*, a specialized cell that can transmit electric current. Neurons are not just passive conduits for electricity; they also receive, integrate, transform, and send signals to other neurons. Most neurons in the PNS are unipolar, connecting to just one other target neuron or muscle cell. Neurons in the CNS can be multipolar, often making connections with thousands of other neurons.

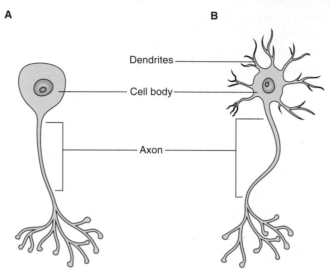

(*A*) unipolar and (*B*) multipolar neurons.

Action potentials are carefully choreographed electrical events that involve the opening and closing of potassium, sodium, and calcium channels in the neuronal membrane and that propagate down the neuron, creating an electric current. The ability of neurons to conduct action potentials is enhanced by an external insulating layer called *myelin*, produced by specific types of *glial cells* (these are called Schwann cells in the periphery and oligodendrocytes in the brain), which effectively prevents current from leaking out of the neurons and thereby significantly speeds up nerve conduction.

Neurons talk to each other across a space called the *synapse*, and this conversation is carried on by chemicals called *neurotransmitters*, which are released by the arrival of an action potential at the synapse. There are many types of neurotransmitters; most of the ones you know already are small peptides such as acetylcholine, GABA, glutamate, serotonin, and the catecholamines (dopamine, epinephrine, and norepinephrine).

Box 1.2 Voltage-Gated Sodium Channel Toxins

Voltage-gated sodium channels are a crucial component of action potentials and therefore fundamental for neuronal functioning. As you might imagine, ingestion of toxins that block these channels can have a devastating effect. *Tetrodotoxin*, present in pufferfish and other animals, is a potent sodium channel blocker that, when ingested, prevents neurons from communicating with each other. Symptoms develop rapidly and include paresthesias, dizziness, nausea, vomiting, tremor and, if severe, seizures, paralysis, cardiac arrhythmias, and even death. Treatment consists of activated charcoal (to bind the toxin) and gut lavage (to get it out of the body). There is no known specific antidote.

In disease, things can go wrong at any of these locations—the nerve cell, myelin sheath, or synapse.

But keep in mind, as we move from one disorder to the next, that our neurologic system is also what makes life worth living. It's not all about disease. Our ability to sense pleasure and beauty are all rooted in our neurons. With so much at stake, it is no wonder neurologic disease can be so catastrophic.

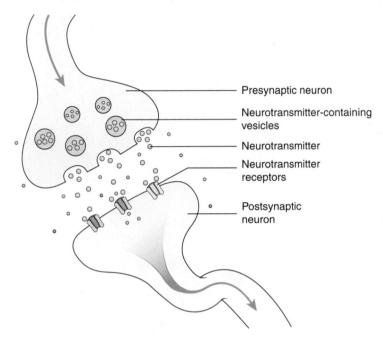

The synapse is the place where neurons communicate with each other.

 ## *The Good News!*

With our neurologic system responsible for so much, it would be easy to throw up our hands and proclaim that it must be impossible to figure out what is going on when things go haywire. But our neurologic toolbox—the instruments we have at our disposal to diagnose neurologic disorders—is compact and, with the help of this book, something that you will soon grow comfortable applying to any and all neurologic issues. Learn how to use these tools and the world of neurology will unfold before you. The most essential elements of our neurologic toolbox are:

- History
- Neurologic examination
- Lumbar puncture (for CSF analysis)
- Electroencephalography (EEG)
- Imaging (CT and MRI, among others)
- Nerve conduction studies (NCS) and electromyography (EMG)

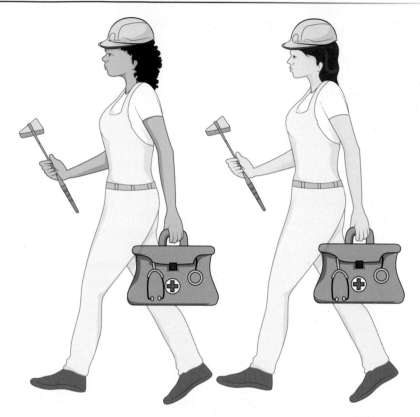

So let's get familiar with each item in our toolbox, and then we can move on to discussing the neurologic disorders you will need to be familiar with. We are going to take each item one by one, starting with the neurologic history.

 ## The Neurologic History

Before picking up a spinal needle or ordering an MRI, neurologists, arguably more than in any other field of medicine, rely on a good history to guide their differential diagnosis and subsequent management. A common misconception is that taking a good neurologic history needs to take *War and Peace*-length amounts of time. It does not. We would in fact argue that the more skilled at this you become, the more concise and directed your history can be. You've almost certainly already learned the gist of it in your previous training.

Step 1: Your Basic OPQRST. Do not skimp on this step!

Box 1.3

Thank goodness for mnemonics (the only word, besides mnemophobia [yes, this is a word], in the English language that begins with an "m" followed by an "n"; the term is derived from Mnemosyne, the Greek goddess of memory). OPQRST is the first but far from the last mnemonic you will encounter in this book.

OPQRST is a guide to the key items in your history that will help you tease out the details of a patient's illness and help with the diagnosis and subsequent management:

- **O: Onset**—Did the symptom come on suddenly or gradually, and what was happening when the symptom began?
- **P: Provocation**—What makes the symptom better, what makes it worse?
- **Q: Quality**—Ask the patient to describe the symptom. This can be difficult for even the most articulate patient, so be patient.
- **R: Region or Radiation**—Where is the symptom located? Is it localized or generalized? Does it move to other areas of the body?
- **S: Severity**—How bad is the symptom? If the symptom is weakness, for instance, is it subtle, complete paralysis, or something in between? If the symptom is pain, many clinicians use a pain scale of 0 to 10, but a good verbal description is often more helpful.
- **T: Time**—How long has this been going on? Has it happened before? Has the pain/sensation changed over time?

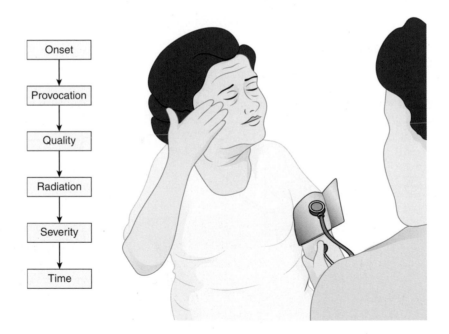

When neurologic disease affects the brain, it may be impossible for your patient to give a coherent history. In that case, enlist family members, friends, home health aides—anyone you can find!—to help out.

Step 2: Start Localizing. This is the bread and butter of neurology. While you're OPQRST-ing, start thinking about where in the nervous system you could situate your patient's chief complaint. Start at the top and work your way down, tracing your way from the brain all the way down into the muscles. Why not the other way—from bottom to top? Anatomically, "top-down" is the simple, tried-and-true way of making sure you don't miss anything. But perhaps the best reason to start thinking in this way is that most of the more serious "do not miss" diagnoses localize to higher up in the neuraxis. For instance, a paretic (*i.e.*, weak) hand can be caused by both "lower down" (*e.g.*, peripheral nerve injury) and "higher up" (*e.g.*, stroke or brain tumor) lesions. All are important diagnoses, but the higher up etiologies are the more dangerous and the more pressing to rule out.

This top-down approach works best for motor complaints (you are essentially tracing the motor pathway from start to finish; see page 18), but it can be used for just about any neurologic complaint. For example, hand numbness, a sensory issue, can be caused by exactly the same lesions as mentioned above (peripheral nerve injury, stroke or brain tumor); just be aware that you are tracing the anatomic pathway backward (from finish to start, so to speak; this will make sense in a few pages, see page 23).

The basic localization pathway

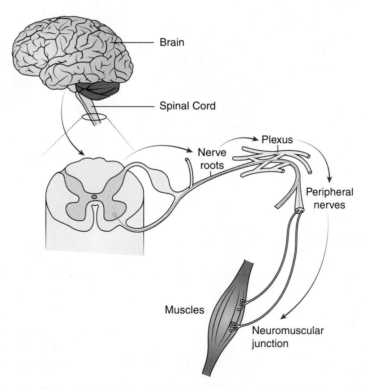

The basic localization pathway: Brain → Spinal Cord → Nerve roots → Plexus → Peripheral Nerves → Neuromuscular Junction → Muscles.

Let's take an example of how you might localize a neurologic lesion. Don't be discouraged by all the neuroanatomy in this paragraph. We are just making a point here and will get into all the messy details later. Let's say that your patient is presenting with acute left-sided face, arm, and leg weakness. You start as high as possible, in the right-sided motor strip of the cerebral cortex. You next follow those motor fibers down through the subcortical white matter and into the brainstem, but once you hit the cervical spinal cord, you're done. Why? Because your patient has facial involvement, the symptoms cannot be due to a lesion lower down in the cord. Now stop and think. If your patient has a lesion in the brain, where could it be? Is it more likely to be superficial, in the cortex, or deeper in the brain?[1] Could your patient have had a stroke? A tumor? An infection? Your subsequent evaluation can now be geared toward figuring this out.

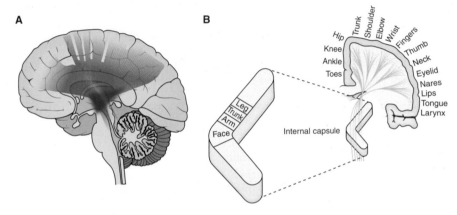

The motor pathways converge as they descend, from the cortex down into the internal capsule and brainstem. You can see that it would require a very large cortical lesion but a relatively small internal capsule lesion to result in face, arm and leg weakness.

The Neurologic Examination

The neurologic examination is the pride and joy of neurology. This is not because it's complicated or because it requires a bag full of tools (a pen light, reflex hammer, tuning fork, safety pins, *etc.*) but because it *works*: when properly utilized and performed, the neurologic examination can tell you things that even the most meticulously obtained history and highest-resolution MRI cannot. In the right context, a downward drift of an extended arm can prompt emergent thrombolytic therapy to dissolve a blood clot; subtle weakness

---

[1]The answer, by the way, is that the lesion is most likely located in the subcortical white matter of the brain. Because the motor pathways converge as they descend (see the picture above), it is much easier to "knock out" the face, arm, and leg all together by a single lesion in the internal capsule, for instance, than it is in the cortex, where the face, arm, and leg motor fibers are much more spread out. If this doesn't make any sense to you just yet, don't worry: it will soon!

in neck flexion can raise red flags for the impending need for intubation; a dropped reflex or asymmetric smile can dramatically change a patient's differential diagnosis, management, and treatment.

Yes, the neurologic examination can seem intimidating. So let's walk through it, one step at a time.

The components of a comprehensive neurologic examination include:

1. **Mental status:** level of consciousness, intellectual function, language, and praxis (praxis refers to the cognitive ability to perform learned motor tasks, from writing to throwing a curveball)

2. **Cranial nerves:** 2 to 12 (why not 1? Cranial nerve 1 is the olfactory nerve, and most of the time you won't need to test smell)

3. **Motor system:** bulk, tone, and strength

4. **Somatosensory system:** light touch, pain, temperature, vibration, and proprioception

5. **Reflexes:** six common reflexes are tested: the brachioradialis, biceps, triceps, patellar, Achilles, and plantar (also known as the Babinski sign)

6. **Coordination:** rapid alternating movements, finger-nose-finger and heel-to-shin testing

7. **Gait:** stance, balance, arm swing, and ability to heel, toe, and tandem walk

Now let's look at each of these seven domains individually, stressing the way each is evaluated during your neurologic examination. We've included just enough neuroanatomy so that you can understand the context and importance of each examination finding. We readily admit: it is a lot of material, so take your time. You don't have to master it all at once, although you are certainly welcome to try, and the relevance of much of it to neurologic diagnosis will become apparent to you as we go through the various neurologic disorders that comprise the bulk of this book.

Mental Status

The mental status examination tests a multitude of mental capacities and functions, but it is often easy to determine someone's mental status within the first minute of meeting them. Is your patient awake and alert, acknowledging you, smiling appropriately? Can your patient hold a coherent conversation? If so, you're likely good to go.

However, the mental status examination can be highly nuanced and detect subtle abnormalities you might miss on first impression. We've simplified it here to include only the most relevant and clinically useful components.

1. *Level of consciousness.* You need to recognize the terms listed below because you'll hear them used, but be aware that, because there are no standardized, agreed-upon definitions of these terms, the best way to describe a patient's level of consciousness is simply to specify what you see. If the patient is groggy and not responsive to vocal stimuli, for instance, just say that. Everyone uses and defines these terms slightly differently, but here are some of the more common definitions:

   a. Awake and alert: Normal.

   b. Lethargic: Groggy, but responsive to vocal stimuli.

    c. Obtunded: Briefly arousable to painful stimuli, then falls back to sleep.

    d. Comatose: Unarousable.

2. ***Intellectual function***. A few simple tests will establish a patient's cognitive function:

    a. Orientation to person, place, and time.

    b. Attention and concentration. This can be tested by asking your patients to spell the word "WORLD" backward or subtract serial 7's from 100. You must take educational background into account here.

    d. Memory. Test 3-item recall: Give your patients 3 words to remember, then ask them to repeat the words back to you after several minutes. More in-depth memory and cognitive testing, such as the *Mini-Mental State Examination (MMSE)* and the *Montreal Cognitive Assessment (MOCA)*, will be discussed later (see Chapter 7).

3. ***Language.*** This covers expression and comprehension[2]:

    a. Naming. Start with "high-frequency" (easy) objects such as "finger," and progress to "low-frequency" (more difficult) objects such as "nail."

    b. Comprehension. Start with simple one-step commands: "stick out your tongue," or "close your eyes." Progress to more complex commands that require your patients to "cross the midline." For example, ask your patient to "take your left hand and touch your right ear."

    c. Repetition. Ask your patient to repeat a phrase: we like "it's a sunny day in New York City," and "no ifs, ands or buts."

4. ***Praxis***. Praxis is the cognitive ability to perform learned motor tasks. Ask your patients to show you how they brush their teeth or comb their hair. If they are unable to do so despite normal motor function, they are "apraxic."

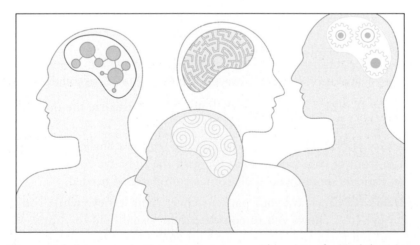

The mental status examination encompasses a wide variety of critical domains.

---

[2]See Chapter 2, page 59 for a comprehensive review on language components and localization.

Cranial Nerves

Cranial Nerve (CN) Anatomy 101. This can get complicated, and we will be digging deeper into cranial nerve anatomy in Chapter 18, but for now all you need to know is that the cranial nerves (with the exception of CN1 and 2, which arise from the nasal cavity and the retina, respectively) originate in the brainstem, the part of the CNS that connects the cerebrum to the spinal cord and includes the midbrain, pons, and medulla. The cranial nerves are involved in most of the noncognitive things we do with our head, from seeing, smelling, hearing, and tasting to moving our eyes, turning our head, chewing, and swallowing. Each nerve can contain, in varying degrees, sensory, motor, and autonomic fibers.

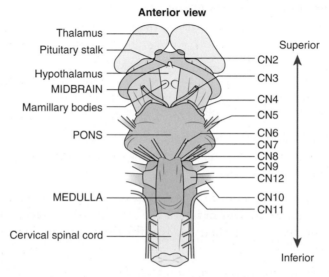

The entrance and/or exit of the cranial nerves into or out of the brainstem. The sensory fibers of the cranial nerves are afferents: they enter the brainstem (in other words, they receive sensory information from the environment and relay it to the brainstem). The motor fibers are efferents: they exit the brainstem (they receive motor commands from the brainstem and relay the instructions out to the target muscles).

When you test cranial nerve function, always go in order, 2 to 12, so you don't miss anything.

- **Funduscopy (CN2).** Use your ophthalmoscope to visualize the optic disc and surrounding vessels.
- **Visual acuity (CN2).** Hold a visual acuity card (called a Snellen chart) approximately one foot in front of your patient's left eye with the right eye covered. Then test the other eye. Patients should wear their contacts or glasses if needed.
- **Visual fields (CN2).** Have your patients cover their left eye while you cover your own right eye (this allows you to compare their visual field to yours). Face them directly and tell them to keep their eyes on your nose. Quickly flash some fingers in each visual quadrant and ask them to tell you the number of fingers that they see. Then test the other eye.
- **Pupillary reflexes (CN2, CN3).** Reduce the light in the room as much as possible. Swing your penlight back and forth several times between your patient's eyes, assessing pupil size as well as the degree and rate of constriction.

- **Extraocular movements (CN3, 4, 6).** Tell your patients to follow your index finger with their eyes while keeping their head still. Draw an "H" in the air to bring their eyes up, down, and side-to-side. Assess for full and symmetric eye movements as well as eyelid drooping (ptosis) and nystagmus (rapid, involuntary jerking movements that will be discussed in more detail later on). We'll sort out the specific contributions of each of these three cranial nerves in Chapter 18 when it becomes important.

- **Facial sensation (CN5).** Lightly touch both sides of your patient's forehead, cheeks, and chin, and ask if the left and right sides feel the same. You're testing the first (V1), second (V2), and third (V3) branches of the fifth cranial nerve, respectively. Testing jaw strength (the "muscles of mastication") by having patients open and close their jaw against resistance also assesses V3.

- **Facial movements (CN7).** Ask patients to close their eyes tightly, raise their eyebrows, puff out their cheeks, and smile. You're looking predominantly for symmetry. Facial weakness may be obvious at first glance or may require "activation"—smiling, raising eyebrows—to be appreciated. Nasolabial fold flattening is a subtle sign of smile weakness.

- **Hearing (CN8).** Rub your fingers together in front of your patient's ear. Each ear should be tested separately.

- **Uvula deviation (CN9, 10).** Ask your patient to say "ahh" so you can assess the movement and position of the palate and uvula.

- **Shoulder shrug and neck turn (CN11):** Have your patients turn their head all the way to the left, place your hand on the left side of the face, and ask them to resist you as you try turning their head to the right. Test both sides. Ask your patients to shrug their shoulders while you resist with your hands.

- **Tongue movements (CN12).** Ask your patients to stick out their tongue and move it side to side. To test strength, ask them to push the tongue against the cheek from inside the mouth while you push against it from outside.

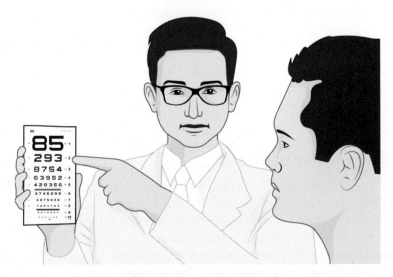

Using a Snellen chart to evaluate cranial nerve 2.

What happened, you may ask, to cranial nerve 1? That is the olfactory nerve, and it is often unnecessary to evaluate it. If you think it is relevant—for example, in a patient with suspected COVID-19 (loss of smell—*anosmia*—is a common complication of this disease)—you can use whatever stimulus you can find (we like strong coffee!) to test one nostril at a time.

The Motor System

Motor System Anatomy 101. The *corticospinal tract* is the major motor pathway, responsible for voluntary movement of the limbs and body. The fibers originate in the motor cortex (which is located within the precentral gyrus of the brain—see the figure below) and descend through the subcortical white matter (including the corona radiata), the internal capsule, and brainstem. They decussate (or cross) in the medulla at the medullary pyramids, right where the brainstem meets the spinal cord; this is why the left side of the brain controls movement on the right side of the body, and vice versa.

These neurons, the *upper motor neurons*, continue to descend through the cord (on the contralateral side from their site of origin) in the lateral corticospinal tract. They synapse just before they leave the cord on *lower motor neurons* (also called anterior horn cells), which exit the cord and travel to their target muscles.

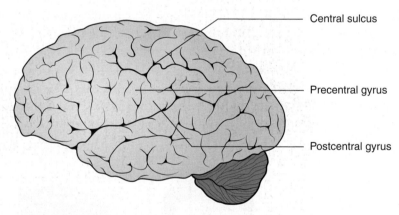

Central sulcus

Precentral gyrus

Postcentral gyrus

The central sulcus divides the frontal and parietal lobes. The gyrus just anterior to it is called the precentral gyrus and functions as the primary motor cortex; the gyrus just posterior to it is called the postcentral gyrus and functions as the primary sensory cortex.

Box 1.4 The Pyramidal Tracts

You'll hear the term *pyramidal tract* used as a synonym for the corticospinal tract, but in fact there are two pyramidal tracts: (1) the *corticospinal tract*—as just discussed, these are upper motor neurons that originate in the motor cortex and terminate on lower motor neurons in the spinal cord and (2) the *corticobulbar tract*—these upper motor neurons also originate in the motor cortex but terminate in the brainstem on the motor nuclei of the cranial nerves.

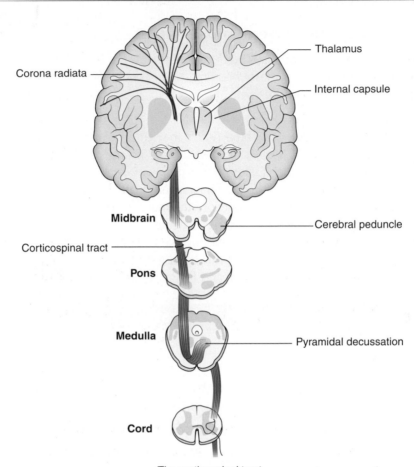

Corona radiata

Thalamus

Internal capsule

Midbrain

Cerebral peduncle

Corticospinal tract

Pons

Medulla

Pyramidal decussation

Cord

The corticospinal tract.

- A second motor system, the *extrapyramidal system*, runs outside the medullary pyramids (hence *extrapyramidal*) and includes neurons within the basal ganglia and cerebellum, among other locations. Unlike the neurons of the pyramidal system, these neurons synapse all over the place and are important for indirect, largely *involuntary*, modulation, coordination, and regulation of movements. Lesions of the extrapyramidal system therefore result in abnormal, dysregulated movements. Dopamine depletion within the basal ganglia, for instance, as in Parkinson disease, can result in tremor and bradykinesia (slowness of movement). Antipsychotic medications (which act as dopamine receptor antagonists) can also cause extrapyramidal symptoms, including parkinsonism, dystonia (abnormal posturing that's often associated with repetitive twisting movements), and akathisia (a movement disorder characterized by restlessness and inability to sit still). We will get to all of this in Chapter 13.

Box 1.5 Upper and Lower Motor Neurons

Damage along the motor pathways produces different types of deficits depending upon whether upper or lower motor neurons are involved. It is therefore important for localization to know the difference:

- *Upper motor neurons* (UMNs) include all neurons that run in the motor pathways above the lower motor neurons. These include the neurons in the corticospinal and corticobulbar tracts. Classic findings of UMN damage include weakness, increased tone and spasticity, hyperreflexia, and upgoing toes (aka the Babinski sign ; see page 28).
- *Lower motor neurons* (LMNs) are the final nerves in the motor pathways that innervate (via the neuromuscular junction) the muscles. These include the anterior horn cells in the spinal cord and the cranial nerves with motor components (*i.e.*, all of the cranial nerves except 1, 2, and 8). Like UMN disease, LMN disease presents with weakness, but unlike UMN disease it can also cause muscle atrophy, decreased muscle tone, hyporeflexia, and fasciculations (or muscle twitching).

Lower Motor Neuron Deficit	Upper Motor Neuron Deficit
Hyporeflexia	Hyperreflexia
Marked muscle atrophy	Less significant atrophy
Muscle fasciculations and fibrillations	Fasciculations and fibrillations are not seen
Decreased tone (muscles are flaccid)	Increased tone (muscles are spastic)
Absent Babinski sign	Present Babinski sign

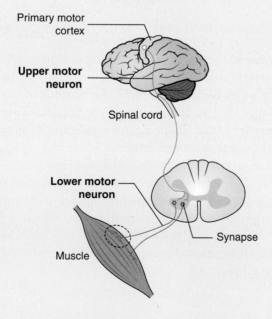

Upper and lower motor neurons. Damage to one or the other can cause very different symptoms.

The motor system is complicated, but for now this is pretty much all you need to know to understand what you are doing and why you are doing it during your neurologic examination. We will get into more detail later when it becomes important to dig a bit deeper.

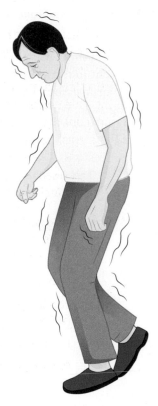

Extrapyramidal dysfunction is responsible for many of the manifestations of Parkinson disease, including tremor, abnormal posture, and gait dysfunction.

The Motor Examination. The motor examination is broken down into 3 components:

1. ***Muscle bulk.*** Inspect and palpate for evidence of atrophy. Keep in mind that "normal bulk" for a college athlete means something different than normal bulk for an elderly grandparent.

2. ***Muscle tone.*** Ask patients to relax and let you manipulate their limbs. Assess for:

   a. *Hypotonia*: Decreased resistance to passive manipulation.

   b. *Hypertonia*: Increased resistance to passive manipulation. This comes in a couple of flavors:

i. *Spasticity*, usually due to pyramidal tract disease (*e.g.*, after a left-sided middle cerebral artery stroke; see Chapter 2), is velocity dependent; the tone increases as the limb is moved more quickly.

ii. *Rigidity*, usually due to extrapyramidal disease (*e.g.*, Parkinson disease; see Chapter 13), is velocity independent; the tone does not change, regardless of movement.

3. ***Muscle strength.*** Test one muscle at a time, using one hand to provide resistance and the other to stabilize the adjacent joint, while asking patients to push or pull as hard as they are able toward or against you. This is called "*confrontation testing.*" Neurologists use a 5-point grading scale, with additional pluses and minuses to further specify the degree of strength (*e.g.*, 4+ is stronger than 4, but not quite as good as 5):

0: No contraction

1: Flicker of movement

2: Able to move in a horizontal plane but not against gravity

3: Able to move against gravity, but not against resistance

4: Able to move against some resistance

5: Normal

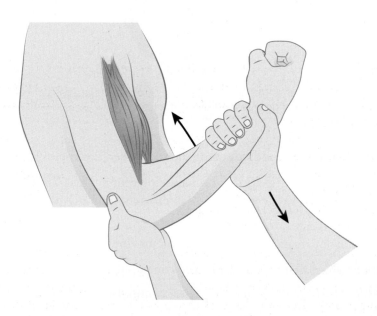

Evaluating motor strength with confrontation testing.

Box 1.6 Pronator Drift

This term refers to a pathologic sign that indicates subtle arm weakness and may be the only motor abnormality you detect. Even (and especially) in isolation, it is an important physical finding, so *look for this in all your motor examinations*. Have your patients extend both arms out in front, palms up, eyes closed. If both arms remain in place, strength is intact. If one arm begins to drift downward and pronate such that the palm begins to turn toward the ground, your patient has mild weakness that you could easily miss on formal confrontation testing. This is a test of *upper motor neuron* weakness.

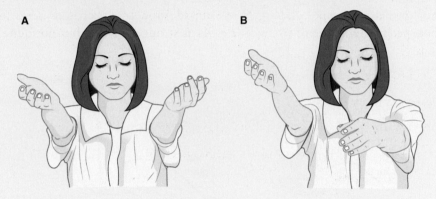

Pronator drift in a patient with small stroke involving the motor pathways.

The Somatosensory System

Somatosensory System Anatomy 101. The somatosensory system arises in the periphery. There are several sensory modalities, including *light touch*, *vibration*, *pain*, *temperature*, and *proprioception* (also known as joint position sense, proprioception enables you to know where your body is in space).

We sense these various modalities via different sensory receptors that are located in our skin and muscles. Neurons extend from these receptors into the spinal cord, where they ascend via various pathways into the brain. The cell bodies of these "first-order" neurons (*i.e.*, the first neurons in the sensory pathways) are located in the dorsal root ganglia (DRG), which are clusters of cell bodies located alongside the cord.

There are two major pathways to know:

- *The **dorsal column/medial lemniscus pathway** carries pressure, vibration, and proprioception fibers. The first-order neuron enters the cord and ascends ipsilaterally in the dorsal column tract, then synapses in the ipsilateral medulla. The second-order neuron immediately decussates, ascends contralaterally in the medial lemniscus tract, then synapses in the thalamus. The third-order neuron extends from the thalamus to the primary somatosensory cortex, located in the postcentral gyrus.

- *The **spinothalamic tract** carries pain and temperature fibers. Unlike the dorsal column/medial lemniscus tract, the first-order neuron enters the cord and then immediately synapses in the ipsilateral dorsal horn. The second-order neuron then decussates (through the anterior white commissure), ascends contralaterally in the spinothalamic tract and then synapses in the thalamus. The third-order neuron then joins the neurons from the dorsal column/medial lemniscus tract as it rises to the somatosensory cortex.

These tracts are less complicated than they sound. Spend a minute going through these diagrams, and you'll know all you need to know.

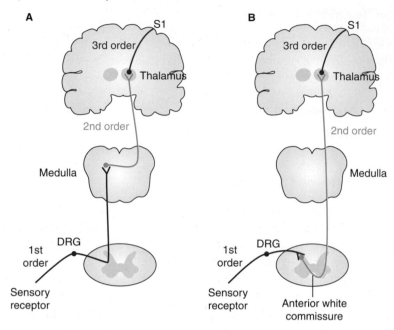

(A) The dorsal column/medial lemniscus tract and (B) the spinothalamic tract. Note that, although the pathways cross at different levels in the neuraxis, both end up on the contralateral side from where they began. This is why the left side of the brain is responsible for sensory input from the right side of the body, and vice versa. DRG: dorsal root ganglia.

Box 1.7 Lissauer Tract

The first-order neuron of the spinothalamic tract actually runs up alongside the cord—in what's known as Lissauer tract—for about 2 vertebral segments before it enters the cord. Knowing about the Lissauer tract can be important when trying to localize spinal lesions, so file it away and we'll come back to it later (see Chapter 10).

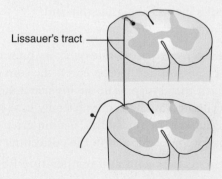

There are several other pathways that carry sensory information, but we won't worry about them for now. Light touch fibers are dispersed throughout several of these pathways, and thus loss of light touch cannot be localized to any particular tract.

The Sensory Examination. Here's how to test the various sensory modalities:

1. *Pain.* Test with a clean safety pin or the jagged, pointy side of a toothpick snapped in half.

2. *Temperature.* Test with the side of a metal tuning fork.

3. *Vibration.* Test with a tuning fork.

4. *Proprioception* (joint position sense). Tell your patients to close their eyes. Then, with your fingers, move one of their big toes up and down. Your patients should know, without looking, which direction the toe is pointing. Be sure to place your fingers on the sides of the toe and not the top and bottom; you're effectively allowing the patient to "cheat" if he or she can feel the pressure from your fingers pushing up or down.

5. *Light touch.* Test with the beds of your fingertips.

Box 1.8 The Romberg Test

The *Romberg test* is another way to evaluate proprioception. Tell your patients to stand up with their arms hanging loosely by their side, feet close together and eyes closed, making sure that you are positioned to catch them if they fall. Then watch them to see how steady they are. Are they able to maintain perfect posture, do they sway from side to side, or do they begin to fall? Balance requires intact proprioception as well as visual function and vestibular function.[3] With eyes closed, patients can only rely on proprioception, so if proprioception is impaired, they will lose their balance.

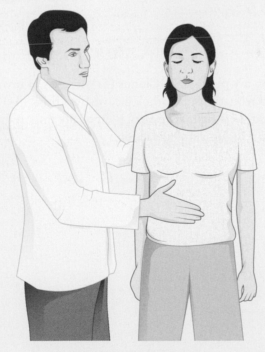

Performing the Romberg Test.

[3]If vestibular function is impaired, patients will sway with their eyes open *and* closed; thus, for patients with *vestibular* dysfunction, a "positive" Romberg is not diagnostic of *proprioceptive* dysfunction.

Reflexes

Deep tendon reflexes are simple circuits made up of one sensory neuron and one motor neuron (and sometimes an intervening "interneuron" between the two; see the picture below) that synapse within the spinal cord. The sensory afferent nerve, activated by the light tap of a reflex hammer, activates the motor efferent nerve, which subsequently causes muscle contraction. There are multiple types of reflex hammers and everyone has their favorite, but don't be fooled: it's all in the wrist!

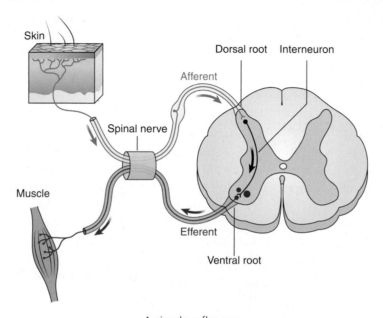

A simple reflex arc.

Reflexes are graded on a 4-point scale. Clonus (4+), a series of involuntary, rhythmic muscle contractions and relaxations, is pathologic, whereas brisk (3+) can be normal or not, depending on the context. Left-right symmetry is especially important here, because any asymmetry may indicate a focal neurologic lesion.

- 0: No response
- 1+: Slightly diminished
- 2+: Normal
- 3+: Brisk
- 4+: Clonus

Box 1.9 Nerve Roots

The spinal cord gives off paired nerve roots at each vertebral level. The dorsal root (containing the sensory afferent fibers) and ventral root (containing the motor efferent fibers) join to form a spinal nerve as shown in the figure on page 26. Specific nerve roots are responsible for specific reflexes. These are important to know, because they can help you localize the damage when a reflex is abnormal.

- Brachioradialis: C5-6
- Biceps: C5-6
- Triceps: C7-8
- Patellar (knee jerk): L2-4
- Achilles (ankle jerk): S1

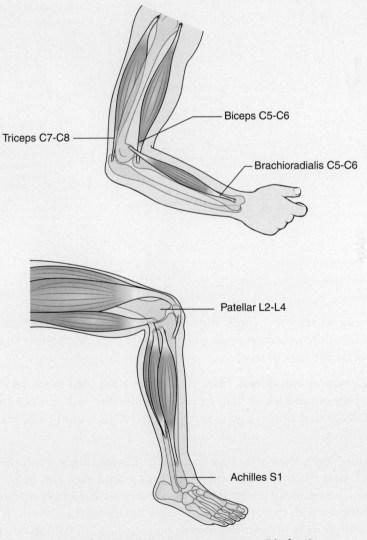

The basic reflexes and the nerve roots responsible for them.

Box 1.10 The Plantar and Hoffmann Reflexes

The plantar and Hoffmann reflexes are indicative of upper motor neuron damage. The plantar reflex (commonly referred to as the Babinski reflex, although the term Babinski actually refers to a physical sign that is present when the plantar reflex is extensor and absent when it's flexor) is present at birth but normally extinguished by about 1 year of age. It is elicited by stroking the sole of the foot (see picture). If the reflex is present, the big toe will move upward (extensor response); if not, the toe flexes down toward the (flexor response). The Hoffmann reflex is the upper extremity equivalent and is elicited by flicking the tip of the middle finger downward. If present, the thumb and index finger on the same hand will flex together. In persons over the age of 1 year, the presence of either of these reflexes is abnormal.

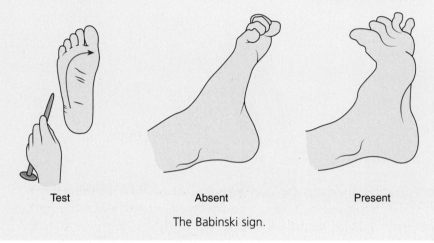

Test   Absent   Present

The Babinski sign.

Coordination

Coordination tests are tests of *cerebellar* function. There are many of these tests; we've selected a handful of the ones most commonly used. Try them all, because abnormalities can be extremely subtle and easy to miss.

1. ***Rapid alternating movements.*** Have your patients rest their hands on their lap, then flip their palms from back to front repeatedly. Difficulty with this task, manifested by the inability to maintain a good rhythm of front-back-front-back, is called *dysdiadochokinesia.*

2. ***Finger-nose-finger.*** Have your patients take their index finger, touch their nose and then touch your finger such that they must fully extend their arm in front of them. Do this repeatedly, moving your finger so that they are constantly reaching for a new target. Difficulty with this task—if their finger zigzags back and forth, is unable to reliably land precisely on your fingertip or on their nose, or consistently points past your fingertip—is called *dysmetria.*

3. ***Heel-to-shin.*** Have your patients place their left heel on their right knee, then drag their left leg straight down and then back up their right leg repeatedly, staying directly on top of their tibia. They should be able to do this smoothly. Any incoordination (typically manifested by a zigzagging motion similar to what can be seen with finger-nose-finger testing) can be indicative of a cerebellar lesion.

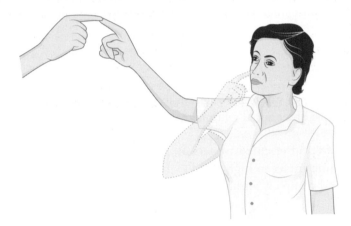

Finger-to-nose testing.

Gait

The gait examination is perhaps the hardest part of the examination to interpret.

Abnormalities in gait and balance can be due to almost anything, with both neurologic (motor, sensory, vestibular, cerebellar) and non-neurologic (orthostasis, deconditioning) causes. That said, gait is incredibly important to observe because the ability to walk *matters*. Let's say you're deciding whether or not to give thrombolytic therapy to a stroke patient who, in the stretcher, seems to have mild left leg weakness. If the patient can walk normally despite this, the risks of therapy may outweigh the benefits. But if they try to walk and cannot, it is likely that this patient will want you to do everything in your power to make them better.

Whenever you're able to do so, test regular walking, toe- and heel-walking, and tandem gait (with one foot placed directly in front of the other, heel-to-toe).

A couple of specific gait disorders to know:

1. ***Ataxic gait.*** Most often due to cerebellar pathology, ataxic gait is characterized by a wide-based stance and staggering, unsteady, and uncoordinated movements. These patients can sometimes be mistaken for being inebriated.

2. ***Shuffling gait.*** Classic for Parkinson disease, this type of gait can also be seen in normal pressure hydrocephalus. It is characterized by small short steps with very little foot elevation off the ground.

So, this was certainly a lot of information, and you're probably thinking that performing a comprehensive neurologic examination will take at least a week! In reality, the entire examination often takes only several minutes. As you get more experienced, you can pick and choose from the various domains; for instance, you likely don't need to test every aspect of mental status in a healthy 25-year-old presenting with a 10-year history of migraine. However, especially at the beginning, it's important to go in order through each component of the examination so that you don't miss anything along the way.

Note Template: An Example of How You Might Document a Normal Neurologic Examination

If you're wondering how all of the information in a neurologic examination is documented, check out this example of a normal neurologic evaluation:

Mental Status. Alert and oriented to person, place, and time (AOx3), attention intact, speech fluent, naming intact to high and low frequency objects, repetition intact, able to follow simple and complex commands across the midline, recognition and recall intact.

Cranial Nerves. Discs sharp bilaterally, visual fields full (VFF) to finger counting, pupils equally round and reactive to light and accommodation (PERRLA), extraocular muscles intact (EOMI) without nystagmus, facial sensation intact to light touch (V1-3 intact to LT), face symmetric with equal activation, hearing grossly intact, tongue/uvula/palate midline (t/u/p midline), sternocleidomastoid (SCM) and shoulder shrug symmetric.

Motor. Normal bulk and tone, 5/5 throughout, no pronator drift (PND).

Sensory. Sensation intact to light touch (LT), temperature, pinprick (PP), vibration and joint position sense (JPS), no extinction to double simultaneous stimulation (DSS; see Box 1.11), Romberg negative.

Reflexes. 2+ and symmetric, toes down.

Coordination. Finger-nose-finger (FNF), rapid alternating movements (RAM), and heel-to-shin (HTS) intact.

Gait. Steady narrow-based gait, able to heel/toe/tandem without difficulty.

Not so bad, right? The hardest part can be sorting through all of the abbreviations scribbled by busy students, residents, and fellows; we've included many of them here so later on you won't feel like you're reading a foreign language.

Box 1.11 Hemineglect and Extinction to Double Simultaneous Stimulation

Hemineglect is a neurologic condition in which patients lose awareness of one side of space. Hemineglect can be dramatic, such as when patients fail to recognize their own arm or only appropriately dress half of their body, or more subtle, such as when patients extinguish to double simultaneous stimuli. *Extinction*, in the world of neurology, is defined as the impaired ability to perceive two stimuli of the same type simultaneously, and it indicates a relatively subtle form of neglect.

Here's an example: let's say a patient has developed mild left-sided numbness and neglect from a right-sided stroke. If you touch the patient's left hand, with his or her eyes closed, the patient will be able to tell you that you're touching the left hand; it feels "less" than if you touch the right hand, but the patient is able to perceive the stimulus. If, however, you touch both hands at once (again while the patient's eyes are closed), the patient will consistently "extinguish" the stimuli on the left and tell you that you're only touching the right hand. The patient has proven to you that he or she can feel the stimulus on the left, but with "double simultaneous stimuli," reliably neglects that side of the body. Extinction to visual stimuli can be tested as well.

Because there is no a stand-alone category for "neglect" within the neurologic examination, if you find sensory extinction on examination, you can document it as part of the sensory examination; visual extinction can be documented under cranial nerves (right next to visual fields); the inability to recognize one's own arm can go under mental status. However you choose to document neglect, the important takeaway here is to remember to test for it. It's one example of how important the neurologic examination can be: you can detect a very subtle but serious deficit that, almost by definition, the patient is not aware of.

Is it Neurologic?

One of the biggest challenges of neurology is how to distinguish neurologic complaints and diseases from nonneurologic ones. If, for example, a patient presents with new-onset confusion, what would make you think that the *primary* problem is with the brain and not, say, with the kidneys (uremia) or the liver (hepatic encephalopathy)?

The most honest answer is that we often don't know. The distinction can be hard, and even the most experienced neurologists will tell you that you should have a low threshold to consider any and all neurologic possibilities. The more satisfying answer is that there are findings—really only a handful of findings—that we look for to help guide us. Like flashing stop signs stuck to the patient's forehead, these findings should make us stop in our tracks and feel confident that a primary neurologic diagnosis is likely.

Number One: FOCALITY. A focal neurologic deficit is a symptom that can be localized to a particular anatomic site in the nervous system. Unilateral weakness or sensory loss are classic focal symptoms. Changes in speech, language, vision, hearing, and coordination can also be focal symptoms. The remainder of this book will help clarify these symptoms—how they typically present and where, anatomically, they come from (or, in neurologist speak, "localize to"). Focal neurologic symptoms are usually the result of neurologic disease, but there are exceptions. For example, severe hypo- and hyperglycemia can cause focal symptoms as well.

Number Two: GAZE PREFERENCE. A patient with a right gaze preference will prefer to look to the right. If the gaze preference is mild, the patient may occasionally voluntarily look to the left. If it's a little worse, they will only look to the left when adequately stimulated (*e.g.*, if you wave a familiar item or yell out to the patient from their left visual field). If it's severe, they may never look to the left, no matter how loud you shout from their left side. When you see a gaze preference, you should have little doubt that the patient has an underlying neurologic problem.

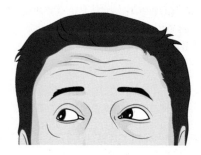

A patient with a right gaze preference.

Number Three: LACK OF AN ALTERNATE EXPLANATION. Let's go back to our confused patient. What if he is an end-stage renal patient, and we discover that he has missed his last three dialysis sessions? In all likelihood, this patient is confused due to uremic encephalopathy, and he will improve with time and dialysis. There is no urgent need to consider primary neurologic etiologies unless he fails to improve or—and this is critical—if he also has either FOCALITY or a GAZE PREFERENCE. But what if your confused patient is not medically ill? What if he or she has been completely healthy up until today? Without an obvious medical trigger to explain the confusion, we have to think a little harder. Often a lot harder. Here is where a good neurologic examination and additional neurologic testing become essential.

Box 1.12 Tip-Offs to a "Functional" Neurologic Examination

Some patients, either consciously (factitious disorders) or unconsciously (conversion disorders), feign neurologic disorders when they do not have one. The neurologic symptom can be anything: they may claim that they can't see out of one eye or insist that they cannot move both legs. The importance of identifying patients with functional examinations isn't to catch them in a lie, but rather to spare them needless neurologic testing and address the real issue, which may be a psychiatric one.

Box 1.12 Tip-Offs to a "Functional" Neurologic Examination (Continued)

There are specific tests for specific complaints, but a couple of basic principles will serve you well. Here is one from the sensory side of things and one from the motor side that are often helpful:

- **Splitting the midline.** Patients may complain that their sensation is abnormal or decreased on one side of their face, and evaluation will reveal a precise split down the midline of their nose between the good side and the affected side. This is not physiologic. The cutaneous branches of the trigeminal nerves are simply not wired that way; they overlap some to the contralateral side, so that organic neurologic deficits actually cross the midline, usually by several centimeters.
- **Give way weakness.** Strength testing can be both pain- and effort-limited, and patients often require significant encouragement to demonstrate full strength. Occasionally, however, a patient will initially, briefly, offer full resistance and then suddenly collapse, or "give way" and provide no further effort. This is not characteristic of true motor weakness.

 Diagnostic Tools

The diagnostic possibilities can feel endless when you are confronted with a patient with a neurologic disorder. In many cases, the history and examination will tell you all you need to know, but not always. There are a few (just a few!) questions you need to ask yourself after you've taken your history and completed your examination in order to figure out your immediate next step:

1. Would this patient benefit from imaging?

2. Would this patient benefit from a lumbar puncture (LP)?

3. Would this patient benefit from an electroencephalogram (EEG)?

4. Would this patient benefit from electromyography (EMG) or nerve conduction studies (NCS)?

These four questions, once your history and examination have been completed, are prompting you to consider the remaining items in your neurologic toolbox. Various other tests, such as serum markers for infection, inflammation, and immunologic disease, and urine studies for toxicology, can be helpful as well, but these four—imaging, LP, EEG, and EMG/NCS—form the crux of the diagnostic toolbox for neurologic disease. They may be used acutely in urgent settings to determine the best and potentially life-saving intervention, or more leisurely to establish the diagnosis in a patient with a complex, chronic presentation.

But don't use these tests haphazardly, like throwing darts at a dartboard and hoping to hit the center. Every test carries certain risks, not least among them the risk of false positives (leading to more, often invasive testing and a huge amount of anxiety for the patient) and overdiagnosis (uncovering actual lesions but ones that may never prove harmful to the patient). Use these tests wisely and well, and only in appropriate circumstances. What are those circumstances? Well, that's why you are reading this book!

A Quick Overview of Head Imaging

CT Scan. CT scans are fast and relatively inexpensive. They expose the patient to ionizing radiation, but a head CT delivers no more radiation (~1.5 mSv) than a series of back x-rays. Nevertheless, this factor should be taken into consideration, particularly when deciding to image children and pregnant women.

CT scans do not provide the same degree of anatomic detail as MRIs, but they can detect structural abnormalities and signs of elevated intracranial pressure and are actually more sensitive than MRI for identifying acute blood.

You should examine all CT scans for:

1. **Density.** Acute blood is bright white or "hyperdense," whereas infarction from an ischemic stroke is darker or "hypodense" compared with normal brain tissue. Calcium deposits also appear hyperdense and are often seen within the choroid plexus of the ventricles (these are normal!).

2. **Gray-white differentiation.** Normal CT scans of the brain show clear delineation between the gray matter of the cortex and the subcortical white matter. Blurring of this distinction can indicate stroke or other anoxic brain injury.

3. **Symmetry.** As with all brain imaging, symmetry is key. If you see something on one side of the brain that you don't see on the other, it is in all likelihood abnormal.

4. **Shift.** The falx cerebri, the crescent-shaped dural fold that separates the two cerebral hemispheres, should be midline. If it's shifted to one side, pushed over by blood or a mass, you should be immediately concerned about the risk of herniation, that is, brain tissue being forced into places that it shouldn't go.

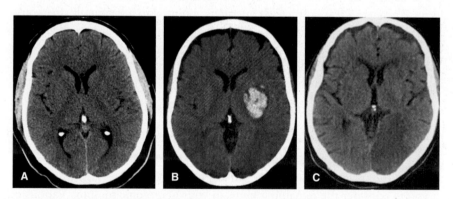

(A) A normal CT scan of the head. You can see choroid calcifications within the temporal horns of the lateral ventricles (a common, physiologic finding). (B) A deep left-sided intraparenchymal bleed. (C) A large left-sided posterior cerebral artery (PCA) infarction. (A, reprinted from Herzog E. *Herzog's CCU Book*. Wolters Kluwer; 2017; B, reprinted from Kollef MH, Isakow W, Burks AC, Despotovic V. *The Washington Manual of Critical Care*. 3rd ed. Wolters Kluwer; 2017; and C, reprinted from Cheng-Ching E, Baron EP, Chahine L, Rae-Grant A. *Comprehensive Review in Clinical Neurology*. 2nd ed. Wolters Kluwer; 2016.)

MRI. MRI scans are more expensive and take more time than CT scans, but they can also provide significantly more information.

Radiologists use the term "intensity" as opposed to "density" to describe brightness on an MRI: things that appear bright are referred to as "*hyperintense*" (or "increased signal"), and things that appear dark are "*hypointense*" (or "decreased signal").

There are several basic sequences of MRI imaging (*i.e.*, different ways of modifying the magnetic field, resulting in specific image appearances) that you should be familiar with. These are listed below. T1-weighted sequences are thought of as the most anatomical, best at showing the gross anatomy of the brain. T2-weighted sequences showcase pathology, because edema and gliosis (scarring) appear bright. Fluid-attenuated inversion recovery (FLAIR) sequences are T2-based, but with the CSF signal suppressed. This helps to highlight abnormal increased signal elsewhere.

	T1	T2	T2 FLAIR
CSF	Dark	Bright	Dark
Gray matter	Dark	Bright	Bright
White matter	Bright	Dark	Dark

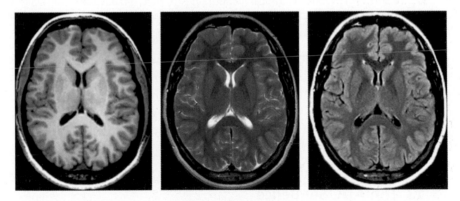

T1, T2, and FLAIR sequences. (Reprinted from Louis ED, Mayer SA, Rowland LP. *Merritt's Neurology*. 13th ed. Wolters Kluwer; 2015.)

Two additional important MRI sequences you should know are *susceptibility-weighted imaging* (SWI) and *diffusion-weighted imaging* (DWI).

SWI is used to detect blood, which appears dark (calcium will appear dark, as well). The process of determining how long the blood has been around (*i.e.*, is it acute or chronic) on MRI is complicated, and beyond the scope of this book. *Gradient-echo (GRE)* sequences are similar to SWI sequences but are less sensitive for detecting blood.

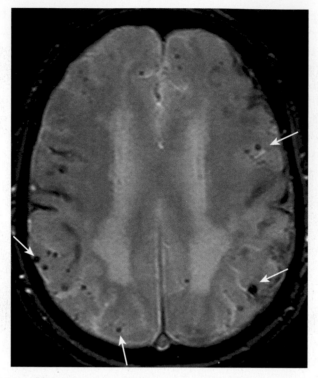

SWI sequence showing multifocal cortical hemorrhages (the little black dots; see white arrows), consistent with cerebral amyloid angiopathy (see page 79 for details). (Courtesy of E. Mark Haacke, PhD.)

DWI is the first sequence to look at when you are concerned about stroke. It is used to detect cytotoxic edema and infarcted tissue, which appear bright white. Here, the term "restricted diffusion" is used to denote bright white. This sequence is derived from measuring the random motion of water molecules within a given volume of tissue. When cells die, they swell, making it difficult for water to move around: thus, infarcted tissue "restricts" water diffusion.

Box 1.13 The ADC Sequence

Yet another sequence, the *apparent diffusion coefficient (ADC)* sequence, is calculated from the DWI scan and can be used to confirm that what appears bright on DWI is in fact true restricted diffusion and not what is referred to as "T2 shine-through," that is, when bright T2 signal "shines through" to DWI.

Acute infarction will be bright on DWI and dark on ADC (we refer to this as an "ADC correlate"). If you see a bright lesion on DWI but no corresponding dark lesion on ADC (*i.e.*, no ADC correlate), the DWI lesion is most likely T2 shine-through and not acute infarction. Shine-through is most often attributed to subacute (older than 1 week) infarctions, but can also be caused by other lesions such as cysts.

Note that stroke stays bright on DWI for about 1 month after it occurs, but stays dark on ADC for only about 1 week.

Box 1.13 (Continued)

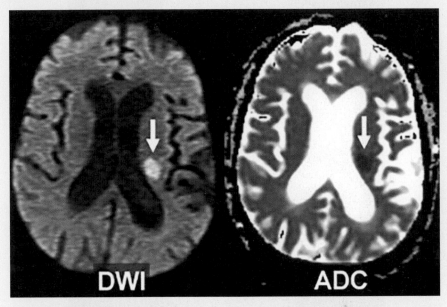

An acute infarct of the left corona radiata (the subcortical bundle of white matter fibers that continue inferiorly as the internal capsule and carry the descending motor fibers; see Motor System Anatomy 101), bright on DWI (*left*) with dark ADC correlate (*right*). (Reprinted from Klein J, Vinson EN, Brant WE, Helms CA. *Brant and Helms' Fundamentals of Diagnostic Radiology*. 5th ed. Wolters Kluwer; 2018.)

Box 1.14 Diffusion-Restricting Lesions

This goes a bit beyond the scope of this book, but just so you know, lesions other than infarction can restrict diffusion. When you see bright white on DWI with corresponding dark on ADC, always think "stroke" first, but keep in mind that hypercellular tumors (such as lymphoma and meningiomas) and bacterial abscesses, among other lesions, can restrict diffusion as well. Clinical context and other MRI sequences are often sufficient to help you figure out what's going on.

Vessel Imaging. No need to go into the details, but you should know that there are both CT-based and MR-based angiography studies. These scans enable us to look specifically at the blood vessels within the neck and head. They are frequently utilized in acute stroke to detect vessel occlusions. They can also help diagnose dissection, vasculitis, and other angiopathies. CT angiography (CTA) always requires intravenous (IV) contrast; MR angiography (MRA) does not.

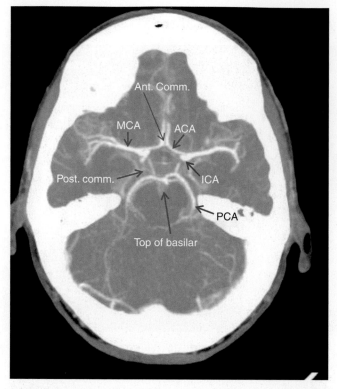

The circle of Willis, as visualized on a CTA of the head. (Courtesy of Jonathan Howard.)

Box 1.15 A Quick Note on Contrast

IV contrast can be used with both CT and MRI to help visualize and enhance specific abnormalities. Neurologists often order contrast-enhanced studies when they're concerned about malignancy or abscess, as both of these lesions typically enhance on imaging. CT uses iodinated contrast; MRI uses gadolinium. Both can cause allergic reactions, and patients should always be asked prior to contrast administration if they have any history of reactions to contrast, including rash and shortness of breath. Iodinated contrast can cause contrast-induced nephropathy (CIN), which presents as an acute kidney injury (AKI) within 24 to 48 hours of contrast administration, and is generally reversible with supportive treatment. Gadolinium can cause nephrogenic systemic sclerosis (NSF), characterized by thickening and hardening of the skin that can cause joint contractures and diffuse fibrosis affecting vital organs. NSF *only* occurs in patients with advanced kidney disease; likewise CIN, most of the time. Thus, especially in patients with kidney disease, the benefits and risks of administering contrast must always be taken into account before ordering testing.

Box 1.15 A Quick Note on Contrast (Continued)

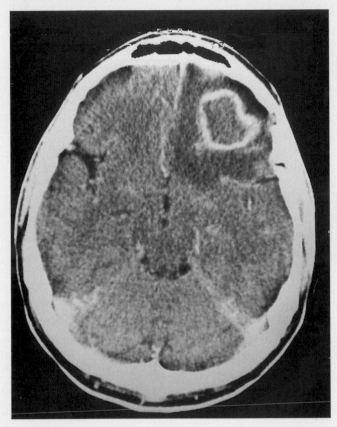

A left frontal ring-enhancing abscess seen on CT with contrast. Modified from Daffner RH. *Clinical Radiology*. 3rd ed. Wolters Kluwer; 2007.

Lumbar Puncture

An LP provides access to the CSF. Indications for an LP include:

1. ***CSF analysis:*** to detect bleeding, infection, inflammation, malignant cells, and so forth

2. ***CSF pressure measurement:*** a normal adult "opening pressure" is 10 to 18 cm H_2O; this can only be accurately obtained with the patient lying in the lateral decubitus position

3. ***CSF removal:*** this can be indicated for both diagnosis and therapy in conditions such as normal pressure hydrocephalus and idiopathic intracranial hypertension

4. ***Medication injection:*** such as anesthesia or chemotherapy

An LP can be performed at the patient's bedside. We typically position patients on their side (the "lateral decubitus position"), with their knees curled into their chest to help open up the spaces between the vertebrae. The spinal cord ends somewhere around the L1-L2 vertebrae, so we aim to insert our needle between the L3-L4 or L4-L5 vertebrae to avoid potential injury to the cord.

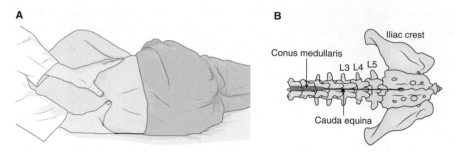

Position patients on their side in the lateral decubitus position. Place your fingers on the tops of the iliac crests, which lie at approximately the L4 level, and stretch your thumbs midline to the spine. You can then palpate the vertebrae and the spaces in between, to determine the best place—between the bones of the vertebrae, so you'll have access to the subarachnoid space—to insert your needle.

Complications from an LP are rare. *Post-LP headache* is the most common adverse effect and is due to rapid CSF removal and the subsequent "low pressure" situation. We tell patients to lie flat for 1 to 2 hours after the procedure, which is more than enough time for the body to replace the CSF that has been removed. This makes logical sense, but, just so you know, there is no clear evidence that doing so actually prevents the headache. Other complications include lower back discomfort, bleeding at the needle insertion site or, rarely, into the epidural space, and—incredibly rarely, now that we use sterile technique—infection.

Box 1.16

Adults have about 150 mL of CSF at any given time, but turn it over rapidly. CSF is produced by the choroid plexus at about 20 mL/hour, or approximately 500 mL/day. To put these numbers in perspective, we typically remove anywhere from 5 to 20 mL of CSF when performing an LP.

Box 1.17 LP Contraindications

1. Patient cannot lie flat (*e.g.*, in a patient with decompensated heart failure)
2. Concern for elevated intracranial pressure and risk of herniation (CSF removal in the presence of elevated intracranial pressure can cause downward displacement of the brain and compression of the brainstem)
3. High risk for bleeding (*e.g.*, low platelets, current use of anticoagulation)
4. Presence of an epidural abscess (risk of seeding the CSF)
5. Significant prior lumbar surgery (with distorted anatomy)

Electroencephalography

EEG detects electrical activity in the cerebral cortex by using small, sticky electrodes attached to the scalp. What exactly an EEG is recording (whether the electrical activity is derived from action potentials, chronic depolarizations, postsynaptic potentials, or other sources) is complicated and not entirely understood, although it is believed at the very least to originate from neurons. Regardless, the electrocortical activity is very small and must be amplified by a factor of one million to be detected on a computer screen.

EEG is most often used to diagnose epilepsy. Seizures are bursts of abnormal electrical activity, and different seizure disorders have different characteristic patterns on EEG (see Chapter 6).

There are four main frequencies of EEG waves, each of which is associated with different states of normal brain functioning. Each frequency can also, under specific circumstances, be the result of underlying disease (excessive delta activity, for instance, can be indicative of encephalopathy). The table below is by no means comprehensive, but it will be useful for you to have seen these words—delta, theta, alpha, and beta—and have a basic understanding of what they mean.

Frequency	Hz	Brain State	Notes
Delta	<4	Deep sleep	Can occur focally, in the general distribution of underlying brain lesions (*i.e.*, you can see "delta slowing" over an area of an old stroke); or excessively and diffusely, indicative of encephalopathy of nonspecific etiology
Theta	4–8	Drowsiness, sleep	Diffuse theta is normal in awake children; it can be seen in awake adults, but it may also be completely absent during wakefulness
Alpha	8–12	Relaxed, with eyes closed	You'll hear the term "posterior dominant rhythm": this is the normal alpha rhythm that's seen over the posterior region of the brain when patients are relaxed with their eyes closed (when they open their eyes, the "PDR" attenuates or even disappears)
Beta	12–30	Awake and active	Various drugs (including benzodiazepines and barbiturates) can increase beta activity

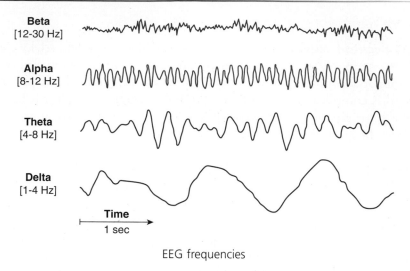

EEG frequencies

Nerve Conduction Studies and Electromyography

These are predominantly outpatient tests that can help diagnose various neuromuscular disorders. These include diseases involving the peripheral nerves (for example, diabetic neuropathy), neuromuscular junction (myasthenia gravis), or muscles (dermatomyositis). EMG measures muscle response to nerve stimulation via needles inserted into the muscles. NCS, often done at the same time, measures how well and how fast peripheral nerves send signals.

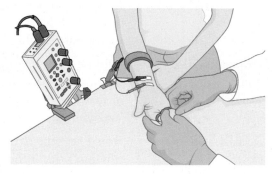

Obtaining an NCS and EMG. We will show you what the tracings look like in Chapter 12.

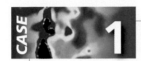

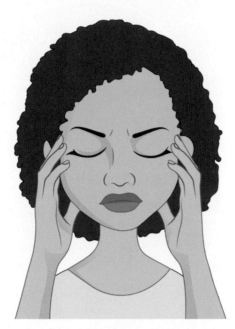

Your Patient's Follow-up: Hailey presented with a headache that had been worsening over several days and is now much improved after receiving pain medication. Your attending has asked you if she can go home, but you feel uneasy. You were only able to spend a few minutes with her because you had to prioritize other more acutely ill patients. You tell your attending to give you five more minutes, and you return to Hailey's bedside.

On further questioning, she tells you that this headache was right-sided (unlike her typical headaches, which are bilateral) but denies any other associated symptoms such as nausea, vomiting, or light or sound sensitivity. You repeat a quick neurologic examination and this time notice just the slightest downward drift and pronation of her left hand when you test pronator drift. You do the test again, and yet a third time, and convince yourself: it's subtle, but it's there. She has noticed no weakness but she is right handed, and you wonder if she may not have been aware of this subtle change. Given this new information (a new headache feature in the setting of a focal finding on examination) you order a CT of the head which is suggestive of a right frontal mass, followed by an MRI to better evaluate the lesion. The MRI is shown on the next page, and the moment you see it you know that those extra 5 minutes you took to talk to her and thoroughly examine her may have saved her life.

Hailey is ultimately diagnosed with a low-grade glioma and is quickly scheduled for surgery.

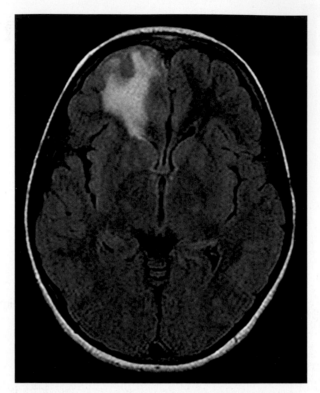

Hailey's MRI (FLAIR sequence) shows right frontal vasogenic edema. The postcontrast images (not pictured) confirm an underlying mass. (Reprinted from Fisher RG, Boyce TG, Correa AG. *Moffet's Pediatric Infectious Diseases.* 5th ed. Wolters Kluwer; 2017.)

You now know:

- | Basic neuroanatomy. There's more to come but, believe it or not, you have now learned the bulk of it. Have you memorized it all? Of course not, but you can keep coming back to these pages to refresh your learning.
- | How to take a focused and useful neurologic history.
- | How to perform a comprehensive neurologic examination.
- | How to distinguish neurologic diseases from non-neurologic diseases. This isn't always easy, even for experienced neurologists.
- | The basic principles of the diagnostic tools at our disposal: imaging tests, LP, EEG, and EMG/NCS.

You now have all the tools that you will need to understand, diagnose, and evaluate virtually all of the neurologic disorders you will encounter in the chapters to follow. We will make you this promise: it gets a lot more interesting from here!

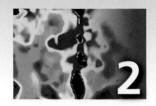

Stroke and Cerebrovascular Disease

2

In this chapter, you will learn:

1 | The many causes of ischemic stroke, and how to divvy them up into a manageable handful of categories

2 | How to recognize the most common ischemic stroke syndromes

3 | The evaluation and treatment of acute ischemic and hemorrhagic strokes

4 | The presentation, management, and complications associated with subarachnoid hemorrhage (SAH)

5 | The most clinically relevant and useful essentials of other important cerebrovascular disorders, including arterial dissection, reversible cerebral vasoconstriction syndrome (RCVS), cerebral venous sinus thrombosis, and central nervous system (CNS) vasculitis

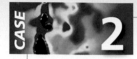

2

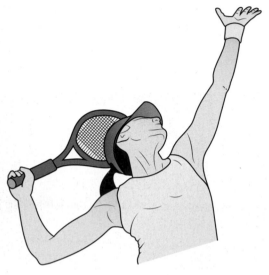

Your Patient: Laura, a 27-year-old professional tennis player, presents to the emergency department 2 hours after experiencing the sudden onset of left face and arm numbness and weakness. The triage nurse activates a stroke code, and you meet Laura as she is being taken for a CT scan. She tells you that she has no past medical history and takes no medications. On examination, you find mild sensory loss involving her left face and arm with extinction to double simultaneous stimulation on the left (see page 31), left nasolabial fold flattening, subtle weakness of her left wrist extensors and left-hand clumsiness. Her NIH stroke scale (NIHSS) is 3. A CT of her head is normal. What is the next step in your management?

Bad News But Good News Too

Someone in the United States has a stroke every 40 seconds. Every 4 minutes, someone dies from stroke. It is the fifth leading cause of death in the United States and is second only to cardiac disease worldwide. It is also a leading cause of serious long-term disability. Conservatively, stroke costs the United States over 30 billion dollars each year.

So, yes, cerebrovascular disease is common and can be devastating, but the pace of scientific discovery and clinical advances over the past few decades—and especially over the past few years—has been breathtaking. This is nowhere more evident than in our rapidly escalating ability to halt and reverse the effects of stroke *while it is in progress*, thereby preventing disability and saving lives. In addition, global awareness efforts and aggressive risk factor control have led to significant reductions in both the incidence of and mortality from stroke.

The Basics

As complicated as stroke care has become, there are two (only two!) major categories of stroke, and—from an etiologic standpoint—they are diametrically opposite conditions:

- *ischemia*, which is caused by blocked or severely narrowed blood vessels resulting in inadequate tissue perfusion, and
- *hemorrhage*, due to extravasation of blood from a damaged vessel.

In other words, *too little versus too much blood*. About 85% of all strokes are ischemic.[1]

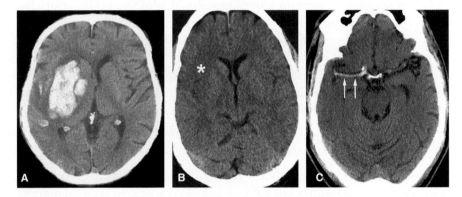

Examples of acute (*A*) hemorrhagic and (*B*) ischemic strokes. Acute blood is bright white, or "hyperdense," on computerized tomography (CT), and easy to recognize. Acute ischemia is more subtle, characterized by the loss or blurring of gray/white differentiation (see image B, star) and effacement of the sulci. Sometimes you may be able to visualize the clot itself as a hyperdense segment of a vessel: (*C*) shows a clot in the right middle cerebral artery (MCA, known as the "dense MCA" sign). (*A*, reprinted from Louis ED, Mayer SA, Rowland LP. *Merritt's Neurology*. 13th ed. Wolters Kluwer; 2015. B, reprinted from Daffner RH, Hartman M. *Clinical Radiology*. Wolters Kluwer; 2013. C, reprinted from Pope TL Jr, Harris JH Jr. *Harris & Harris' The Radiology of Emergency Medicine*. 5th ed. Wolters Kluwer; 2012.)

Stroke is, first and foremost, a clinical diagnosis, defined as the **acute onset of focal neurologic symptoms** caused by brain, spinal cord, or retinal cell death.

Box 2.1 Transient Ischemic Attack (TIA)

TIAs are "almost-strokes," more precisely defined as brief episodes of neurologic dysfunction due to focal brain, spinal cord, or retinal ischemia *without permanent tissue infarction*. Most TIAs last less than 1 hour. They are important to recognize because approximately 10% of patients with a TIA will go on to have a stroke within the next few months. The risk is highest in the immediate 24 hours following the TIA, and most patients should be hospitalized for evaluation and careful monitoring even though their neurologic symptoms have resolved.

---

[1]This number is for adults in the United States, and it changes based on geographic location and age; in children, for instance, hemorrhagic stroke is much more common than ischemic stroke.

Before we go any deeper into detail, a quick review of cerebrovascular anatomy is crucial. Only by knowing the vascular anatomy of the central nervous system (CNS) will you be able to recognize specific stroke syndromes, conceptualize the underlying stroke etiology, and understand the subsequent management. We promise to make this as concise, clinically relevant, and painless a review as possible.

Cerebrovascular Anatomy

The cerebral blood supply is divided into two components:

- *The anterior circulation* supplies approximately 75% of the brain. It originates from the common carotid arteries (left and right), which bifurcate into the internal and external carotid[2] arteries at approximately the level of the C4 vertebrae. The internal carotid arteries then travel up the neck, enter the skull at the petrous part of the temporal bone, pass through the cavernous sinus, give off the ophthalmic arteries (which supply the eyeball and ocular muscles), and then split into the anterior and middle cerebral arteries.

- The *anterior cerebral arteries (ACAs)* supply the majority of the frontal lobe, the anterior limb of the internal capsule, the anterior basal ganglia, and most of the corpus callosum.

- The *middle cerebral arteries (MCAs)* supply the majority of the lateral surface of the hemispheres, including both Broca and Wernicke's areas, which are responsible for the production and comprehension of speech, respectively (see page 59). They also give off countless microscopic arteries called lenticulostriates that supply the internal capsule and the basal ganglia.

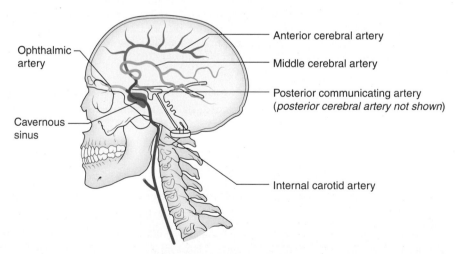

The anterior circulation to the brain.

- *The posterior circulation* supplies the remaining ~25% of the brain. It originates from the vertebral arteries (again, there are two—left and right; the vertebral arteries arise from the subclavian arteries), which travel superiorly, looping in

---

[2]We will not be talking anymore about the external carotid artery, but in case you are interested, it supplies blood to the face and neck, not the brain. External carotid artery disease does not cause stroke.

and out of the transverse foramina of the vertebrae, enter the skull through the foramen magnum, and then merge at the pontomedullary junction to form the basilar artery. The basilar artery runs up the pons then splits into the two posterior cerebral arteries (PCAs) at the junction of the pons and the midbrain.

- The *vertebral arteries* each give off three important branches: the *posterior* and *anterior spinal arteries* (which supply the spinal cord), and the *posterior inferior cerebellar artery* (PICA, which supplies the posterior inferior cerebellum and lateral medulla).

- The *basilar artery* also gives off three important branches: the *anterior inferior* and *superior cerebellar arteries* (AICA and superior cerebellar artery [SCA], which together supply the rest of the cerebellum) and the PCAs (see the next paragraph). The basilar artery also gives off many microscopic *pontine perforator* branches, which supply the pons.

- The posterior cerebral arteries (PCAs) supply the occipital lobe, medial temporal lobe, thalamus, midbrain, and posterior limb of the internal capsule.

Posterior circulation

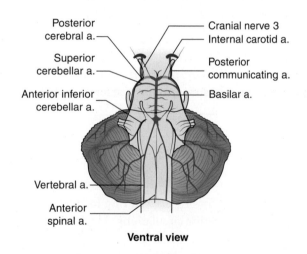

Posterior cerebral a. — Cranial nerve 3 — Internal carotid a.
Superior cerebellar a. — Posterior communicating a.
Anterior inferior cerebellar a. — Basilar a.
Vertebral a.
Anterior spinal a.

Ventral view

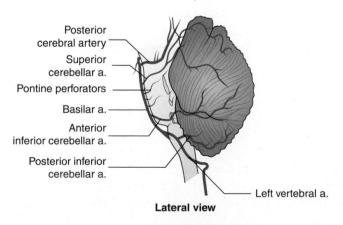

Posterior cerebral artery
Superior cerebellar a.
Pontine perforators
Basilar a.
Anterior inferior cerebellar a.
Posterior inferior cerebellar a.
Left vertebral a.

Lateral view

The posterior circulation to the brain. Note the proximity of the posterior communicating artery to the third nerve; this is why posterior communicating artery aneurysms can cause third nerve palsies!

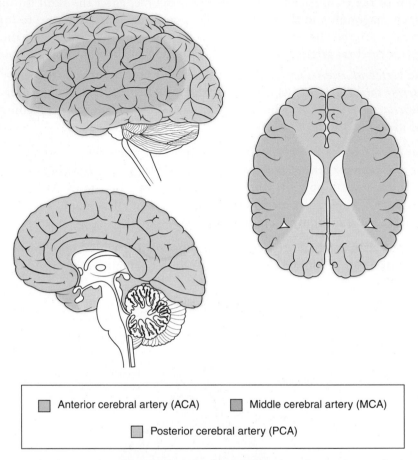

Anterior cerebral artery (ACA), middle cerebral artery (MCA), and posterior cerebral artery (PCA) territory distributions.

The circle of Willis is an anastomotic arterial ring formed at the base of the brain that ties together the anterior and posterior circulations. The *anterior communicating artery* (Acomm) joins the two ACAs, and the *posterior communicating arteries* (Pcomm; there are two of them) connect the internal carotid arteries (ICAs) to the PCAs.

The importance of this circle cannot be overstated, because it can maintain cerebral perfusion despite major vessel blockages. For an extreme example, there are people who live asymptomatically despite two blocked internal carotid arteries; their cerebral blood flow is derived entirely from the posterior circulation which, via the two Pcomm arteries, is able to supply the entire brain.

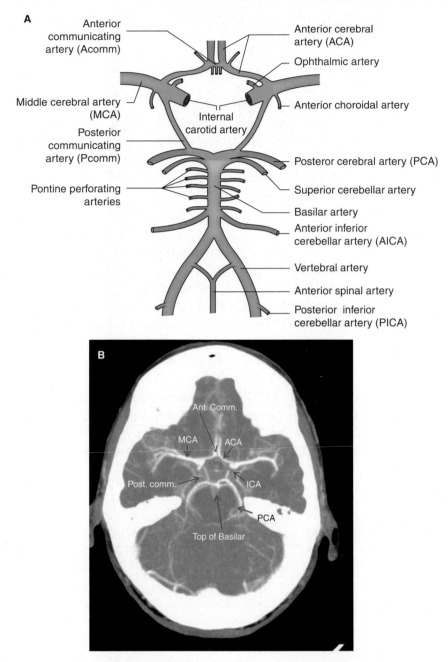

(*A*) The circle of Willis, highlighted in pink, and (*B*) A computerized tomography (CT) angiogram of the circle of Willis.

There are nearly as many anatomical variants in the cerebral circulation as there are people. It's not uncommon, for instance, for the PCAs to be fed predominantly from the anterior circulation via the Pcomms, with only weak or even absent connections to the basilar artery (these are known as **fetal PCAs**). But for our purposes, it's enough to be aware that variation exists and that it can be important in determining both stroke etiology and management.

Ischemic Stroke

Etiology

Ischemic stroke is the result of critically decreased blood flow to an area of brain tissue (or spinal cord or retinal tissue). Many things can cause this; the categories below should help you keep things simple. This is known as the **TOAST classification**—the acronym does not refer to burnt bread but rather to the *Trial of Org 10,172 in Acute Stroke Treatment*, which helped set the framework for this categorization system.

- *Cardioembolism.* Cardioembolic infarcts are due to thrombi that form within the heart and then embolize into the cerebral circulation. *Atrial fibrillation* is the most common cardiac source of emboli. Other cardiac sources include *intracardiac tumors or thrombi, infective endocarditis* (with septic emboli originating from affected valves), *a severely reduced ejection fraction*, and *aortic arch atheroma* (although not technically of cardiac origin, these emboli act the same as if they came from the heart). A *patent foramen ovale* (PFO) is also considered a cardioembolic source, because it can allow for thrombi that form in the deep veins of the legs to pass through the heart via right-to-left shunting and ultimately lodge in the cerebral circulation.

Cardioembolic strokes can be big, knocking out entire vascular territories, or so tiny that they cause virtually no neurologic compromise at all. Either way, they tend to involve the cerebral cortex. Clinically, the neurologic symptoms they cause are often maximal at onset but can also rapidly resolve—embolic clots are unstable and can sometimes dissipate before causing any significant damage.

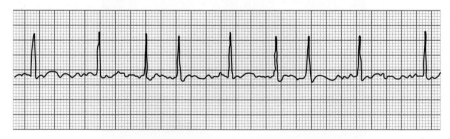

An electrocardiogram (EKG) showing the classic irregularly irregular rhythm of atrial fibrillation, a potential source of cardioembolic stroke.

- *Large artery atherosclerosis.* The specific vessels that qualify as "large" remain debatable, but for our purposes we're talking about the big vessels that bring blood into the brain, including the common and internal carotid arteries, the vertebral and basilar arteries, and the proximal portions of the ACAs, MCAs, and PCAs. These vessels are predisposed to atherosclerotic narrowing at sites of bifurcation (*e.g.*, where the common carotid artery splits into the internal and external carotid arteries) and sites of origin (*e.g.*, at the take-off of the vertebral arteries from the subclavian arteries), but atherosclerosis can—and often does—occur wherever it likes. There are three major mechanisms by which this process can cause ischemic stroke:

  1. *Artery-to-artery embolism.* Just as emboli can shoot up from the heart into the brain, bits of atherosclerotic plaque can break off from the walls of large vessels, travel to and ultimately block the more distal circulation.

  2. *Thrombotic occlusion.* At some point, an atherosclerotic lesion can become sufficiently large that it occludes the lumen of the vessel. These strokes tend to be less severe than those caused by embolism. Because atherosclerotic lesions do not develop overnight, the brain has often had time to adjust, forming well-developed collateral vessels that supply the at-risk tissue and can help maintain perfusion in the setting of thrombotic occlusion.

  3. *Hypoperfusion.* Under normal conditions, a large vessel must be more than 99% narrowed in order to cause ischemia from hypoperfusion alone. However, in the setting of sepsis, cardiac arrest, or even severe dehydration—that is, conditions causing significantly lowered blood pressure—tight vessels can result in **watershed infarcts**, defined as strokes that affect areas located at the border zone between two vascular territories. These areas are the farthest from the vascular supply and thus most vulnerable to reduced perfusion.

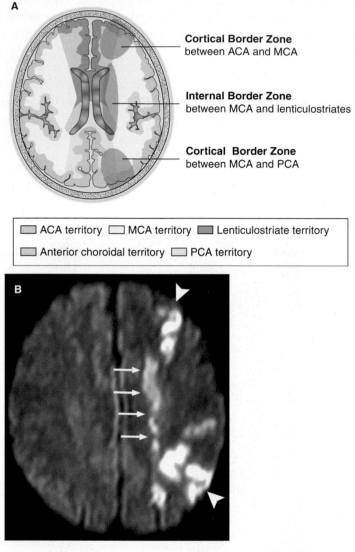

(A) Classic watershed areas, (B) Acute watershed infarcts corresponding to the cortical border zones (between ACA/MCA and MCA/PCA territories; big arrows) and internal border zones (between the MCA and its lenticulostriate branches; small arrows). (B, reprinted from Pope TLJr, Harris JHJr. *Harris & Harris' The Radiology of Emergency Medicine.* 5th ed. Wolters Kluwer; 2012.)

- *Small vessel occlusive disease.* Small vessel disease is often caused by lipohyalinosis of the small penetrating arteries, a process characterized by thickening, weakening, and degeneration of the vessel wall with eventual vessel occlusion, most often the result of long-standing poorly controlled cardiovascular risk factors such as hypertension and diabetes. Smoking is also an important risk factor. Microatheroma is another cause of small vessel disease—essentially the same atherosclerotic process we talked about with large arteries but affecting the smaller vessels. Infarcts due to microatheroma tend to be a little larger and more ovoid than those due to lipohyalinosis. Hyperlipidemia is an important risk factor. In either case, the small arteries that can be affected are:

- The *perforating arteries of the MCA* (the lenticulostriates, which supply the basal ganglia and internal capsule)

- The *perforating arteries of the PCA* (which predominantly supply the thalamus)

- The *perforating arteries of the basilar artery* (the pontine perforators, which supply the pons).

The territories at risk of small vessel disease are therefore the internal capsule, basal ganglia, thalamus, and pons. Small, deep infarcts in these areas caused by small vessel disease are referred to as **lacunar strokes**.

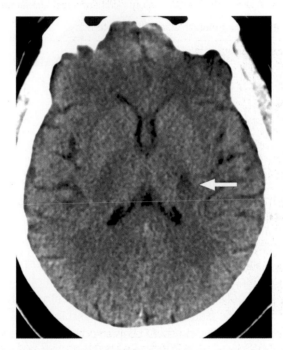

A subacute left internal capsule lacunar infarct. (Reprinted from Pope TLJr, Harris JHJr. *Harris & Harris' The Radiology of Emergency Medicine.* 5th ed. Wolters Kluwer; 2012.)

- *Stroke of other determined etiology.* We can divide this category up into three less common but important etiologic groupings: (1) nonatherosclerotic vessel disease (such as vasculitis, vasospasm, and dissection), (2) hypercoagulability (such as antiphospholipid syndrome), and (3) genetic syndromes that predispose to stroke (such as cerebral autosomal dominant arteriopathy with subcortical infarcts and leukoencephalopathy [CADASIL] and moyamoya; more on these later).

- *Stroke of undetermined etiology.* Despite all of the preceding categorizations, nearly one-third of all strokes are ultimately classified as "cryptogenic."

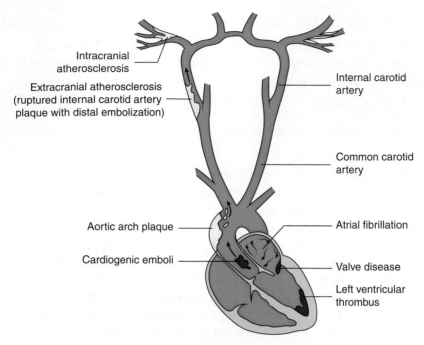

Intracranial
atherosclerosis

Extracranial atherosclerosis
(ruptured internal carotid artery
plaque with distal embolization)

Internal carotid
artery

Common carotid
artery

Aortic arch plaque

Cardiogenic emboli

Atrial fibrillation

Valve disease

Left ventricular
thrombus

A diagram summing up some of the potential etiologies of ischemic stroke.

Box 2.2 Embolic Stroke of Undetermined Source (ESUS)

ESUS is a subcategory of cryptogenic stroke. It is defined as an image-positive (*i.e.*, it can be visualized on CT or MRI) nonlacunar stroke for which no high-risk cardioembolic source, significant large artery stenosis, or other nonembolic source (such as dissection or vasculitis) has been identified. These look like embolic strokes, but without a known embolic source. Occult paroxysmal atrial fibrillation, atrial cardiopathy,[a] and nonstenotic plaque in the cervical and intracranial arteries are thought to be the most likely etiologies. ESUS is important to recognize because it may require different management than "non-ESUS" cryptogenic strokes; the jury's still out, but ongoing studies are assessing the efficacy of anticoagulation in this patient population. At the time of this writing, however, there is no concrete evidence supporting the use of anticoagulation in the management of patients with cryptogenic stroke. Only proven (as opposed to suspected) atrial fibrillation, for instance, is an officially approved indication for anticoagulation.

[a]Atrial cardiopathy is defined as a structural abnormality of the left atrium in the absence of atrial fibrillation; it is thought to increase the risk of stroke either as a precursor to atrial fibrillation or as an independent risk factor for the formation of atrial thrombi.

Box 2.3 Stroke in the Young

The typical culprits that increase the risk of ischemic stroke—hypertension, hyperlipidemia, atrial fibrillation, *etc.*—are far less common in young patients, which in this context is anyone less than 50 years of age. When young patients—like our patient, Laura—present with stroke, they often require a bit more thinking and a more extensive work-up to determine the underlying cause. In this population, the most common etiologies to consider are:

- *Arterial dissection* (see page 84)
- *Hypercoagulability*: Keep in mind that in the setting of stroke we need to consider conditions that predispose to *arterial* thromboembolism, such as antiphospholipid syndrome, underlying malignancy, and the use of estrogen-containing birth control pills when combined with cigarette smoking. Conditions that predispose *only to venous* thromboembolism, such as protein C or S deficiency, are relevant to stroke only in the setting of a PFO or some other type of atrial septal defect.
- *Cardioembolism:* Unlike in older patients, cardioembolism is less often the result of atrial fibrillation and more often the result of conditions such as congenital heart disease, dilated cardiomyopathies, infective endocarditis, intracardiac tumors, and a PFO.
- *Vasculitis:* These can be infectious, autoimmune, and drug related; see page 88.
- *Genetic syndromes:* Specific syndromes that predispose to stroke include sickle cell disease, CADASIL, and moyamoya, see Box 2.4.
- *Illicit drug use:* Cocaine, methamphetamines, and other stimulants can cause rapid elevations in blood pressure, cardiac arrhythmias, and diffuse vasospasm.

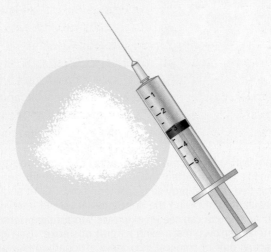

Drugs, such as cocaine, are among the more common precipitants of stroke in those under the age of 50.

Box 2.4 Genetic Syndromes

CADASIL is a small vessel arteriopathy associated with mutations in the NOTCH3 gene on chromosome 19. It classically presents in young adults with some combination of migraine with aura, cognitive decline, and stroke (most often lacunar infarcts involving the external capsule and anterior temporal lobes). There is no specific treatment.

Moyamoya is another nonatherosclerotic progressive arteriopathy. The incidence is highest in the Asian population. Although the etiology is unknown, there appears to be a strong genetic component. Moyamoya typically presents in children or young adults with ischemic or hemorrhagic strokes. Angiography is diagnostic, demonstrating progressive vessel narrowing affecting the arteries around the circle of Willis associated with the growth of prominent but flimsy new vessels (or "neovascularization") that is often referred to as "hazy" or "smoky" (moyamoya actually means "puff of smoke" in Japanese). Surgical revascularization with direct external-to-internal carotid artery bypass or indirect bypass (the procedure is called encephaloduroarteriosynangiosis; EDAS for short—you're welcome), is often necessary.

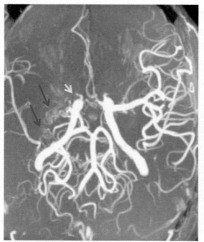 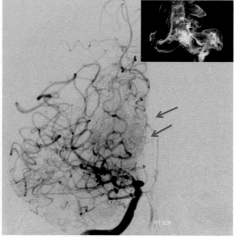

(*A*) An MR angiogram (MRA) from a patient with moyamoya, demonstrating occlusion of the proximal right middle cerebral artery (MCA, yellow arrow) with significantly dilated lenticulostriate vessels (red arrows) providing collateral flow. (*B*) An angiogram demonstrating significant vessel irregularities involving the right internal carotid artery (ICA) bifurcation and right proximal MCA. Again, you can see an extensive surrounding network of thin and flimsy lenticulostriate collaterals (arrows) resembling a "puff of smoke" (see image insert in upper right corner for an actual puff of smoke!). (Courtesy of Jonathan Howard.)

Stroke Syndromes

The ability to rapidly recognize various stroke syndromes is essential because acute stroke treatment is a highly time-sensitive endeavor. The faster you intervene, the better the outcome for the patient.

Cortical Signs. The first strokes that we'll discuss—and the most important to recognize—are those that affect the cerebral cortex. Cortical strokes are most often due to large vessel occlusion (LVO), which in turn is most often the result of either cardioembolism or artery-to-artery embolism. These blood clots are often retrievable via endovascular thrombectomy (*i.e.*, mechanical removal of the clot, see page 73). Urgent head CT *and* CT angiogram are therefore essential, because if an LVO is identified and the patient is eligible, he or she can be whisked off to the operating room for mechanical thrombectomy.

What makes you suspect a cortical stroke? There are only a few signs you need to know.

- *Aphasia.* Both Broca and Wernicke's areas (see the discussion that follows) are part of the dominant cerebral cortex.

Box 2.5

The *dominant cerebral hemisphere* is defined as the hemisphere that controls language. In right-handed people, this is invariably the left hemisphere. In left-handed people, it's about 80/20, right versus left-dominant.

Aphasia is an acquired disorder of language comprehension and/or production. Don't get this confused with *dysarthria*, which is a motor deficit characterized by the impaired ability to control the muscles used for speech, resulting in unclear articulation of speech (often described as "slurred") that is otherwise normal. There are two main language centers in the brain that cause two distinct language deficits when damaged:

1. **Broca's area** is located in the inferior frontal gyrus of the frontal lobe and is responsible for language production. Broca aphasia (also known as *expressive*, or nonfluent, aphasia) is characterized by halting and effortful speech, often with long pauses and difficulty naming objects. The ability to repeat words spoken to them is also lost but *comprehension remains intact*. Damage to the cortex surrounding Broca's area produces a similar expressive aphasia but with preserved repetition (called **transcortical motor aphasia**).

2. **Wernicke's area** is located in the superior temporal gyrus of the temporal lobe and is responsible for language comprehension. Patients with Wernicke aphasia (also known as *receptive*, or fluent, aphasia) demonstrate fluent speech with intact syntax and prosody but devoid of content or meaning. Listening to a patient with Wernicke aphasia speak is like listening to someone speaking in a foreign language that you don't understand; it can be pretty but it is meaningless. Patients are unable to follow spoken commands and, like those with Broca aphasia, lose the ability to repeat. Damage to the cortex surrounding Wernicke's area produces a similar receptive aphasia but with preserved repetition (called **transcortical sensory aphasia**).

Few patients actually present with a pure Broca or Wernicke aphasia. Most aphasias are mixed, although they tend to favor one or the other, meaning they present with either predominantly expressive or receptive deficits.

The arcuate fasciculus is the bundle of nerves that connects Broca and Wernicke's areas and is responsible for repetition; thus, damage here results in the inability to repeat, with preserved fluency and comprehension.

Global aphasia is most often seen in the setting of big left-sided MCA infarcts (somewhere between 70% and 95% of the population is right-handed), which knock out components of the arcuate fasciculus, Wernicke's area and Broca's area, resulting in impaired ability to repeat, understand and produce language.

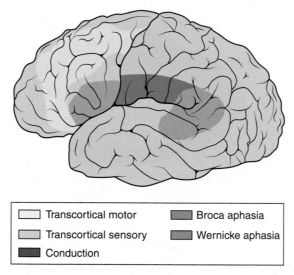

☐ Transcortical motor	▨ Broca aphasia
☐ Transcortical sensory	▨ Wernicke aphasia
▨ Conduction	

Major domains of the brain, illustrating the regions that, when damaged, produce Broca and Wernicke aphasia.

Type of Aphasia	Location of the Lesion	Presentation
Broca aphasia	Inferior frontal gyrus	Expressive (nonfluent) aphasia, with retained comprehension
Transcortical motor aphasia	Cortex surrounding Broca's area	As above, with preserved repetition
Wernicke aphasia	Superior temporal gyrus	Receptive (fluent) aphasia, with retained fluency
Transcortical sensory aphasia	Cortex surrounding Wernicke's area	As above, with preserved repetition
Conduction aphasia	Arcuate fasciculus	Isolated inability to repeat
Global aphasia	Some component of all of the above	Inability to speak fluently, comprehend, or repeat

- *Neglect.* Neglect is the second classic sign of a cortical stroke. It usually localizes to the *nondominant* parietal cortex but can occur with dominant as well as nondominant cortical lesions. Neglect can be dramatic, such as when patients fail to recognize their own arm or only appropriately dress half of their body, or—a much more subtle finding on examination—when patients (like Laura, whom we met at the beginning of this chapter) extinguish to double simultaneous stimuli (see page 31 for a review on neglect and extinction).

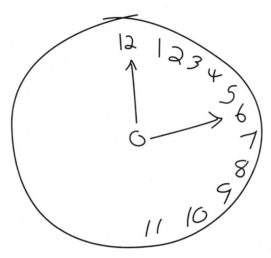

A drawing of a clock by a patient with neglect due to a stroke in the nondominant parietal cortex.

- *Visual field cuts.* Visual field cuts in which the entire contralateral visual field is lost (homonymous hemianopia), or in which the upper or lower quadrant of the contralateral visual field is lost (homonymous quadrantanopia) are due to lesions that involve the visual cortex in the occipital lobe or lesions impacting the optic radiations, which are also by and large cortical pathways.

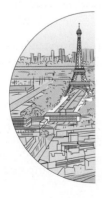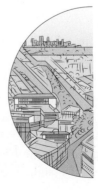

Paris as seen through the eyes of a patient with a right homonymous hemianopia.

• *Gaze preference.* Gaze preference (see page 32) is most often due to involvement of the frontal eye fields, which are tracts located in the frontal cortex. For instance, when stimulated (as in seizure), the left frontal eye field pushes the eyes to the right, and vice versa. When knocked out (as in stroke), the left frontal eye field loses its influence and the right frontal eye field "wins," pushing the eyes to the left. The result is that patients who are seizing "look away from the lesion," and patients with stroke "look toward the lesion."

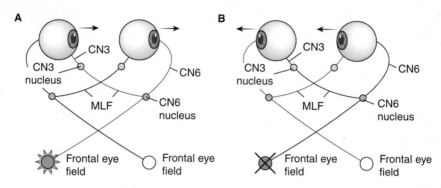

The frontal eye fields. (*A*) When the left frontal eye field is stimulated, the right sixth nerve nucleus and (via the medial longitudinal fasciculus [MLF]; see page 232) the left third nerve nucleus are stimulated, resulting in right gaze. (*B*) When the left frontal eye field is knocked out, the right frontal eye field takes over, and the eyes deviate to the left.

Again (because this is important!): **aphasia, neglect, visual field cuts, and gaze preference are the four major cortical signs you need to know.** There are other cortical signs to be aware of that are not part of the official NIH stroke scale (NIHSS) used to assess stroke severity (see the next page) but which can be equally as helpful. Listed below, these tend to localize to the parietal lobe.

• *Apraxia*—the inability to execute a previously known motor task, not explained by other deficits (such as weakness or blindness). To test for various apraxias, you can ask your patients to show you how they brush their teeth, comb their hair, or button their shirt.

• *Astereognosis*—the inability to recognize objects through touch alone. Ask your patients to close their eyes and then place an object—a penny or a paper clip—in their hand. If they cannot figure out what the object is, they have astereognosia.

• *Agraphesthesia*—the inability to recognize writing on the skin. Ask your patients to close their eyes, but this time draw a letter or number on the palm of the hand. If they cannot figure out what you've written, they have agraphesthesia.

• *Anosognosia*—a condition in which patients do not recognize—or have significantly reduced insight into—their own deficit.

Box 2.6 The NIHSS

The NIHSS became the gold-standard scale for rating stroke severity following the publication of the National Institute of Neurological Disorders and Stroke (NINDS) trial in 1995.[a] It ranges from 0 (no deficits) to 42. It can be useful in an acute setting to get a quick sense of just how bad a patient's symptoms are but should not be substituted for a real neurologic examination. It significantly underrepresents both right-sided and posterior circulation symptoms, and—although high scores are meant to convey more severe symptoms—low scores can hide devastating deficits: pure aphasia, for instance, may result in only a 1, 2, or 3 on this scale.

1a. Level of Consciousness	0 - Alert
1b. What is month/age	0 - Answers both correctly
1c. Open/close eyes and hand	0 - Performs both correctly
2. Best gaze	0 - Normal
3. Visual fields	0 - No visual loss
4. Facial palsy	1 - Minor
5a. Motor—left arm	0 - No drift
5b. Motor—right arm	0 - No drift
6a. Motor—left leg	0 - No drift
6b. Motor—right leg	0 - No drift
7. Limb ataxia	0 - Absent
8. Sensory	1 - Mild to moderate loss
9. Best language	0 - No aphasia
10. Dysarthria	0 - Normal
11. Extinction/inattention	1 - Extinction to one modality

Our patient Laura's NIHSS result. Although you picked up on subtle left upper extremity weakness on your examination, Laura is able to hold her left arm up against gravity for a full 10 seconds without any downward drift; thus, she scores 0 for left arm weakness. As is often the case, the NIHSS does not capture the full extent of her deficits.

[a]see National Institute of Neurological Disorders and Stroke rt-PA Stroke Study Group. TPA for acute ischemic stroke. *N Engl J Med*. 1995;333(24):1581-1587.

ACA, MCA, and PCA Strokes. MCA strokes are by far the most common, but ACA and PCA strokes are not rare. The table below is far from comprehensive but gives a good overview of the most important and most frequent signs and symptoms to recognize. You'll note that all of these syndromes include the cortical signs we just discussed above.

	Symptom	Localization
MCA	Contralateral hemiparesis (face/arm > leg)	Motor cortex
	Contralateral hemisensory loss (face/arm > leg)	Sensory cortex
	Contralateral homonymous hemianopia	Optic radiations
	Aphasia (dominant MCA)	Broca or Wernicke's areas
	Neglect (either dominant or nondominant MCA)	Parietal cortex
ACA	Contralateral hemiparesis (leg > face/arm)	Motor cortex
	Contralateral hemisensory loss (leg > face/arm)	Sensory cortex
	Abulia—*i.e.*, apathy (inability to act willfully), often associated with decreased spontaneous speech and movement	Uncertain; thought to involve the cingulate gyrus
	Aphasia (dominant ACA)	Transcortical motor area
	Gait apraxia—*i.e.*, difficulty initiating gait	Frontal cortex
PCA	Contralateral homonymous hemianopia	Visual cortex
	Contralateral hemisensory loss	Thalamus
	Memory impairment (dominant or bilateral PCA)	Hippocampus
	Alexia without agraphia (dominant PCA)—*i.e.*, the inability to read with the retained ability to write	Temporal/Occipital cortex
	Prosopagnosia (nondominant PCA)—*i.e.*, the inability to recognize faces	Fusiform gyrus

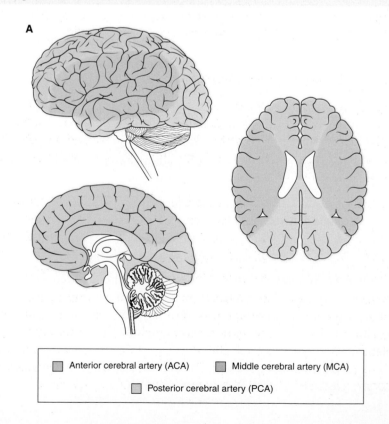

A

▢ Anterior cerebral artery (ACA)	▢ Middle cerebral artery (MCA)
	▢ Posterior cerebral artery (PCA)

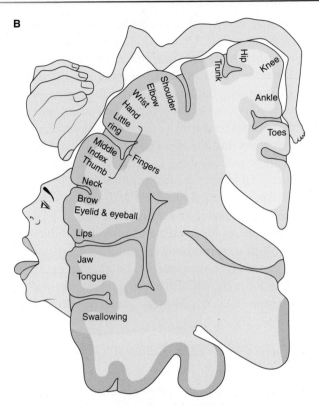

(*A*) A reminder of the anterior cerebral artery (ACA), middle cerebral artery (MCA), and posterior cerebral artery (PCA) territories. (*B*) The homunculus (*i.e.*, "small human") is a topographic representation of the cortical motor areas dedicated to different parts of the body (a similar version exists for the cortical sensory areas). As you can see, ACA strokes will predominantly affect the lower extremities, whereas MCA strokes will affect the upper extremities and face.

Box 2.7 A Few Stroke Syndromes to Know

Gerstmann syndrome is characterized by the clinical tetrad of left/right confusion, finger agnosia (the impaired ability to discriminate among one's own fingers), acalculia (the inability to perform mathematical calculations), and agraphia (the inability to write). It is caused by lesions in the dominant parietal cortex, typically MCA (but occasionally PCA) territory.

Balint syndrome is caused by lesions in the bilateral parieto-occipital cortex, corresponding to the MCA/PCA border zone. It presents with oculomotor apraxia (the absence of controlled, purposeful eye movements, often causing significant trouble with reading), optic ataxia (poor visual-motor coordination), and simultagnosia (the inability to perceive more than one object at a time).

Anton Syndrome is a form of cortical blindness associated with anosognosia, in which the patient is unaware that he or she is blind. Patients will continue to insist—often quite adamantly, and in the face of clear evidence to the contrary—that they can see, and will often confabulate (meaning they will fabricate imaginary information) when asked about objects or images placed in front of them. This is caused by bilateral damage to the occipital cortex, a result of bilateral PCA or top-of-the-basilar artery occlusion.

Basilar Artery Stroke. Basilar artery occlusions can be devastating due to thalamic, brainstem, and cerebellar involvement. Unlike ACA, MCA, and PCA strokes, they can be difficult to recognize given their highly variable and often stuttering presentation. Symptoms range from isolated oculomotor palsies to locked-in syndrome or coma. Importantly, unlike most ACA, MCA and PCA strokes, basilar occlusions can present with a decreased level of consciousness, a result of involvement of the reticular activating system (RAS).

The "top of the basilar" syndrome is a stroke caused by a clot lodged at the very top of the basilar artery, just before it splits into the two PCAs. The pontine perforators are spared, but both PCA territories are at risk, resulting in ischemia of the bilateral thalami, midbrain, posterior temporal and occipital lobes. Classic symptoms include a decreased level of consciousness, vertical gaze palsy, cortical blindness and—if the superior cerebellar arteries are involved—vertigo, nausea, vomiting, and ataxia.

Locked-in syndrome is a catastrophic condition caused by bilateral pontine ischemia due to basilar artery embolism or thrombosis (pontine hemorrhage, usually related to hypertension, is another cause). It is characterized by quadriplegia and the inability to speak or swallow, but consciousness, cognitive function and vertical eye movements are spared. Patients are effectively "locked in"—wide awake but only able to communicate by blinking.

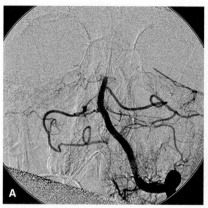 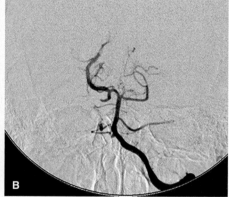

Anteroposterior (AP) angiographic view showing a top of the basilar occlusion pre- (*A*) and post- (*B*) thrombectomy. In figure A, blood flow is blocked and you can't see the posterior cerebral arteries (PCAs); but in figure B, following thrombectomy, the PCAs fill with blood and can now be clearly visualized. (Reprinted from Barkovich AJ, Raybaud C. *Pediatric Neuroimaging.* 6th ed. Wolters Kluwer; 2018.)

Brainstem Stroke Syndromes. The brainstem structures—the midbrain, pons, and medulla—are small but important: they contain the majority of the cranial nerve nuclei as well as the sensory and motor tracts that run to and from the cortex and the spinal cord. The result is that a very small brainstem stroke can have very big consequences. There are dozens of specific brainstem stroke syndromes, but if you keep the following principles in mind you won't need to memorize much at all.

- Crossed symptoms, a term referring to ipsilateral cranial nerve deficits (affecting the face) and contralateral sensorimotor deficits (affecting the body), are a classic feature of brainstem strokes. Remember, the cranial nerves (CNs) do not decussate (with the exception of CN4 and the branch of CN3 that innervates the contralateral superior rectus; don't worry about this!), but the motor and sensory pathways do (*i.e.*, the corticospinal tracts and dorsal column medial lemniscal tracts in the medulla and the spinothalamic tracts in the cord; see pages 18 and 23).

- The major motor pathway (the corticospinal tract) runs medially in the brainstem.

- The pain/temperature pathway (the spinothalamic tract) runs laterally in the brainstem, often side-by-side with the sympathetic tract.

- Cranial nerves 3 through 12 exit from the brainstem (CN3 and 4 exit from the midbrain; 5, 6, 7, and 8 exit from the pons; and 9, 10, 11, and 12 exit from the medulla; see the picture below). Thus, among other symptoms, midbrain strokes often present with CN3 and 4 involvement, pontine strokes with some combination of CN5, 6, 7, and 8 involvement, and medullary strokes with CN9, 10, 11, and 12 involvement. Keep in mind that the trigeminal nerve (CN5) nucleus is the largest of the cranial nerve nuclei and actually extends from the midbrain through the pons and medulla into the high cervical spinal cord. Ipsilateral facial numbness is therefore not a particularly helpful localizer, as it can be seen in strokes affecting any of the above mentioned structures.

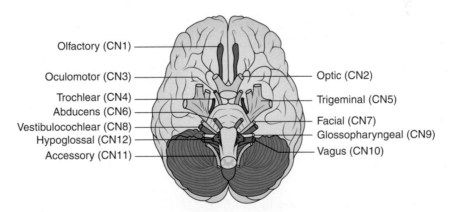

The cranial nerve nuclei.

Keeping these few points in mind, here are a few brainstem stroke syndromes you should know. These are clinically important, and come up frequently on rounds and even in real life—often not in complete form but certainly in a recognizable presentation. The italicized font on the next page helps highlight the key distinguishing features of each syndrome.

Box 2.8

Jean-Dominique Bauby was the editor-in-chief of the French edition of *Elle* magazine in 1995 when he suffered a brainstem stroke that left him locked in. *The Diving Bell and the Butterfly* is his memoir, published several years later and written entirely—with the help of a transcriber who repeatedly recited the alphabet—by blinking, selecting one letter at a time. The film adaptation premiered in Cannes in 2007.

- *Wallenberg syndrome*
  - Location: lateral medulla
  - Vascular supply: PICA
  - Presentation:
    - *Hoarseness, dysphagia, hiccups* (nucleus ambiguus: CN10, 11)
    - Ipsilateral pain/temperature loss to face (CN5)
    - Contralateral pain/temperature loss to body (spinothalamic tract)
    - Ipsilateral Horner syndrome (sympathetics)
    - Ataxia (inferior cerebellar peduncle)
    - Vertigo (vestibular nuclei)
- *Dejerine syndrome*
  - Location: medial medulla
  - Vascular supply: vertebral artery, anterior spinal artery
  - Presentation:
    - *Ipsilateral tongue weakness* (CN12)
    - Contralateral hemiparesis (corticospinal tract)
    - Contralateral vibration/proprioception loss to body (dorsal column medial lemniscus tract)
- *Marie Foix syndrome*
  - Location: lateral pons
  - Vascular supply: AICA, pontine perforators
  - Presentation:
    - Ipsilateral pain/temperature loss to face (CN5)
    - *Ipsilateral facial droop* (CN7)
    - *Ipsilateral hearing loss* (CN8)
    - Contralateral pain/temperature loss to body (spinothalamic tract)
    - Ipsilateral Horner syndrome (sympathetics)
    - Ataxia (middle and inferior cerebellar peduncles)

Lacunar Stroke Syndromes. Lacunar strokes account for approximately 25% of all ischemic strokes and are most often due to small vessel disease of the perforating arteries of the MCA, PCA, and basilar artery (see page 54). There are five classic lacunar syndromes. The first three characteristically involve the face, arm, and leg; all five are usually, but not always, devoid of any cortical signs.

- Pure motor—weakness of the contralateral face, arm, and leg. This is the most common lacunar syndrome, usually due to infarcts in the internal capsule or basal ganglia.
- Pure sensory—sensory loss of the contralateral face, arm, and leg; almost always due to thalamic infarcts.
- Sensorimotor—some combination of the above; most often due to infarcts involving both the thalamus and the internal capsule (termed thalamocapsular infarcts).
- Ataxic hemiparesis—characterized by weakness and ataxia of the involved limb(s). Localization varies.
- Clumsy-hand dysarthria—characterized by dysarthria as well as by clumsiness and mild weakness of one hand. Localization varies.

CT misses most lacunes (particularly those in the brainstem), so MRI is often necessary for diagnosis.

Box 2.9 Internuclear Ophthalmoplegia (INO)

INO, a disorder of conjugate lateral gaze in which one eye is unable to fully adduct even as the other abducts completely, is caused by damage to the medial longitudinal fasciculus (MLF; a tract of fibers located in the paramedian area of the midbrain and pons). Although it is most often due to multiple sclerosis in young patients, brainstem stroke is the most common cause in the elderly. INO is described in greater detail in Chapter 9 (see page 232).

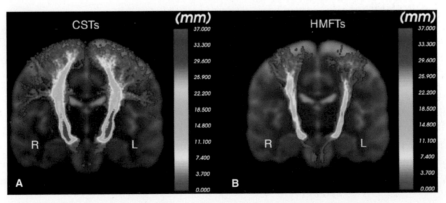

A heat map of the corticospinal fibers, which start out widely dispersed in the motor cortex and then gather together, as they descend through the corona radiata into the internal capsule and brainstem, into a tightly bound bundle. The result is that cortical damage to these fibers tends to affect only part of the hemibody (either the face, arm, or leg), whereas deeper damage—as occurs in lacunar infarcts—affects the entire hemibody. (Reprinted from Dalamagkas K, Tsintou M, Rathi Y, et al. Individual variations of the human corticospinal tract and its hand-related motor fibers using diffusion MRI tractography. *Brain Imaging Behav.* 2020;14(3):696-714.)

Ischemic Stroke Etiologies	Ischemic Stroke Syndromes
Cardioembolism	ACA, MCA, PCA stroke
Large artery atherosclerosis	Basilar artery stroke
Small vessel occlusive disease	Brainstem stroke
Stroke of other determined etiology	Lacunar stroke
Stroke of undetermined etiology	

A quick summary of what you've learned so far about ischemic stroke—see, it's not that bad!

Management

Not long ago, stroke was treated as a chronic condition. Management focused solely on rehabilitation and secondary prevention. Then, in 1996, tissue plasminogen activator (tPA) was approved for the acute treatment of ischemic stroke. Because tPA must be given quickly to be effective, the arrival of this drug resulted virtually overnight in the transformation of ischemic stroke from a chronic condition into a neurologic emergency. With the advent of endovascular thrombectomy in 2015, the time window in which we could treat ischemic stroke was expanded, and today, with ongoing trials utilizing new imaging techniques that help us identify salvageable brain tissue, that window continues to grow.

Acute stroke care moves fast. There is a clear association between time to treatment and meaningful recovery. Thus, when a patient presents with an acute onset of a focal neurologic deficit, in order to provide the best care possible, it becomes a true team effort, often involving the patient's family members, coworkers, and even bystanders, as well as emergency medical services, nurses, and physicians.

When a patient with a likely stroke shows up at an emergency setting, there are two decisions that must be made as quickly as possible.

- Is the patient a candidate for tPA?
- Is the patient a candidate for endovascular thrombectomy?

These questions are independent of each other; the answer to one in no way affects the answer to the other.[3] If the answer to both is "no," the urgency of the stroke code is over. But let's walk through what happens when the answer to both is "yes."

IV Thrombolytic Therapy. Thrombolytics break up blood clots. tPA, the first and still most commonly used IV thrombolytic[4] in acute stroke care, does this by catalyzing the conversion of plasminogen into plasmin, which in turn lyses the fibrin clot. It was Food and Drug Administration (FDA) approved in 1996 to be given within a 3-hour time window; since then, that window has expanded to 4.5 hours[5] from what we refer to as

---

[3]This is true as of this writing, but ongoing research is currently investigating the risks and benefits of giving tPA prior to thrombectomy.

[4]Tenecteplase (TNK) is another thrombolytic that can be used. It is similar to tPA but has a higher fibrin specificity and a longer half-life; its time window and contraindications are the same. Ongoing research is evaluating its efficacy for acute stroke.

[5]The recent publication of several large clinical trials has resulted in further expansion of the tPA window in carefully selected patient populations with specific imaging characteristics suggestive of significant salvageable brain tissue. Perhaps most excitingly, patients with "wake-up" strokes (*i.e.*, patients who fall asleep "normal" and wake up the following morning with neurologic deficits) are now potential tPA candidates if their imaging meets specific criteria.

Box 2.10 Capsular Warning Syndrome

Motor lacunes occasionally present with a burst of dramatic, hemiplegic TIAs, in which the motor deficit repeatedly appears and then—usually after 10 to 15 minutes or so—fully resolves. Unfortunately, about 50% of these patients go on to develop fixed deficits within a day or so.

"last known well," or the time at which the patient was last definitively seen at his or her neurologic baseline.

When a stroke code is activated, the last known well is the first piece of information you need to obtain. If the patient is within the therapeutic window, all of your follow-up questions should then be geared toward determining whether or not the patient is eligible for tPA. The list of relative and absolute contraindications for tPA is long and complicated but can be simplified by asking two questions.

1. *Is the patient likely to bleed?* tPA breaks up clots and thus predisposes to bleeding. There are only three objective measures that must always be checked prior to tPA administration: blood pressure, a finger-stick glucose, and a CT of the head. Severely elevated blood pressure (systolic blood pressure [SBP] >185 or diastolic blood pressure [DBP] > 110, according to the most recent guidelines) is a contraindication to tPA, but can often be rapidly reduced with IV antihypertensive therapy. Glucose levels below 50 or above 400 are also contraindications (hypo- and hyperglycemia are common stroke mimics; see page 75), but again can often be rapidly corrected and, if the neurologic deficits persist despite correction, do not preclude tPA administration. Finally, a CT of the head must be completed to rule out intracranial hemorrhage.

   Significant surgery, head trauma, or stroke within the preceding 3 months are all relative tPA contraindications, determined on a case-by-case basis by weighing risks and benefits. The presence of an intra-axial brain tumor or active use of an anticoagulant (including heparin, Lovenox, dabigatran, apixaban, and rivaroxaban) are also contraindications. Warfarin is its own story: if the patient is on warfarin, a stat international normalized ratio (INR) must be checked, and if it's greater than 1.7, tPA is contraindicated.

2. *Are the patient's symptoms disabling?* Isolated sensory symptoms, for example, tend to be considered nondisabling, and thus tPA is not recommended; the risk/benefit ratio favors withholding treatment. That said, one person's minor neurologic deficit is another's entire world. Mild finger weakness, for instance, may not affect the quality of life of a 90-year-old patient who lives in a nursing home but could end the career of a young pianist or surgeon. In the case of our patient, Laura, the numbness and weakness involving her left arm are subtle findings but ultimately deemed disabling given her career as a professional tennis player. These decisions must be individualized, with risks and benefits weighed as appropriate.

If there are no contraindications, tPA is relatively safe. The two immediate concerns are *symptomatic intracerebral hemorrhage (ICH)* and *orolingual angioedema.*

Symptomatic ICH (seen in approximately 6% of patients in the original trials; it is more common in older patients with larger infarcts) occurs as a consequence of reperfusion injury (*i.e.*, bleeding and tissue damage caused by the rapid return of blood flow to weakened blood vessels following a period of ischemia). If your patient's examination begins to worsen after you've started tPA, symptomatic ICH must be at the top of your differential. Stop the tPA infusion, obtain a stat CT, and if significant bleeding is identified, reverse the tPA with either cryoprecipitate or tranexamic acid.

Orolingual angioedema is most often seen in patients previously or currently on an angiotensin-converting enzyme inhibitor. It is typically asymmetric and can cause significant airway compromise. If the symptoms are severe, the tPA infusion must be stopped, intubation considered, and steroids and an antihistamine given as soon as possible.

tPA works (*i.e.*, it opens, or recanalizes, the occluded vessel) between 5% and 30% of the time. It is more effective at breaking up smaller clots than bigger ones; the rate of success with large vessel occlusions (LVOs) is only around 10%.

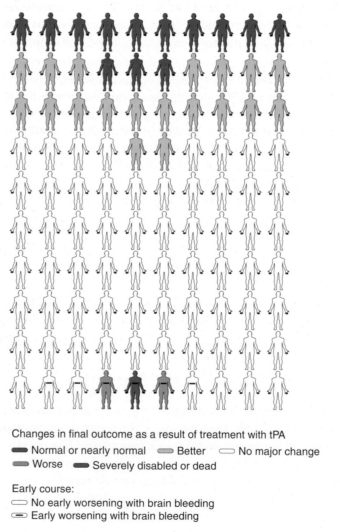

Changes in final outcome as a result of treatment with tPA
- Normal or nearly normal   - Better   - No major change
- Worse   - Severely disabled or dead

Early course:
- No early worsening with brain bleeding
- Early worsening with brain bleeding

For every 100 patients who receive tissue plasminogen activator (tPA), about one-third improve, most are unaffected, and a few do worse.

Box 2.11 Last Known Well

The moment when a patient was last known well may be equivalent to the time of symptom onset (*e.g.*, if the patient is able to tell you that he or she was fine at 11:45 pm and became acutely weak on the left side at 11:46 pm, then he or she was last known well at 11:45 pm), but it's often not so straightforward. Aphasic patients, for instance, may not be able to tell you when their symptoms began, and thus you must rely on collateral input, often from family members or home health aides, to determine last known well. So-called "wake-up" strokes are also common: patients go to sleep "well" and then wake up with new neurologic deficits. In these cases, we can't know what time the stroke happened and the last known well will be the time at which the patient fell asleep.

Endovascular Thrombectomy. The need to develop effective endovascular therapy was prompted by the tight time window and long list of contraindications associated with tPA; although groundbreaking, tPA is ultimately able to treat only a fraction of patients with acute ischemic stroke.

The road to the development of safe and effective mechanical thrombectomy was a rocky one, with multiple failed trials along the way. But the pivotal moment came in 2015 with the publication of the MR CLEAN trial, a randomized controlled trial out of the Netherlands that showed clear benefit of mechanical thrombectomy in patients with acute ischemic stroke and LVO presenting within 6 hours of symptom onset. This trial prompted a flurry of others which not only confirmed positive outcomes but continued to expand the time window. Today, with the help of perfusion imaging techniques that allow us to distinguish dead from dying tissue (see Box 2.12), we routinely treat patients up to 24 hours after symptom onset, and that window continues to grow.

So what is mechanical thrombectomy? The techniques and devices continue to evolve, but the general idea is to mechanically remove the clot and thereby restore blood flow to the affected area of the brain.

The clot must be retrievable, and therefore only patients with LVOs (*i.e.*, with a clot in the ICA, proximal MCA, ACA, PCA, or basilar artery) that are visualized on angiographic imaging are eligible. There are otherwise no absolute contraindications. Decisions for eligibility are determined on a case-by-case basis, taking into account the patient's baseline functional status, symptom severity, and, in cases that push the limits of the time window, specific perfusion imaging characteristics.

The "number needed to treat" for one patient to regain functional independence is around 3, making mechanical thrombectomy one of the most effective quality-of-life and disability-saving procedures that we have.

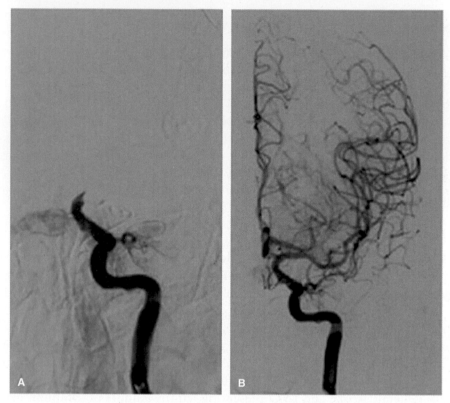

Pre- and postoperative angiogram. (*A*) Preoperative angiogram demonstrating a left internal carotid artery (ICA) occlusion, and (*B*) postoperative angiogram, showing complete reperfusion of the ICA, anterior cerebral artery (ACA), and middle cerebral artery (MCA) branches. (Reprinted from Ikeda H, Yamana N, Murata Y, Saiki M. Thrombus removal by acute-phase endovascular reperfusion therapy to treat cerebral embolism caused by thrombus in the pulmonary vein stump after left upper pulmonary lobectomy: case report. *NMC Case Rep J.* 2014;2(1):26-30.)

Box 2.12 Perfusion Imaging

The idea behind perfusion imaging, which can be either CT or MR based, is to distinguish dead from dying brain tissue (referred to as *core* and *penumbra*, respectively). There are various parameters, including *cerebral blood flow* (CBF, the total blood volume moving through a given imaging parameter per unit time), *cerebral blood volume* (CBV, the total blood volume within a given imaging parameter), and *time to peak* (TTP, also known as *mean transit time*, and defined as the time from the start of contrast injection to maximal tissue enhancement), that help determine the extent of dead versus dying tissue.

Box 2.12 Perfusion Imaging (Continued)

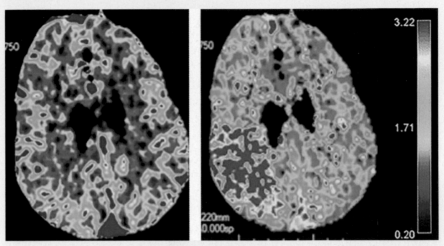

A computerized tomography (CT) perfusion scan in a patient with a right middle cerebral artery (MCA) stroke. The scans are "mismatched" in that the area of increased time to peak (TTP; image on the right) has no correlate on the cerebral blood volume (CBV; image on the left) map. This patient would be a candidate for thrombectomy, because there is significant penumbral tissue to save. (Modified from Saremi F. *Perfusion Imaging in Clinical Practice*. Wolters Kluwer; 2015.)

Why does this distinction matter? It turns out that time, used for so long as a surrogate for salvageable brain tissue, isn't always the most reliable indicator. There are patients who have a completed infarct (*i.e.*, 100% dead tissue) within an hour of their stroke, and others who have significant salvageable tissue (*i.e.*, a large penumbra) days after their stroke. There is no benefit—and very real potential harm—in performing mechanical thrombectomy in patients with a large core infarct: there is no tissue to save, and the dead tissue is at high risk of bleeding if perfusion is suddenly restored. But the reverse is also true: there is often significant benefit with little potential harm in performing thrombectomy in patients with a substantial penumbra. Perfusion imaging can therefore be extraordinarily useful in helping to select patients—particularly those at the outer limits of the currently-accepted time windows—for endovascular intervention.

Long-Term Management and Secondary Prevention of Stroke. Antiplatelet therapy (most often with aspirin, clopidogrel, or, in specific cases, some combination of the two) and lipid-lowering therapy (with statins, *i.e.*, the 3-hydroxy-3-methyl-glutaryl-coenzyme A [HMG CoA] reductase inhibitors) are mainstays of secondary stroke prevention. Anticoagulation is indicated when atrial fibrillation is found.

Risk factor control is essential. After the acute period following stroke, during which we sometimes allow "permissive hypertension" to help maintain tissue perfusion, we aim for strict blood pressure control. Management of diabetes, weight loss, and smoking cessation are also critical.

Box 2.13 Stroke Mimics

There are many things that can cause the acute onset of focal neurologic deficits besides stroke. Some of these disorders—such as migraine with aura—can often be clinically distinguished from stroke, but many cannot, at least not rapidly and with 100% confidence. If you aren't sure, and if the patient is eligible for tPA, give the tPA. The risk is low, especially in patients without underlying brain pathology. It is almost always better to treat a patient with a stroke mimic than to miss the opportunity to treat an ischemic stroke.

Common stroke mimics include:

- *Seizure/postictal paralysis* (see page 166)
- *Brain tumors.* We tend to think of brain tumors as presenting gradually, with headache, systemic symptoms such as weight loss and fatigue, and the insidious onset of focal neurologic deficits, which they usually do (see Chapter 16). But it isn't uncommon for patients to present more acutely. Whether this is because the tumor has bled, has finally crossed some symptomatic threshold or because the patient has previously been unaware of the deficit until he or she is finally prompted to recognize it, we often don't know.
- *Hypertensive encephalopathy.* Sudden rises in blood pressure can cause cerebral edema due to failure of cerebral autoregulation resulting in rapid rises in cerebral blood flow. This condition typically presents with the gradual onset of headache, nausea, vomiting, and confusion, but can present with focal neurologic symptoms as well.
- *Migraine with aura* (see page 96)
- *Stroke recrudescence.* Recrudescence refers to the re-emergence or unmasking of prior stroke-related neurologic deficits. Such symptoms can last hours to days and are often triggered by infection, hypotension, metabolic derangements, and even severe stress. Deficits should gradually improve with resolution of the provoking factor.
- *Hypo- or hyperglycemia.* Severe abnormalities in the levels of blood glucose can both trigger stroke recrudescence and cause new focal symptoms all on their own, without any underlying brain pathology.

Some specific stroke etiologies also require specific treatments. Infective endocarditis, for instance, is treated with long-term intravenous antibiotics. Symptomatic extracranial carotid stenosis (*i.e.*, narrowing of an extracranial portion of a carotid artery that is thought to have caused the stroke) can be treated surgically if the patient is eligible and the stenosis is severe, with either angioplasty and stenting or open endarterectomy.

 Intracerebral Hemorrhage (ICH)

Congratulations, you've made it to stroke type number two! Hemorrhage is more straightforward than ischemia (we promise), both in terms of etiology and management. Although it remains significantly less common than ischemic stroke, the incidence of intracerebral hemorrhage (ICH) is rising, likely due to the aging population and to the increasingly widespread use of antiplatelet and anticoagulant medications.

Symptoms

Hemorrhagic and ischemic strokes are clinically indistinguishable. The tissue is damaged either way, either from a blocked or ruptured blood vessel, and the consequent neurologic deficits will be identical.

So how do you distinguish between hemorrhage and ischemia in a patient presenting with new, acute-onset focal symptoms? Easy: get a CT scan. Every single stroke patient needs a CT, because the CT is the only way to know for sure.

Prior to imaging, you should suspect ischemic stroke based on the numbers alone (remember, over 85% of strokes are ischemic), with only two exceptions. These are not hard-and-fast rules, only tip-offs to make you think of hemorrhage instead of ischemia:

- *Worst headache of life.* Patients who present with "the worst headache of my life" have a subarachnoid hemorrhage until proven otherwise (see page 81).

- *Decreased level of alertness.* This is nearly always seen with large bleeds, presumably due to elevated intracranial pressure and subsequent diffuse compression of the RAS, the network of thalamic and brainstem neurons that mediate arousal and alertness. Ischemic strokes that affect these RAS neurons can also cause a decreased level of consciousness, but the majority of ischemic strokes—even the really big ones—do not, and patients are usually wide awake. Basilar strokes are the big exception; see page 66.

Box 2.14 Ischemic Stroke and Altered Level of Consciousness

There are three ischemic stroke locations that can result in altered consciousness: the thalamus, brainstem, and bilateral cerebral hemispheres. *Strokes that affect the thalamus or brainstem* can do it as a result of direct damage to the reticular activating system (RAS). *Bilateral hemispheric strokes*—often in the setting of an embolic shower, when tiny emboli are shot up from the heart and scatter into the cerebral circulation— can also be responsible. Finally, *any big stroke* that swells, causing midline shift, ventricular compression, and elevated intracranial pressure will also cause a decreased level of consciousness via the same pathophysiologic mechanism as large bleeds.

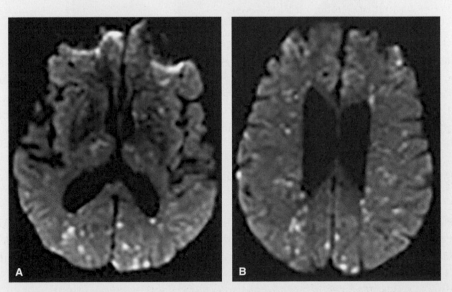

A diffusion-weighted imaging (DWI) MRI sequence showing numerous bilateral, embolic-appearing strokes. (Modified from Atlas SW. *Magnetic Resonance Imaging of the Brain and Spine.* 5th ed. Wolters Kluwer; 2016.)

Both ischemic and hemorrhagic stroke can, and often do, present with elevated blood pressure. In the setting of ischemia, this is the result of the body's attempt to keep pumping blood to the dead or dying oxygen-deprived brain tissue (a phenomenon colloquially known as "auto-pressing"). In the setting of hemorrhage, acute hypertension is often the cause, not the consequence, of the stroke.

Etiology

The majority of ICHs are the result of uncontrolled hypertension which over time can lead to the formation of tiny Charcot-Bouchard aneurysms that are prone to rupture. The blood vessels that are affected are generally the same as those affected by small vessel occlusive disease that causes lacunar infarcts. Thus, with one notable exception, hypertensive hemorrhages tend to occur in the same anatomic locations as lacunar infarcts: the basal ganglia, internal capsule, thalamus, and pons.

The major exception is the cerebellum, which is not affected by lacunar infarcts but is commonly affected by hypertensive bleeds. Cerebellar hemorrhages usually present with occipital headache, nausea, vomiting, vertigo, and gait dysfunction due to ataxia. Direction-changing nystagmus and dysmetria are often present on examination.

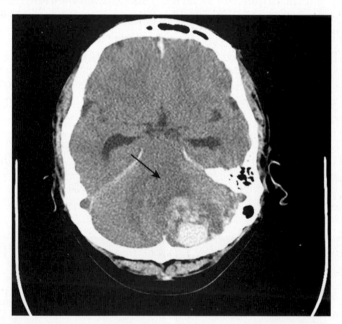

A CT of a patient with a cerebellar hemorrhage and surrounding edema causing complete effacement of the fourth ventricle (arrow) and developing hydrocephalus of the lateral and third ventricles. (Reprinted from Biller J. *Practical Neurology*. 5th ed. Wolters Kluwer; 2017.)

Other less common but important causes of ICH include:

- *Cerebral vascular malformations*
  - *Arteriovenous malformations (AVMs)* account for nearly half of ICHs in patients younger than 40. AVMs are tangles of intraparenchymal arteries and veins that lack the normal intervening capillary bed. The result is that arterial pressures are

directly transmitted to venous structures, causing increased blood flow, venous dilation, and, ultimately, ICH. They can be visualized on MRI but are best diagnosed by cerebral angiography. Treatment, when indicated, is with surgical resection or stereotactic radiosurgery.

- *Cavernous malformations* are composed of clusters of abnormal blood vessels with defective and leaky tight junctions. Unlike AVMs, these are best diagnosed on MRI (they are often described as "popcorn"-like, with varying intensities reflecting thrombosis, blood, and calcification); because of minimal blood flow, they are often missed on angiography. If symptomatic, these can be treated surgically.

- *Cerebral amyloid angiopathy (CAA).* CAA is due to amyloid deposition within the walls of the cerebral vessels, causing weakening, degeneration, and predisposition to rupture. The amyloid material is biochemically similar to that comprising the plaques associated with Alzheimer disease, but the two diseases are not inextricably linked; although they frequently coexist, it's possible to have CAA without Alzheimer disease and vice versa. The bleeds associated with CAA tend to be cortical (as opposed to the subcortical and deep gray matter bleeds associated with hypertension). Age is the most important risk factor; CAA is uncommon in patients under the age of 50, and the incidence rises with each decade thereafter. Because of the high rate of recurrent bleeding, it is preferable to keep these patients off anticoagulation and antiplatelet agents if possible.

- *Inflammatory and infectious conditions. Vasculitis* (see page 88) and *encephalitis* (most often associated with herpes simplex virus) can both cause ICH. ICH is also a relatively common complication of *endocarditis*, due to septic emboli or ruptured mycotic aneurysms.

- *Brain tumors.* Any brain tumor can bleed. The most common brain tumors in adults are metastases: those associated with the highest risk of hemorrhage are metastases from renal cell carcinoma, lung carcinoma, melanoma, thyroid carcinoma, and choriocarcinoma (see Chapter 16).

- *Bleeding diathesis.* Common causes include severe *thrombocytopenia* associated with hematologic malignancies and hepatic failure, *iatrogenic coagulopathy* due to anticoagulation, and *disseminated intravascular coagulation* (DIC). These patients can bleed spontaneously, without any underlying brain pathology.

- *Illicit drugs. Cocaine* and *methamphetamines* are the most common culprits.

- *Head trauma.*

Management

Emergent management of acute ICH is relatively straightforward: control the patient's blood pressure to prevent further bleeding; consider anticoagulant reversal if the patient is taking any such medication; repeat head imaging (typically done at 6-hour intervals) until you confirm that the bleed is no longer expanding; and consider surgical intervention as needed. Angiography and MRI may be indicated (usually nonurgently) to help determine the cause of the bleed.

Anticoagulant/Antithrombotic	Reversal Agents
Heparin	Protamine sulfate
Enoxaparin	Protamine sulfate
Warfarin	4-factor prothrombin complex concentrate (PCC), vitamin K
Direct thrombin inhibitors (dabigatran)	Idarucizumab
Direct oral anticoagulants (apixaban, rivaroxaban)	4-factor PCC, andexanet alfa
Aspirin	Desmopressin (DDAVP)

Common anticoagulants/antithrombotics and their reversal agents. A few things to note. (1) Andexanet alfa is a biologic Xa decoy that binds and inhibits the direct oral anticoagulants. It was FDA-approved in 2018 for reversal of apixaban and rivaroxaban in patients with uncontrolled or life-threatening bleeding, but its use remains limited due to lack of randomized clinical trial data as well as its high cost. Large-scale randomized trials are ongoing. (2) Given that aspirin acts as an antiplatelet agent, one would think that reversal with platelet transfusion would make sense. However, platelet transfusions have not been shown to improve outcomes (and actually may worsen them). As a result, platelet transfusions are typically reserved only for patients on aspirin for whom a neurosurgical procedure is planned.

Patients with big hemispheric bleeds, bleeds that enter the CSF spaces (*i.e.*, intraventricular hemorrhage in which blood can clog up the arachnoid granulations and prevent CSF reabsorption) and posterior fossa bleeds (the posterior fossa is the most confined place in the skull and has a very limited ability to accommodate additional volume) are all at high risk of developing elevated intracranial pressure and herniation. These patients should be admitted to an ICU and considered for surgical intervention, usually with either an external ventricular drain or craniectomy.

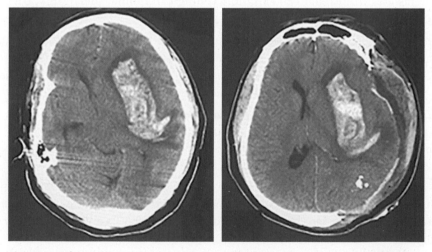

Computerized tomography (CT) scan of an intracerebral hemorrhage (ICH) pre- and post-decompressive hemicraniectomy. (Modified from Louis ED, Mayer SA, Noble JM. *Merritt's Neurology*. 14th ed. Wolters Kluwer; 2021.)

Subarachnoid Hemorrhage (SAH)

SAH—bleeding within the space between the pia and arachnoid membranes—accounts for approximately 3% of all strokes. It is a life-threatening event. The majority of nontraumatic SAHs are due to ruptured saccular (or "berry") aneurysms, which often involve the circle of Willis arteries at the base of the brain (the anterior communicating artery is the most frequent location). Arterial dissections, AVMs, cocaine use, and pretty much any of the other causes of ICH listed above can cause SAH as well.

The most common modifiable risk factors include hypertension, cigarette smoking, and heavy alcohol use. Females are slightly more at risk than males.

Mortality rates are high. An estimated 15% of patients will die before reaching the hospital, and approximately 25% will die within 24 hours of aneurysm rupture.

Presentation

The textbook presentation of SAH is a thunderclap headache, defined as headache that reaches maximal intensity in under a minute (see page 94). In reality, only approximately 20% of patients with SAH present with a thunderclap headache, but nearly 100% report the *"worst headache of my life."* Severity, then, and not acuity of onset, is key. Some patients will report a history of a prior severe headache, usually occurring within the preceding few days. These are referred to as *sentinel headaches* and are thought to represent minor, low-volume aneurysmal leaks. Recognizing them can be lifesaving. Other symptoms can include:

- Nausea, vomiting, and neck pain or neck stiffness (due to meningeal irritation caused by the breakdown of blood products within the CSF)
- Focal neurologic symptoms (these will depend on where the aneurysm is located, but the classic finding is a pupil-involving CN3 palsy due to compression of the nerve by a posterior communicating artery aneurysm)
- Preretinal hemorrhages (known as Terson syndrome, these portend a poorer prognosis)

Diagnosis

A CT of the head is extremely sensitive if performed within the first 6 hours of the subarachnoid bleed. The sensitivity then drops with each passing hour, falling to only ~50% by 1 week out. If the CT of the head is negative—beyond 6 hours or even within 6 hours, if clinical suspicion is high—a lumbar puncture must be performed. You are looking for red blood cells that do not dilute from tube 1 of collected CSF to tube 4 (dilution is more suggestive of a traumatic tap), pleocytosis (elevated white blood cells within the CSF; blood is irritating and can cause a chemical meningitis, hence the elevated white count), and xanthochromia (a yellowish color due to bilirubin released from red blood cell breakdown; this can be confirmed visually but is more accurately identified by spectrophotometry techniques in the laboratory).

If the CT and/or CSF analysis are positive, vessel imaging (with CT angiography or, if needed, digital subtraction angiography) is indicated to determine the presence of an aneurysm.

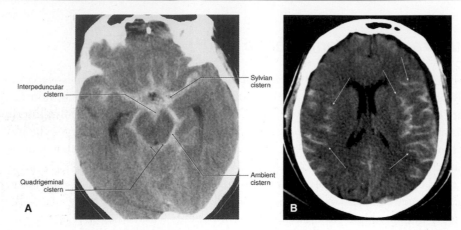

The classic appearance of subarachnoid hemorrhage on CT scan is pooled blood within the basilar cisterns (including the sylvian, ambient, quadrigeminal and interpeduncular cisterns—don't worry about these names; we've included them as a reference, and so you'll recognize them if and when you hear them mentioned) at the base of the brain (*A*). The blood can then spread into the subarachnoid spaces of the cortical sulci (*B*; white arrows are pointing to blood within the sulci). (*A*, modified from Haines DE. *Neuroanatomy Atlas in Clinical Context*. 10th ed. Wolters Kluwer; 2018. *B*, reprinted from Mansoor A. *Frameworks for Internal Medicine*. Wolters Kluwer; 2018.)

Treatment and Complications

Patients should be admitted to an ICU, because both medical and neurologic complications are common. If an aneurysm is found, early repair with either endovascular coiling or clipping is the standard of care.

The risk of *aneurysmal rebleeding* is highest within the first 24 hours after symptom onset. Vasospasm, thought to be due to spasmogenic substances generated during the breakdown of blood, is another early complication, although the highest risk period is a bit later, usually cited as between days 4 and 14. To reduce the risk of vasospasm, all patients should receive nimodipine (a calcium channel blocker) for 21 days, and euvolemia should be maintained. Transcranial Doppler studies (which are done bedside, and can detect increased velocity of flow within the ACA and MCA, which is suggestive of spasm) and angiographic imaging are diagnostic of vasospasm. Treatment is aggressive, with blood pressure augmentation (via fluids or vasopressors) and, if needed, endovascular intervention with either intra-arterial administration of vasodilators or balloon angioplasty.

Hydrocephalus due to obstruction of CSF reabsorption by blood is another complication, and often requires placement of an external ventricular drain.

Seizures occur in 5% to 15% of patients. Although the ideal duration of therapy continues to be debated, most patients receive seizure prophylaxis for several days following their bleed.

Medical complications include hyponatremia (thought to be mediated by hypothalamic injury causing either the syndrome of inappropriate antidiuretic hormone secretion [SIADH] or cerebral salt wasting), fevers, and cardiac abnormalities including electrocardiogram (ECG) changes (most often ST segment depression, deep T wave inversions, and prominent U waves, but can also include ventricular fibrillation with cardiac arrest), troponin leaks, and left ventricular dysfunction (often characterized by apical ballooning that mimics myocardial infarction with ST segment elevation on the ECG that looks just like a typical myocardial infarction; catheterization, however, will reveal clean coronary arteries—this condition is known as *takotsubo, or stress, cardiomyopathy*).

Box 2.15 Subdural and Epidural Hematomas

Subdural and epidural hematomas are not typically classified as "strokes" because they cause focal neurologic symptoms by compression only; that is, the blood itself does not contact brain tissue. Nonetheless, they are important and deserve a quick review here.

Subdural hematomas form between the dura and arachnoid membranes. They result from rupture of the bridging veins that drain from the surface of the brain into the dural venous sinuses. Subdurals are generally seen in two settings: in young patients, following acute shearing trauma or whiplash injury, and in elderly patients (or anyone with significant cerebral atrophy, including alcoholics). Even seemingly trivial head injury—without head impact—can cause subdural bleeds in the elderly. Symptoms are dependent on the location and extent of the bleed and can include headache, encephalopathy, and focal deficits due to mass effect and/or elevated intracranial pressure. Treatment is supportive unless there is significant mass effect with midline shift, in which case surgical intervention may be indicated.

Epidural hematomas form within the potential space between the skull and the dura and are most often due to rupture of the middle meningeal artery. The classic presentation is one of a "lucid interval" followed by progressive neurologic decline into coma; but again, patients can present with almost anything (including headache, declining mental status, and focal deficits) depending on the location and extent of the bleed. Surgical treatment is more common than with subdural bleeds, given the proclivity of epidural bleeds toward rapid expansion (remember, epidural bleeds are *arterial* bleeds). Endovascular treatments, including embolization of the middle meningeal artery, are becoming increasingly widespread.

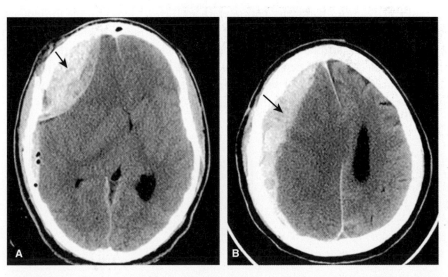

Epidural bleeds (*A*) usually appear convex because they are bound by the skull's suture lines (where the dura firmly attaches to the skull). Subdural bleeds (*B*) can cross suture lines and appear concave on imaging. (Modified from Haines DE. *Neuroanatomy Atlas in Clinical Context.* 10th ed. Wolters Kluwer; 2018.)

A Few Other Cerebrovascular Disorders to Know

Entire chapters could be dedicated to each of the following topics, but we will summarize the salient features of these disorders as concisely as we can.

Cervicocephalic Arterial Dissection

The term dissection refers to a tear in the intimal lining of an artery. The most important thing to keep in mind with cervicocephalic dissection (dissection involving vessels in the neck and head) is that, somewhat counterintuitively, the biggest concern is not bleeding but thrombosis and embolism. Blood collects between layers of the vessel wall, and the subsequently altered pattern of blood flow and exposure of thrombogenic subendothelial material to circulating blood predisposes to intramural clot formation. The clot can then either obstruct blood flow in situ or embolize to block more distal vessels.

The internal carotid and vertebral arteries are most commonly affected. Minor trauma (such as sports injuries and inexperienced chiropractic manipulation) and predisposing genetic conditions (fibromuscular dysplasia, Ehlers-Danlos syndrome, Marfan syndrome, and autosomal dominant polycystic kidney disease) are the most common causes.

Carotid dissection is usually extracranial, occurring near the base of the brain, but can be intracranial as well. Headache is the most common presenting symptom, classically retro-orbital and ipsilateral to the dissected artery. Horner syndrome (due to involvement of the sympathetic nerves running on the surface of the artery, see page 310), retinal artery occlusion or amaurosis fugax (temporary loss of vision), and anterior circulation strokes can also occur (due to thrombus formation and embolization).

Vertebral dissection is also most often extracranial, typically around the C1-C2 vertebrae, where the vertebral arteries are most mobile and least protected. Occipital headache or posterior neck ache are common, as are focal deficits due to brainstem and cerebellar ischemia.

Angiography is diagnostic and can demonstrate an intimal flap, double lumen, and a long, tapered-appearing arterial stenosis or occlusion (referred to as the "flame" sign). Treatment is with either antiplatelet or anticoagulant therapy (the best option remains debatable, and the decision will depend on the specific circumstances of the patient). Treatment is typically continued for several months at the very least until follow-up imaging demonstrates healing or resolution of the tear.

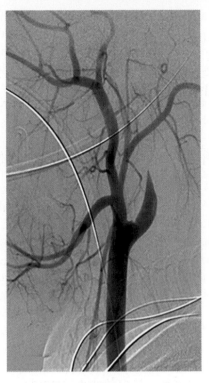

Digital subtraction catheter angiography showing a typical flame-shaped occlusion of the internal carotid artery. (Reprinted from Castillo M. *Neuroradiology Companion*. 4th ed. Wolters Kluwer; 2011.)

Cerebral Venous Sinus Thrombosis

Thrombosis of the cerebral veins or dural venous sinuses is relatively rare but an important do-not-miss diagnosis. The dural venous sinuses (also referred to as cerebral venous sinuses) are venous channels located within the dura that drain both blood and CSF from the brain into the internal jugular vein. Consequently, thrombosis can obstruct drainage of both blood (predisposing to ischemic and hemorrhagic stroke) and CSF (which can result in elevated intracranial pressure).

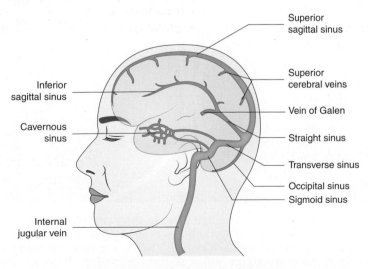

The major cerebral veins and sinuses.

Women are affected more often than men. Risk factors include both genetic and acquired thrombophilia (most notably pregnancy-associated thrombophilia; the risk of cerebral venous sinus thrombosis (CVST) is more than ten times elevated during late pregnancy and the early postpartum period), head injury, and infection involving the ears, sinuses, mouth, and throat.

Symptoms vary widely and include headache (often with features of intracranial idiopathic hypertension; see page 115), seizures, encephalopathy, and focal symptoms dependent on the location of the thrombosed vein.

Cerebral Venous Thrombosis with Vaccine-Induced Immune Thrombotic Thrombocytopenia

The use of the adenovirus-based coronavirus vaccines was briefly suspended in the spring of 2021 given reports of both cerebral and splanchnic venous thrombosis associated with thrombocytopenia and antibodies directed against platelet factor 4 (PF4). Currently, only a handful of cases have been reported among the tens of millions of vaccinated patients, and the benefits of the vaccines have been determined to greatly outweigh the risks. However, early recognition of the signs and symptoms of venous thrombosis in patients recently vaccinated with the adenovirus-based vaccines remains critical, and should prompt testing for anti-PF4 antibodies and treatment with nonheparin (argatroban, fondaparinux) anticoagulation.

MR or CT venograms are the most sensitive techniques for diagnosing venous sinus thrombosis. Occasionally, CT will demonstrate direct visualization of the clot. Infarcts due to venous sinus thrombosis tend to involve multiple arterial territories, because they do not respect the arterial vascular distributions. Treatment is with anticoagulation, which is continued anywhere from several months (in the case of a provoked thrombosis) to lifelong (in patients with severe genetic thrombophilia). Importantly, the presence of venous hemorrhage is not a contraindication to anticoagulation.

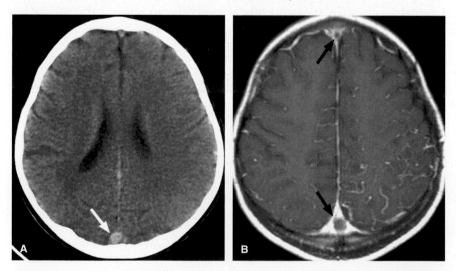

(A) The "dense triangle" sign on noncontrast CT scan demonstrating a hyperdense clot within the superior sagittal sinus. (B) The "empty delta" sign on postcontrast MRI in the same patient, demonstrating a filling defect in the same location. There is also associated leptomeningeal enhancement likely due to venous congestion. (Reprinted from Pope TLJr, Harris JHJr. *Harris & Harris' The Radiology of Emergency Medicine.* 5th ed. Wolters Kluwer; 2012.)

Reversible Cerebral Vasoconstriction Syndrome (RCVS)

RCVS is a syndrome that is characterized by reversible and multifocal constriction of the intracranial cerebral arteries. It is more common in women than men, and risk factors include pregnancy, migraine, and the use of vasoconstrictive and other medications (including triptans, selective serotonin reuptake inhibitors and various immunosuppressants) and illicit drugs (cocaine and methamphetamine).

Recurrent, excruciating thunderclap headaches over the span of days to weeks, with or without associated focal deficits (due to edema, or ischemic or hemorrhagic strokes caused by vasospasm), are the most typical presentation.

Brain imaging is often normal especially early on, but can show small ischemic infarcts (typically in watershed distributions) as well as intracerebral and subarachnoid hemorrhage. The presence of diffuse, segmental vasoconstriction causing a "beaded" appearance on CT or MR angiography is classic and, in the right clinical context, diagnostic, but these scans can be normal early on as well. If the initial scan is negative and clinical suspicion is high, it's a good idea to repeat the scan a few days later.

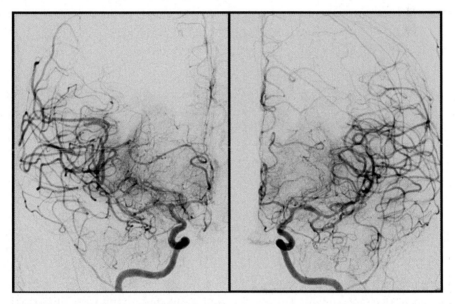

An angiogram showing multifocal arterial narrowing consistent with reversible cerebral vasoconstriction syndrome (RCVS). (Courtesy of Jonathan Howard.)

There is no proven treatment for RCVS, although anecdotal evidence suggests calcium channel blockers may be helpful. Steroids have actually been shown to worsen outcomes and should be avoided. If a causative agent is present (such as a triptan, SSRI, or cocaine), it should be stopped. Most patients recover spontaneously within weeks to months.

Vasculitis

CNS vasculitis refers to diffuse inflammation and breakdown of the blood vessels in the brain and/or spinal cord. The overwhelming majority of cases are secondary to another process, such as a systemic autoimmune or inflammatory disease, infection or neoplasm. When no secondary etiology is found, the condition is referred to as primary angiitis of the CNS (PACNS). PACNS is rare, most often seen in older men, and typically lacks the systemic symptoms associated with most other vasculitides (such as fever and weight loss).

Examples of Secondary Causes of CNS Vasculitis

Systemic vasculitides	Large vessel vasculitis (giant cell arteritis, takayasu arteritis)
	Antineutrophil cytoplasmic antibody (ANCA)-associated small vessel vasculitis (granulomatosis with polyangiitis)
	Immune complex-associated small vessel vasculitis (cryoglobulinemic vasculitis)
Autoimmune disease	Sjögren syndrome
Infection	Viral (HIV, varicella-zoster virus [VZV], cytomegalovirus [CMV])
	Bacterial (TB, lyme, syphilis)
	Fungal (aspergillus, cryptococcus)
	Parasitic (cysticercosis, malaria)
Drug Induced	Cocaine
	Methamphetamines
Neoplastic	Lymphoma
	Paraneoplastic

In general, the presentation of CNS vasculitis is nonspecific and insidious. Headaches, encephalopathy, and seizures are common. Both ischemic and hemorrhagic strokes can occur due to vascular breakdown. Tip-offs on MRI to an underlying vasculitic etiology include a combination of both ischemic and hemorrhagic lesions, small embolic-appearing ischemic strokes affecting both cortical *and* deep gray matter structures (due to involvement of the small and medium vessels) and strokes in odd locations (*e.g.*, the corpus callosum).

Establishing the diagnosis involves confirming vasculitic changes on angiography, which will show segmental narrowing with a beaded appearance. Sound familiar? Distinguishing vasculitis from RCVS can be difficult, but it is critical given the vastly different treatment protocols. CSF analysis is often crucial: you should expect an inflammatory profile with elevated protein and white cells in patients with vasculitis, whereas in RCVS normal CSF is the rule. A battery of both serum and CSF studies should be sent to help determine the presence of a secondary etiology, including various inflammatory, autoimmune, and neoplastic markers.

Treatment is with steroids and should be initiated early, regardless of known or unknown secondary vasculitic etiology. Evidence regarding the optimal duration of therapy is limited, and decisions are most often made on a case-by-case basis.

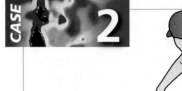

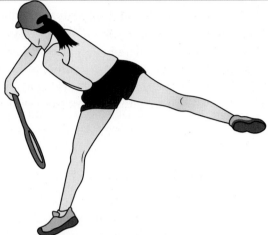

Follow-up on Your Patient: Laura's deficits are subtle but ultimately deemed disabling and, in the absence of any contraindications, she is given tPA. Her CT angiogram is normal, without evidence of an intervenable LVO or any significant stenosis. Her examination improves post-tPA, and several hours later only very mild wrist weakness persists. Her MRI shows an embolic-appearing right-sided frontoparietal infarct. Given her age and lack of cardiovascular risk factors, you order a transesophageal echo, which reveals a large patent foramen ovale (PFO).[5] Lower extremity Dopplers (to look for deep vein thrombosis) are negative, but her hypercoagulability panel returns positive for factor V Leiden. She is started on anticoagulation and discharged home, and after only a week or two of physical therapy, she's back on the court.

---

[5]This is beyond the scope of this book, but in case you are interested, the literature has gone back and forth on the benefits and risks of PFO closure in patients with stroke. Different physicians and institutions have different preferences, but in the case of our patient, most would likely defer closure; because she is positive for factor V Leiden and now has a history of thromboembolism, she will be on lifelong anticoagulation regardless, thus obviating the need for closure.

You now know:

- | The basics of cerebrovascular anatomy and can localize many of the most common stroke syndromes.
- | How to classify ischemic stroke subtypes via the TOAST classification.
- | When to give and—just as important—when not to give tPA for acute ischemic stroke.
- | When to consider endovascular thrombectomy for acute ischemic stroke.

- | How to manage acute intracerebral and subarachnoid hemorrhage.
- | How to recognize and treat several other important cerebrovascular disorders, including cervicocephalic arterial dissection, RCVS, cerebral venous sinus thrombosis, and CNS vasculitis.

Cited statistics here are from:

Virani SS, Alonso A, Benjamin EJ. Heart disease and stroke statistics – 2020 update: a report from the American Heart Association. *Circulation*. 2020;141:e139-e596. https://www.ahajournals.org/doi/10.1161/CIR.0000000000000757
The National Institute of Neurological Disorders and Stroke rt-PA Stroke Study Group. Tissue plasminogen activator for acute ischemic stroke. *N Engl J Med*. 1995;333:1581-1588.

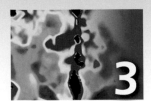

Headache

In this chapter, you will learn:

1 | How to recognize and treat common headache disorders

2 | When to worry (and what to do) about potentially alarming headache etiologies

3 | The differential diagnosis of thunderclap headaches

4 | How to manage acute migraine in an urgent setting

5 | How to manage headache during pregnancy

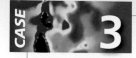

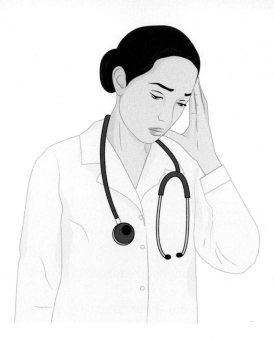

Your Patient: Anna, an otherwise healthy 28-year-old first-year surgical resident, comes to see you because of worsening headaches. She describes a long history of predominantly right-sided, throbbing headaches that used to occur about once a month and resolved with nonsteroidal anti-inflammatory drugs (NSAIDs). But in the past few months, she has been getting these headaches much more frequently, experiencing three this past week alone. NSAIDs take the edge off but no longer fully relieve the pain. She has a hard time working when she has a headache; just looking at a computer screen hurts her eyes, and trying to think feels like "running in a swimming pool," slow and exceedingly effortful. What's the next step in your management?

Headache is one of the most common reasons which send people to seek medical attention. *Primary headache disorders,* such as migraine, tension-type, and cluster headaches, are by far the most frequently encountered. More than one million patients visit emergency rooms in the United States every year for migraines alone. However, *secondary headache disorders*— headaches caused by other underlying, sometimes worrisome, occasionally life-threatening pathologies such as infections, bleeds, and tumors—comprise a significant minority. Distinguishing between primary and secondary headaches is the most important and often the most challenging step in managing patients with headache, so let's start there.

Headache Red Flags

Primary headache disorders can be severe and even disabling, but they are not fatal, unlike some secondary headache disorders. So when do we worry? What sets off alarm bells for a potential secondary etiology? The mnemonic SNOOP is helpful here. As our knowledge base has increased, this mnemonic has gone through multiple iterations (most recently SNNOOPPPPPPPPP—we are not kidding), but for the sake of sanity (yours and ours) and simplicity, we will use SNOOP2.

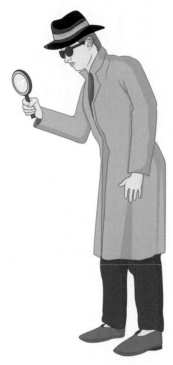

If you know the mnemonic SNOOP2, you won't have to snoop around to quickly identify patients whose headache requires urgent attention.

- **Systemic Symptoms (S):** When headache is associated with fatigue, weight loss, or fever, you must consider underlying systemic or infectious etiologies. Inflammation of the meninges (meningitis), the brain parenchyma (encephalitis), or the intracranial vessels (vasculitis) are important do-not-miss diagnoses.
- **Neurologic Signs and Symptoms (N).** Headache associated with *focal* neurologic deficits is *always* a red flag. Ischemic stroke, intracerebral hemorrhage, and malignancy (along with many other vascular, neoplastic, infectious and inflammatory etiologies) must be considered. But it is important—and perhaps surprising—to note that migraine is actually the most common etiology when headache presents with new focal findings. More on that later.

- **Onset (O).** Thunderclap headaches—headaches that reach maximal intensity within 60 seconds of onset—don't always reflect an underlying catastrophe. Sometimes they are just really bad headaches. That said, they must always be taken seriously and emergently evaluated to rule out subarachnoid hemorrhage (SAH). Once SAH has been excluded, the differential remains broad and includes other potentially life-threatening disorders such as reversible cerebral vasoconstriction syndrome (RCVS, see page 87), and cerebral venous sinus thrombosis (CVST, see page 85).

Box 3.1 Thunderclap Headache: Differential Diagnosis

Vascular Causes	Non-Vascular Causes
Subarachnoid hemorrhage	Spontaneous intracranial hypotension
Intracerebral hemorrhage	Colloid cyst of the third ventricle
Vertebral or cervical artery dissection	Meningitis
Cerebral venous sinus thrombosis	Primary exercise headache
Reversible cerebral vasoconstriction syndrome	Primary sexual headache
Hypertensive emergency	Primary cough headache
Pituitary apoplexy	Primary thunderclap headache
Cardiac cephalalgia	

Don't worry, you will soon learn all you need to know about the diagnoses above.

- **Older Age (O).** Because most primary headache disorders present in younger patients, a new-onset headache in a patient older than 50 raises a red flag for underlying pathology, including neoplasms, infections, and inflammatory disorders such as giant cell arteritis (GCA, see page 112).
- **Positional (P).** Headaches that worsen when the patient lies down or stands up raise concern for abnormalities in intracranial pressure (ICP).
- **Pattern Change (P).** If you remember nothing else from this chapter, remember this: *people who get headaches will get headaches.* Almost any illness, whether neurologic or systemic, including tumors, infections, anemia, thyroid disease, and so many others, can present as worsening of a preexisting headache syndrome in patients already diagnosed with a primary headache disorder. Therefore, any change in the pattern of the patient's "usual" headache (frequency, severity, or character) should always be taken seriously and should prompt close monitoring and further evaluation for potential secondary etiologies.

Primary Headache Disorders

Migraines and tension-type headaches are by far and away the most common causes of headache. If you master the presentation and management of these two conditions, you will be helping countless patients avoid needless imaging and misguided therapies.

Migraine

Odds are, if you yourself don't suffer from migraine headaches, you know many people who do. The classic migraine—as in the case of Anna above—is a unilateral, throbbing, and often disabling headache that is associated with nausea, often vomiting, and sensitivity to light and sound (photo- and phonophobia, respectively).

The more up-to-date way of thinking about migraine, however, is as its own phenotype, meaning a constellation of symptoms (which usually, but not always, includes an actual headache) that also has:

- a predilection for a specific demographic (females in their 20s and 30s),

- a strong genetic component (heritability is estimated to be between 30% and 60%), and

- a predisposition to other medical conditions (such as hypercoagulability and stroke; these connections are still being actively sorted out and studied).

Etiology. What causes migraine? A primary vascular etiology, long believed to be responsible, is no longer the accepted theory. Instead, the pathophysiologic basis is thought to be an electrical phenomenon called *cortical spreading depression*, in which a wave of neuronal depolarization results in brief neuronal activation and vasodilation followed by more sustained neuronal *hypo*activity and vasoconstriction. This self-propagating wave activates trigeminal sensory afferent nerve fibers which in turn cause the release of vasoactive and proinflammatory mediators (including calcitonin-gene-related peptide [CGRP], a target of newer migraine therapies) in the pain-sensitive meninges. Why does this occur in some people and not in others? We still don't know.

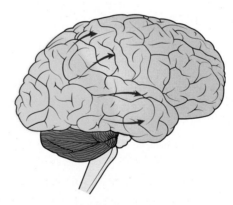

In migraine headaches, a wave of cortical depolarization propagates at approximately 3 mm per minute and is thought to be the pathophysiologic basis of migraine.

Clinical Features. Migraines typically last anywhere from 4 to 72 hours, and can be divided into four phases:

1. *Prodrome.* This can begin hours to days prior to the onset of the headache and consists of nonpainful symptoms such as fatigue, yawning, irritability, food cravings, and frequent urination. People with migraine typically know their prodromal symptoms well.

2. *Aura.* Migraine auras are focal, fully reversible neurologic symptoms that come on gradually, progress over several minutes, and typically resolve within an hour. Not all people with migraine experience an aura; migraine with aura is much less common than migraine without. The symptoms of an aura are classically "positive" (*e.g.*, colorful visual phenomena or tingling of an arm or leg) followed by symptoms that are "negative" (*e.g.*, a visual field cut or numbness of an arm or leg); pathophysiologically this makes sense because the wave of cortical spreading depression induces a transient neuronal activation followed by a more sustained period of *hypo*activity. However, virtually any focal neurologic symptom you can think of, including word-finding difficulty, vertigo, and motor paralysis, can present as an aura. The aura is often, but not always, followed by a headache. When there is no headache—in other words, when we skip phase 3 (see next page)—the patient can be diagnosed (in the most recent iteration of the International Classification of Headache Disorders) with "aura without headache." Importantly, this is still considered a migraine. As you might suspect, these atypical migraines can be difficult to recognize, and can only be diagnosed after careful exclusion of other possible etiologies.

Box 3.2 Migraine with Aura versus Migraine without Aura: Important Clinical Implications

This distinction is an important one because migraine with aura appears to predispose to a number of conditions—such as ischemic stroke and venous thromboembolism—that migraine without aura does not. The reasons underlying these associations are not understood. Smoking and estrogen-containing therapy (in contraceptive pills or hormone replacement treatments, for instance) seem to increase these risks in patients with migraine with aura. Although not absolutely contraindicated in women with migraine with aura, estrogen-containing hormonal therapy should be prescribed with caution and in the lowest possible dose. The absolute risk of stroke and thromboembolic disease is small in patients with migraine with aura, particularly in women who don't smoke and who take low-dose formulations of estrogen, but the benefits and risks of these medications should always be discussed prior to initiation (and, as always, smoking cessation should be strongly encouraged!).

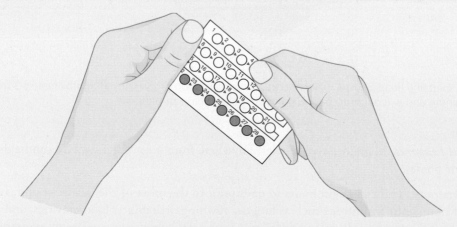

Low-dose contraceptive pills, although not absolutely contraindicated, should be prescribed with caution in patients with a history of migraine with aura.

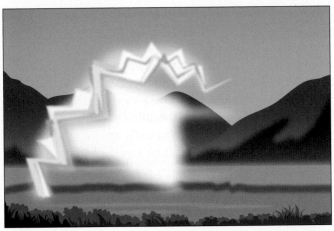

Fortification Spectra. Also known as teichopsia, this is a common form of visual aura. It appears as a shimmering and often brightly colored set of jagged lines that gradually spread across the visual field. The name comes from its resemblance to the battlements or walls of old fortresses.

3. *Headache phase.* The POUND mnemonic is helpful for remembering the typical characteristics of migraine headache. The presence of 4 out of 5 of these features can accurately predict the diagnosis of migraine and often eliminates the need for further diagnostic workup or imaging:

- **P**ulsatile (*i.e.,* throbbing) quality

- **O**ne-day duration

- **U**nilateral location

- **N**ausea or vomiting

- **D**isabling intensity

Other symptoms such as *photophobia* and *phonophobia, neck pain* (which often leads to the incorrect diagnosis of tension-type headache or occipital neuralgia, see pages 104 and 108), and other features that often lead to the mistaken diagnosis of a sinus infection—such as *nasal congestion, runny nose, facial pain, and tearing*—are also frequently present.

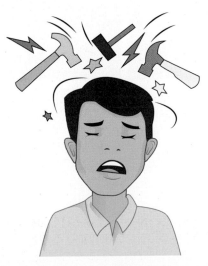

Mnemonics aside, migraine headaches hurt!

4. *Postdrome.* This term describes the period between headache resolution and when the patient feels 100% back to normal. These symptoms are often the same as the prodromal symptoms, and can also last for hours to days.

Box 3.3 MRI Changes Associated With Migraine

Somewhere between 10% and 40% of migraineurs have what are colloquially known as "migraine spots" on their MRI: small nonspecific white matter lesions that, as far as we know, mean absolutely nothing in terms of migraine prognosis or the risk of future neurologic problems. We bring them up for two important reasons:

1. They can look similar to the white matter lesions caused by ischemic vascular disease or multiple sclerosis (MS). Differentiating these etiologies depends largely on clinical context (and knowing the typical lesion locations of MS; see page 242).
2. They are one of many reasons to *think* before you scan every patient with a headache. Although these lesions are ultimately almost always distinguishable from demyelinating diseases such as MS, they can be easily confused by less-experienced physicians, and can then lead to unnecessary and expensive diagnostic evaluation. Perhaps even more importantly, many patients with headache are understandably anxious about their symptoms, and telling them that their brains are, in even the slightest way, "abnormal" does nothing to ease their concern.

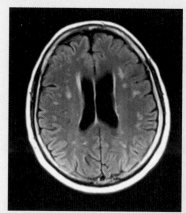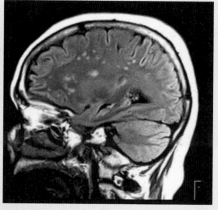

White matter lesions—migraine spots—seen on the MRI of a patient with migraines. (Courtesy of Jonathan Howard.)

Treatment

Lifestyle Management. Migraine treatment begins with lifestyle modifications, often referred to as "headache hygiene." The mnemonic SEEDS (sleep, exercise, eat, diary, and stress) can help you remember the basics. Stability is key: patients should strive to attain a regular amount of sleep each night, exercise frequently, not skip meals, maintain adequate hydration, and avoid their migraine triggers (red wine, aged cheeses and sucralose are common examples). Caffeine intake should be limited or at least maintained at a stable level of consumption. Keeping track of "headache days" in a diary can be useful to monitor the patient's response to lifestyle and pharmacologic interventions.

> ## Box 3.4 "Headache Days"
>
> The best way to track the impact of lifestyle changes on headaches is by asking about and recording "headache days" (*i.e.*, days during which the patient experienced headache), as opposed to headaches themselves. Many patients have headaches that last multiple days at a time, and thus, when they are asked how many headaches they've had over the course of a month, they may say only two or three—which doesn't sound so bad—when in fact they've been symptomatic for significantly longer.

Unfortunately, as in the case of our first-year surgical resident, Anna, who has been waking up at 4 am to preround on her patients and pulling regular 24-hour overnight calls in the hospital, lifestyle stability is not always possible. When lifestyle modifications aren't sufficient, we turn to medications.

Migraine medications are divided into two types: acute medications (also called rescue or abortive medications), which are taken as needed to acutely treat a headache, and preventive (also called prophylactic) medications, which are taken daily to raise the threshold for developing a headache and decrease the number of headaches over time.

Acute Treatment. Acetaminophen and NSAIDs are the most commonly used initial therapies for migraine. Triptans are considered second line and are frequently prescribed for patients who do not respond to anti-inflammatories, cannot tolerate them, or require increasingly high doses (which can be harmful to the liver, kidneys, and gastrointestinal [GI] tract and can potentially trigger medication-overuse headache; see page 111).

Triptans were the first migraine-specific medications, and remain among the most widely used abortive treatments. They act as serotonin receptor agonists (specifically on the 5-hydroxytryptamine receptors, HT1B, and 5HT1D: the "B" receptor vasoconstricts—you can remember "B" for Blood vessels—and the "D" receptor inhibits the trigeminal nerve branches responsible for pain transmission—"D" for Damn nerve). Interestingly, stimulation of these receptors also seems to inhibit release of CGRP (see page 102) and other proinflammatory cytokines.

Triptans, which come in oral, nasal spray, and injectable formulations, are most effective when taken at the onset of headache pain and often work best when combined with an NSAID. Because of their vasoconstricting properties, they are contraindicated in patients with significant vascular disease, including coronary artery disease and peripheral vascular disease, and particularly should be avoided in patients with a prior history of stroke or myocardial infarction.

Two small molecule CGRP antagonists (ubrogepant and rimegepant) have also been approved for acute migraine treatment. Currently, these are most often used in patients with an insufficient response or contraindication to triptans. Unlike triptans, which should be limited to 2–3 per week to avoid potential rebound headaches, these medications can be taken every day if needed.

Antiemetics, such as metoclopramide and chlorpromazine (many of these also have antimigraine properties), and muscle relaxants such as tizanidine are also used to treat migraine.

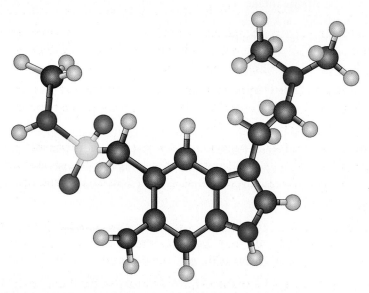

Molecular model of sumatriptan, the first triptan that was available for clinical use.

Preventive Treatment. There is a long list of medications that can work as migraine prophylaxis, none of which—up until the advent of the CGRP inhibitors (see Box 3.5)—were developed specifically for migraine. The efficacy of preventive drugs is not 100%: overall, approximately 50% of patients will experience a 50% reduction in headache frequency with any of these drugs, and thus, expectations must be managed accordingly. The choice of medication is typically made based on the side effect profile.

No specific number of headaches "qualifies" a patient for a prophylactic medication, although the American Headache Society suggests considering prophylactic treatment for patients with four or more debilitating headache days per month (or 6 or more if not debilitating). But the best thing to do is to listen to your patients, and decide if the disability caused by their headache disorder merits the risks of starting a daily medication. Commonly used medications are listed on the following page, grouped by their original intended use.

In the case of our patient Anna, prophylaxis should be offered because of her increasing headache frequency (likely due to stress and lack of sleep, variables she cannot control for now) and the negative impact that her headaches are having on her day-to-day life. The specific medication choice should be a joint decision made with her particular history and preferences in mind.

The table below summarizes some of the more commonly-used medications; it is not a comprehensive list. Note that none of these medications are proven to be completely safe in pregnant women and, as such, are almost always tapered off prior to pregnancy planning.

Common Migraine Preventive Medications

Medications	Notes
Antihypertensives	
Beta blockers (propranolol, metoprolol, timolol, nadolol)	Avoid in patients with low baseline blood pressures and/or heart rates, as well as asthma, decompensated heart failure, and refractory depression. Common side effects include hypotension and exercise intolerance.
Angiotensin-converting enzyme inhibitors, aka ACE inhibitors (lisinopril)	Avoid in patients with low baseline blood pressure, renal failure, hyperkalemia, or a history of angioedema. Side effects include hypotension, lightheadedness, and cough.
Angiotensin II receptor blockers, aka ARBs (candesartan)	Avoid in patients with low baseline blood pressure and a history of hyperkalemia. Side effects include hypotension and lightheadedness.
Calcium channel blockers (verapamil)	Avoid in patients with low baseline blood pressure, a history of cardiac arrhythmias, renal or hepatic impairment, or heart failure. Side effects include hypotension, light-headedness, and constipation.
Antidepressants	
Tricyclics (amitriptyline, nortriptyline)	Avoid in patients with a history of cardiac arrhythmias or suicidal thinking/behavior. Side effects include sedation, weight gain, dry mouth, and constipation.
Serotonin-norepinephrine reuptake inhibitors, aka SNRIs (venlafaxine, duloxetine)	Avoid in patients with a history of renal or hepatic impairment, or suicidal thinking/behavior. Side effects include nausea, light-headedness, insomnia, and sexual dysfunction.
Anticonvulsants	
Divalproex sodium/ sodium valproate	Avoid in patients with hepatic impairment, thrombocytopenia and in women of childbearing age (highly teratogenic; can cause neural tube defects and major congenital malformations). Side effects include weight gain, nausea, tremor, and fatigue.
Topiramate	Avoid in patients with a history of renal impairment, nephrolithiasis, or glaucoma. Side effects include paresthesias, weight loss, and word-finding difficulty (typically only seen at higher doses).
CGRP Monoclonal Antibodies	
Fremanezumab Galcanezumab Erenumab Eptinezumab	Given monthly (or every 3 months). Injectable (Fremanezumab, Galcanezumab, Erenumab) or intravenous (Eptinezumab). These are remarkably well-tolerated; common side effects include constipation (predominantly associated with Erenumab) and injection site reactions. There is little evidence regarding use in children and in women during pregnancy and lactation.
Small Molecule CGRP Antagonist	
Atogepant	This is a daily oral medication that was FDA approved about a week before this book was sent off to the press! Common adverse effects include nausea and constipation. Safety in children and in women during pregnancy is unknown.

Box 3.5 CGRP

Calcitonin gene-related peptide (CGRP) is the newest therapeutic target in migraine treatment. It is a small protein that stimulates release of inflammatory mediators, transmits nociceptive (pain) information from intracranial blood vessels to the CNS, and acts as a potent vasodilator. Levels of CGRP increase in migraineurs during a migraine attack and fall when the attack resolves.

The CGRP monoclonal antibodies are the first migraine-specific preventive medications. Targets include the CGRP molecule itself and the CGRP receptor. Although the available data are still relatively new, these drugs appear to be remarkably safe and well-tolerated. Constipation, along with injection site reactions, are the most commonly reported adverse effects. The CGRP monoclonal antibodies seem to be about as effective as the other prophylactic options.

About a week before this book was sent off to press, a CGRP small molecule receptor antagonist (atogepant) was also approved for migraine prevention. The other two CGRP small molecule receptor antagonists (ubrogepant, rimegepant) are approved for the *acute* treatment of migraine (see page 100).

Galcanezumab, one of the CGRP monoclonal antibodies, is also approved for cluster headache prevention, and another (eptinezumab) is currently in trials for cluster headache.

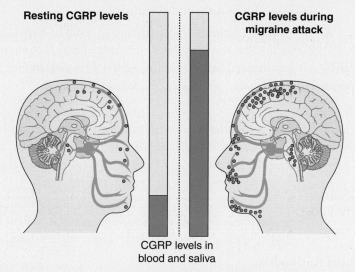

Resting CGRP levels

CGRP levels during migraine attack

CGRP levels in blood and saliva

Calcitonin gene-related peptide (CGRP) levels before and during an acute migraine attack.

Acute Migraine Treatment in the Emergency Department. You can imagine that the emergency department (ED), with its fluorescent lights and beeping monitors, is the last place on earth any patient with migraine wants to be. But the ED is often where they end up when an acute attack fails to respond to treatment and the pain is severe.

Everyone has their preferred "migraine cocktail" of medications to use for these patients. But—big picture—the two most important things to do in these situations are:

1. Manage expectations. We can take the edge off but are unlikely to fully resolve the headache while the patient is in the ED.

2. Arrange close outpatient follow-up. The goal is to establish a solid treatment plan that will hopefully keep the patient far away from the lights and noises of the ED in the future.

Box 3.6 Our ED Migraine Cocktail

First line (given in combination):

IV metoclopramide

IV diphenhydramine (to prevent an acute dystonic reaction from metoclopramide)

IV ketorolac

↓

Second line (when first line fails; but give your first-line medications at least an hour or two to work!):

IV magnesium sulfate and/or

Repeat first-line treatment

↓

Third line (when second line fails):

Option 1: IV valproic Acid + PO valproic acid (then discharge on a quick oral taper)

Option 2: IV levetiracetam

↓

Fourth line (when third line fails):

IV steroids (then discharge on a quick taper; steroids may not decrease pain acutely but have been shown to decrease the risk of headache recurrence)

Notes on a Few Other Treatment Options

Opioids. Opioids carry the highest risk for medication overuse in treating patients for headache. Patients can quickly become dependent, and the more they use them, the worse their headaches are likely to become. Despite this, opioids continue to be prescribed at high rates. There are occasional indications—particularly in patients with multiple comorbidities resulting in their inability to take other medications such as triptans and NSAIDs and in patients with cancer—but in general, opioids should be a last resort (or even a never-resort) treatment for headache.

Alternative Therapies. It's been estimated that approximately 25% to 40% of patients with migraine require preventive therapy, but fewer than half of these patients are able to adhere to these medications for more than a few months. This is likely due to a combination of the side effect burden and the disappointing response to many of these therapies. There has, therefore, been a lot of interest in identifying effective nonpharmacologic therapies, devices, and low-risk interventions that can be offered either as monotherapy or as an adjunct to other treatments.

Acupuncture, meditation and biofeedback are popular alternative therapies. The evidence is limited (although becoming more robust by the day—particularly with regard to biofeedback and meditation), but overall seems to suggest potential benefit with extremely little risk. If a patient is interested, why not try? Nerve blocks and neuromodulation devices (such as transcranial magnetic stimulation, transcranial supraorbital stimulation, and noninvasive vagal nerve stimulation) are other options for patients who cannot tolerate or who fail to respond to pharmacologic therapy.

Tension-type Headache

Tension headaches are the "vanilla" of headache medicine. This is not to belittle them (for those who experience tension headaches, they can wreak havoc on productivity and destroy otherwise good days), but to help you remember that they are effectively "featureless" in that they do not present with any of the symptoms associated with migraine, such as nausea, vomiting, photophobia, or phonophobia. They are most often bilateral, classically described as a tightening "band-like" sensation around the head, and are mild-to-moderate in intensity.

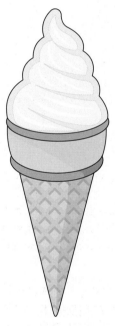

Tension headaches may be devoid of specific defining features, but they can still be unpleasant and distressing if rarely disabling.

The pathogenesis is not really understood. Despite its name, neither nervous tension nor muscular tension has been convincingly identified as an etiologic factor.

Acetaminophen and NSAIDs are the treatments of choice, but you will want to minimize their use as much as possible to avoid potential side effects. Although there is no known causal link between stress and tension headaches, relaxation techniques can be helpful (and what's the downside?). Tricyclic antidepressants (most commonly amitriptyline) can be effective preventive agents.

Although migraine and tension headache are by far the most common causes of primary headache, there are other primary headache disorders that you should be familiar with. These include the trigeminal autonomic cephalalgias (TACs), the neuralgias, and several other disorders that we will touch on briefly.

Trigeminal Autonomic Cephalalgias (TACs)

These are a group of headache disorders characterized by:

1. *Unilateral pain in a trigeminal distribution* (*i.e.*, involving the V1, V2, and/or V3 branches of the trigeminal nerve), and

2. *Ipsilateral autonomic features*, which can include lacrimation, conjunctival injection, nasal congestion, rhinorrhea, eyelid edema, ptosis, miosis, and facial sweating.

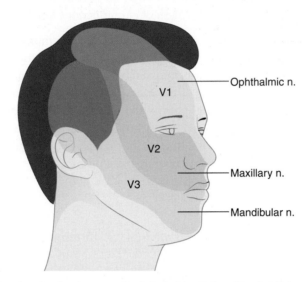

Trigeminal nerve distributions: V1 (ophthalmic), V2 (maxillary), V3 (mandibular).

There are four types of TACs. The easiest way to keep them straight is to classify them by (1) headache duration—with SUNCT/SUNA having the shortest duration and hemicrania continua having the longest duration—and (2) their response to indomethacin (see table on the following page).

1. *SUNCT (short-lasting unilateral neuralgiform headache with conjunctival injection and tearing)* and *SUNA (short-lasting unilateral neuralgiform headache with autonomic symptoms).* Just roll right off the tongue, don't they? These headaches are characterized by sudden attacks of stabbing, unilateral pain that last only a few seconds but can occur hundreds of times a day. The attacks are often triggered by tactile or cutaneous stimuli, such as bathing, brushing one's hair, or shaving. SUNCT presents with both conjunctival injection and tearing; SUNA presents with other autonomic features, and can include either conjunctival injection OR tearing but not both. These headaches are too brief to treat acutely (although IV lidocaine can be used in particularly severe cases). Lamotrigine is first line for prophylaxis.

2. *Paroxysmal Hemicrania.* These attacks are clinically similar to SUNCT and SUNA, but last longer (2 to 30 minutes per attack) and occur less frequently (1 to 40 attacks/day). The headaches are also too brief to treat acutely but are responsive to indomethacin prophylaxis.

3. *Cluster Headache.* This is the most common type of TAC but again is far less common than migraine or tension headache. Compared to paroxysmal hemicrania, cluster headaches can last longer (15 minutes to 3 hours) but typically occur less frequently (1 to 8 attacks/day). They tend to come in cycles lasting 6 to 12 weeks, and often present in a circadian

fashion, with attacks occurring at the same time each day. The pain is severe and is often associated with a sense of restlessness (unlike in migraine, when patients want to lie very still). Acutely, cluster headaches can be treated with oxygen (100% via nonrebreather) and triptans given subcutaneously or via nasal spray. Verapamil is the medication most often used for prevention. Topiramate, valproic acid, lithium, and indomethacin are second-line options. Galcanezumab, one of the CGRP monoclonal antibodies, has also been approved for prophylactic cluster headache treatment. Because it takes these medications a few weeks to kick in, a short steroid course is often used in the interim. Occipital nerve blocks have also been shown to help reduce the length of cluster periods for patients.

4. *Hemicrania Continua.* These headaches persist for days to months at a time. They are characterized by a constant, mild-to-moderate baseline pain that is intermittently punctuated by a more severe, sharp, and stabbing pain. They can be accompanied by a foreign body sensation or itching of the eye, as well as other more typical migrainous features such as nausea, vomiting, photo- and phonophobia. Associated autonomic symptoms are present but are often less prominent than with the other TACs. Hemicrania continua is always indomethacin-responsive: if the headache does not improve with indomethacin, it isn't hemicrania continua.

	SUNCT/SUNA	Paroxysmal Hemicrania	Cluster	Hemicrania Continua
Headache duration	1–600 seconds	2–30 minutes	15 minutes–3 hours	Days–Months
Headache frequency	1–200/day	1–40/day	1–8/day	Continuous
Demographics	M > F, age of onset 40s–70s	F > M, age of onset 20s–40s	M > F, age of onset 20s–40s	F > M, age of onset 20s–40s
Acute Treatment	IV lidocaine	None	O2 SQ/nasal triptans	None
Preventive Treatment	Lamotrigine	Indomethacin	Verapamil, Galcanezumab	Indomethacin

Indomethacin is an NSAID that can be tough to tolerate for long periods of time. Alternative options include melatonin (which has a very similar chemical structure) and topiramate.

Although these are all exclusively clinical diagnoses, an MRI is warranted before making the diagnosis in order to exclude underlying cranial lesions. Pituitary lesions in particular can cause similar trigeminal-distribution pain.

Box 3.7 Cluster versus Migraine Headache

Cluster headaches are often confused with migraines. They shouldn't be. Both are intermittent and severe but in almost all other ways they are distinct. Cluster headaches occur with a predictable pattern over a period of several weeks, whereas migraines come and go with far less regularity. And one of the most useful distinguishing features is one we have already alluded to—migraines make you want to lie down and escape from the world of sensations, whereas cluster headaches typically make you want to move around.

Sinus Headache

Always an iffy diagnosis. Although many patients think of their headaches as "sinus headaches," and many physicians continue to make this diagnosis, in reality very few headaches are directly associated with acute or chronic sinusitis. Stuffy nose, head fullness, and head pressure are actually common features of migraine, which is more often than not the correct diagnosis in these patients.

Does this mean that patients with actual upper respiratory infections don't get headaches? Of course not. The point is that many patients with "sinus"-type headaches do not have upper respiratory infections or acute sinusitis, and are having migraines instead.

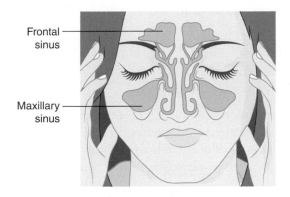

Pain around the sinuses, without evidence of an upper respiratory infection, is rarely a sinus headache, but far more often a manifestation of migraine.

Neuralgias

Neuralgias are characterized by sharp, shock-like pain that follows the course of a nerve. Their presentation is quite distinct and the diagnosis is usually clear from the patient's history. The two most common neuralgias are trigeminal neuralgia (TN) and occipital neuralgia.

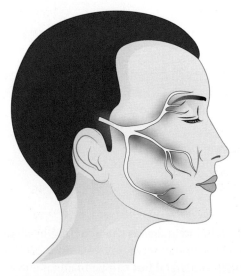

Painful trigeminal nerve irritation.

Trigeminal Neuralgia (TN). TN presents with unilateral, brief episodes of shock-like pain that occur in the distribution of one or more divisions of the trigeminal nerve; the maxillary and mandibular branches (V2 and V3) are more commonly affected than the ophthalmic division (V1). Similar to SUNCT and SUNA, TN can be triggered by innocuous cutaneous stimuli such as brushing one's hair or a light gust of wind. Attacks are short, lasting approximately 10 seconds to 2 minutes; unlike SUNCT and SUNA, however, they are followed by a refractory period during which attacks cannot occur. TN is classified into three broad categories:

1. *Classical TN.* Classical TN is due to neurovascular compression causing morphological changes in the trigeminal nerve root. An abnormal vascular loop compresses the trigeminal nerve around its dorsal root entry zone into the pons, resulting in destructive demyelination and pain.

2. *Secondary TN.* This refers to TN caused by an underlying disease, such as herpes zoster infection and multiple sclerosis (MS) lesions involving the trigeminal nerve root entry zone in the pons. Less common are tumors located at the cerebellopontine angle, arteriovenous malformations, and aneurysms.

3. *Idiopathic TN.* When the workup for TN is entirely normal, it is referred to as idiopathic. Note that contact between a blood vessel and the trigeminal nerve root is a common finding in healthy individuals; if this is seen on MRI but *without morphological changes in the trigeminal nerve*, TN is considered idiopathic.

MRI and MR angiography (MRA) is recommended for all patients in whom you need to rule out a secondary cause, but even in patients at high risk the yield is relatively low (a secondary cause will be found in no more than 15% to 20% of cases).

Carbamazepine and oxcarbazepine are commonly used treatments for classical and idiopathic TN. Oxcarbazepine has fewer side effects, but there is less evidence supporting its efficacy. Lamotrigine, topiramate, valproic acid, and gabapentin are also used. Unfortunately, the response to medication often decreases over time. Surgical intervention (either microvascular decompression or gamma knife therapy) for classical TN is second-line therapy, when feasible. Secondary TN is managed by treating the underlying cause.

Box 3.8 Trigeminal Neuralgia Versus SUNCT/SUNA

	SUNCT/SUNA	TN
Cranial nerve 5 (CN5) division most often affected	V1	V2 and V3
Presence of autonomic features	Yes	No
Presence of refractory period	No	Yes

Occipital Neuralgia. Occipital neuralgia is characterized by sharp, paroxysmal attacks of pain localized to the greater occipital nerve (GON), lesser occipital nerve (LON), or third occipital nerve. Pain is often unilateral but can be bilateral and is felt in the neck rising up to the posterior scalp. Most patients with neck pain will not have occipital neuralgia, but you should consider this possibility when the attacks are short, sharp, and severe (unlike the far-more-common cervical strain and sprain, which is more persistent and usually positional). The diagnosis requires tenderness or allodynia over the symptomatic nerve, as well as elimination of pain with a nerve block over the affected area (which is also the treatment of choice). Most often, occipital neuralgia is due to entrapment of the GON along its path from the C2 vertebrae to the trapezius aponeurosis. Secondary causes include infection (such as herpes zoster) and neoplasm.

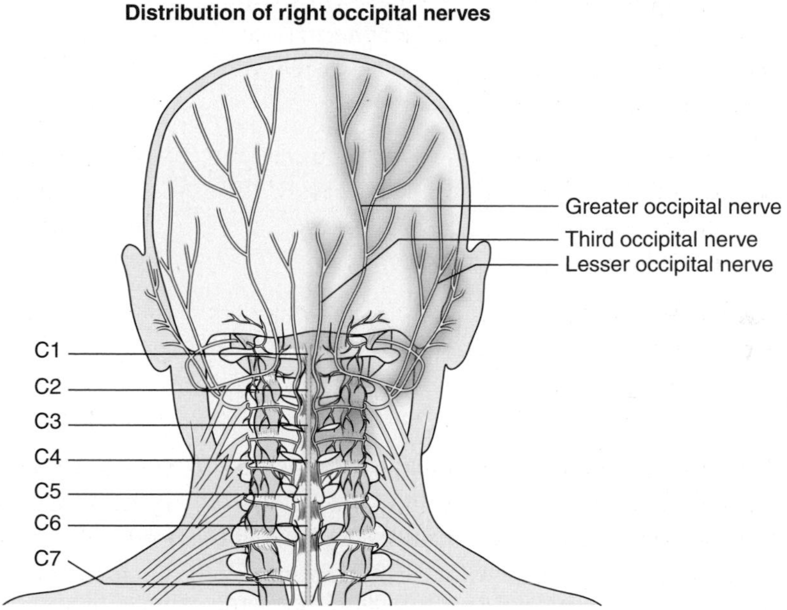

Distribution of right occipital nerves

- Greater occipital nerve
- Third occipital nerve
- Lesser occipital nerve

C1
C2
C3
C4
C5
C6
C7

Irritation of the greater, third, and lesser occipital nerves.

Box 3.9 Less Common (But Important!) Primary Headache Disorders

These are diagnoses to tuck in your back pocket, ready to pull out only when necessary. Usually the history will give the diagnosis away, but no matter how good the history, these are diagnoses of exclusion: you must always consider and often evaluate your patient for other secondary causes.

Primary Stabbing Headache: Short, irregular jabs of pain that usually last 1 to 2 seconds, without any associated migrainous or autonomic features. The location of the pain can be fixed or it can change. This type of headache is most common in children. Treatment is usually unnecessary, but indomethacin is the first-line option in adults.

Nummular Headache: This presents with either episodic or continuous pain confined to a coin-shaped area on the head (*nummular* actually means *coin-shaped*). This diagnosis always warrants a CT or MRI to rule out underlying cranial bone lesions. Acetaminophen or NSAIDs are first-line treatment.

(Continued)

Box 3.9 Less Common (But Important!) Primary Headache Disorders (Continued)

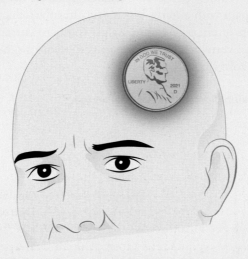

Distribution of pain in a patient with nummular headache.

Primary Headache Associated with Sexual Activity (previously known as Orgasmic Headache): Exactly what it sounds like, this type of headache is hypothesized to be due to brief vasospasm during orgasm. The headache features are variable: sudden or gradual onset, unilateral or bilateral, lasting minutes to hours. Subarachnoid hemorrhage, reversible cerebral vasoconstriction syndrome, arterial dissection, and other vascular disorders must be excluded; imaging is almost always necessary. Indomethacin 30 to 60 minutes before sexual activity is the preferred treatment.

Primary Exercise Headache: A pulsating headache that is consistently precipitated by sustained exercise. Workup is similar to the above. The course is typically self-limited (it resolves within a few months). Treatment involves temporary abstention from exercise or, if that isn't possible, indomethacin taken immediately prior to working out.

Primary Cough Headache: A sudden-onset headache that is consistently provoked by coughing. It is particularly important to rule out structural lesions such as posterior fossa tumors or Chiari 1 malformations (see Box 3.11). Once potential underlying secondary etiologies have been excluded, treatment is with indomethacin—and treating the cough.

Episodic Versus Chronic Headache

Some patients develop a persistent headache pattern that they simply can't shake. *Chronic migraine* can be diagnosed when a patient reports a headache that is present 15 or more days per month for more than three consecutive months. In addition, the headache must meet the acute migraine criteria on at least eight of those days. Episodic migraine is anything less frequent than this. Patients with chronic migraine have generally transitioned—for unknown reasons—from episodic to chronic migraine.

Other forms of chronic headache include:

- *Chronic tension-type headache*: Like chronic migraine, this must be present 15 or more days per month for more than 3 months.
- *New daily persistent headache (NDPH)*: NDPH is a headache that begins one day out of nowhere, then just doesn't go away. Patients will often be able to tell you exactly what they were doing when the headache began (usually something benign like gardening or watching TV). Unfortunately, NDPH is notoriously difficult to treat.
- *Medication overuse headache (MOH, see below)*
- *Hemicrania continua (discussed above on page 106)*

The distinction between episodic and chronic headache matters most in terms of treatment. Once a headache disorder has "transformed" from episodic into chronic, it becomes much more difficult to treat—you can think of it as trying to put out a forest fire as opposed to blowing out a candle. Botox and the CGRP monoclonal antibodies are currently the only Food and Drug Administration (FDA)-approved treatments for chronic migraine. Preventive treatment (see page 101) can be beneficial for these patients.

 ## Secondary Headache Disorders

We have now arrived at the category of headaches for which the SNOOP2 red flags were devised. Not all of these are emergencies but some are. Several of the most serious and dangerous secondary causes of headache—subarachnoid hemorrhage (see page 81), encephalitis, meningitis, and brain malignancies—are discussed elsewhere in this text. Here we will focus on some other secondary etiologies of headache you must know about.

Medication Overuse Headache (MOH)

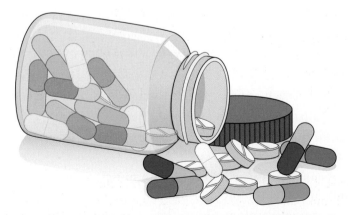

Headache medications come in all sorts of shapes and colors and many can—if overused—cause rebound headaches known as medication overuse headaches.

MOH is not an emergency. It is defined as a headache occurring 15 or more days per month due to regular overuse of symptomatic headache medication(s) for more than 3 months. It is almost always superimposed on top of another headache disorder and often, but not always, resolves with gradual removal of the offending medication. The highest-risk medications are opioids, butalbital-containing analgesics and aspirin-paracetamol-caffeine combination pills, but NSAIDs, acetaminophen, and triptans have been implicated as well.

The validity of MOH as its own clinical entity is being actively debated. Many argue that this diagnosis places blame exclusively on the patient when, in reality, the symptoms may instead be a consequence of the provider's inability to adequately treat the patient's pain.

Box 3.10

Apart from those pain medications that can cause MOH, there are numerous other drugs that can cause headache as a side effect of their use for another condition. Foremost among these are hormonal contraceptives, beta-adrenergic agonists, stimulants (e.g., amphetamines), nitrates (almost universally), and phosphodiesterase inhibitors (used to treat erectile dysfunction). Other drugs and substances can cause headaches during withdrawal, such as caffeine and many antidepressants.

Giant Cell Arteritis (GCA)

Also known as temporal arteritis, GCA is a medium-to-large vessel vasculitis that affects the aorta and most of its major branches. Diffuse vascular inflammation can lead to scarring, stenosis, and eventual occlusion. GCA is seen almost exclusively in patients older than 50, with a peak incidence between 70 and 80 years of age. Women are affected 2 to 3 times more often than men. This diagnosis should always be considered in patients over 50 who present with new-onset headaches.

The headache itself can be unilateral or bilateral and is often but not exclusively temporal. Associated features may include:

- Systemic symptoms such as fever, fatigue, weight loss, and myalgias;
- Tenderness to palpation over the temporal artery;
- Jaw claudication (pain and fatigue with chewing due to involvement of the maxillary artery);
- Polymyalgia rheumatica (which presents with muscle pain, weakness, and stiffness predominantly affecting the shoulders); and
- The most concerning symptom—visual loss, typically due to ischemia of the retina or optic nerve.

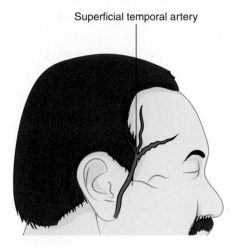

Superficial temporal artery

An inflamed temporal artery in a patient with giant cell arteritis (GCA).

Inflammatory markers, including the erythrocyte sedimentation rate (ESR) and c-reactive protein (CRP), are generally elevated (the CRP has a sensitivity of >95%), but normal values—while uncommon—do not exclude the diagnosis. Nevertheless, if you suspect the disease in any adult over 50, check an ESR or CRP.

Temporal artery biopsy remains the gold standard for diagnosis but can be falsely negative because the inflammation is not uniform but rather "skips," leaving some areas of the temporal artery unaffected. Bilateral biopsy improves the diagnostic yield. Although the diagnosis can be hard to make, maintaining a low threshold to screen for and empirically treat GCA is essential, because 15% to 20% of patients will ultimately suffer from rapid and often irreversible vision loss if not promptly treated. It is important to stress this last point—if you suspect your patient has GCA based on your clinical assessment, start treatment at once; *do not wait for the biopsy results*. High-dose steroids are first-line treatment.

Spontaneous Intracranial Hypotension (SIH)

Also known as "low-pressure" headaches, these are caused by cerebrospinal fluid (CSF) leakage through a tear in the dura. There is often an obvious precipitating event (*e.g.*, a lumbar puncture that pokes a hole in the dura, epidural anesthesia that ever-so-slightly misses its target, a motor vehicle accident or sports injury) or an underlying connective tissue disease (such as Ehlers-Danlos or Marfan syndrome) that predisposes to a flimsy dura that is at high risk of tearing.

The headache is classically "orthostatic" in that it worsens on standing and resolves on lying down, but this feature can resolve with time. Worsening with any Valsalva maneuver is common, a result of elevated venous pressure that forces increased CSF leakage through the tear. Other features can include tinnitus (typically nonpulsatile), nocturnal awakenings, neck pain, and migrainous features such as photophobia, phonophobia, and nausea.

SIH is diagnosed based on these clinical features in conjunction with either specific imaging findings or direct evidence of low CSF pressure obtained via lumbar puncture. However, recent evidence suggests that low CSF pressure is actually relatively uncommon in these patients, and that low CSF *volume* is more important; regardless, the utility of a lumbar puncture is now debatable. MRI of the brain (yes, the brain, even though the site of the leak is usually at the level of the spinal cord) is usually the first imaging test that is obtained and is abnormal approximately 75% of the time.

Potential abnormalities on a brain MRI are numerous and are summed up by the mnemonic SEEPS:

- Subdural fluid collections
- Enhancement of the dura (sometimes referred to as the pachymeninges)
- Engorgement of venous sinuses
- Pituitary hyperemia
- Sagging of the brain and cerebellar tonsil displacement

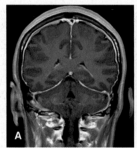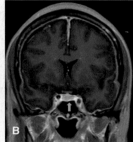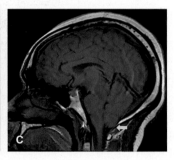

MRI of a patient with spontaneous intracranial hypotension (SIH) shows (*A*) enhancement of the dura (red arrows), (*B*) pituitary hyperemia (blue arrow), and (*C*) mild sagging of the brain (yellow arrow). (Modified from Louis ED, Mayer SA, Noble JM. *Merritt's Neurology*, 14th ed. Wolters Kluwer, 2021.)

Spinal imaging (either with traditional MRI or CT myelography, an invasive imaging technique in which contrast is injected into the CSF space) is also often obtained in order to help visualize the tear.

Depending upon the severity of the symptoms, treatment can begin conservatively with bed rest, caffeine (*e.g.*, 2 to 3 cups of coffee 2 to 3 times a day; it may work via its action as an arterial vasoconstrictor), hydration, and time. If this doesn't work, you'll need to arrange for an epidural blood patch, a procedure that involves epidural injection of autologous blood to tamponade the leak and hopefully repair the tear.

Box 3.11 Chiari Malformations

Chiari malformations are anatomic abnormalities characterized by the downward displacement of the cerebellum, either alone (Chiari 1) or together with the lower brainstem (Chiari 2), below the foramen magnum and into the spinal canal.

Chiari 1 malformations (which are most relevant to this chapter) are often asymptomatic, but in certain cases can cause headaches, most often characterized by prominent occipital pain and neck soreness. Lower cranial nerve palsies causing dysarthria, nystagmus, hoarseness, and/or sleep apnea can also occur, as well

Box 3.11 Chiari Malformations (Continued)

as sensory loss and even scoliosis due to syringomyelia (*i.e.*, the formation of a fluid-filled cyst in the spinal cord, commonly found in association with Chiari 1 malformations). In general, symptoms don't present until young adulthood.

Spontaneous intracranial hypotension can cause a secondary Chiari 1 (*i.e.*, brain sag due to low CSF volume) (see image C on page 114).

Chiari 2 malformations are usually diagnosed prenatally, since they are almost always associated with a myelomeningocele (a neural tube defect characterized by protrusion of a section of spinal cord and its meningeal covering through the child's back). Symptoms can include weakness, dysphagia and apnea due to medullary compression. Progressive hydrocephalus (due to obstruction of CSF outflow) is a common complication.

The need for surgery (usually with posterior fossa decompression or a shunt to treat hydrocephalus) depends on the extent of cerebellar and brainstem displacement and the degree of neurologic impairment.

Pseudotumor Cerebri

Pseudotumor cerebri is characterized by a constellation of signs and symptoms that are the result of *elevated* ICP, which develops because of CSF build-up and subsequent ventricular expansion (otherwise known as hydrocephalus) that puts pressure on the surrounding brain tissue. It can therefore mimic some of the features of a brain tumor—hence the name.

The best way to think about intracranial hypertension is to divide it into 2 categories, idiopathic (colloquially the category referred to as pseudotumor cerebri) and secondary.

Idiopathic Intracranial Hypertension. Idiopathic intracranial hypertension (IIH), as its name indicates, has no known cause. Overweight women of childbearing age are the most commonly affected. Risk factors include recent weight gain, various systemic conditions (including anemia, polycystic ovary syndrome, and systemic lupus erythematosus), and medications (especially tetracyclines, growth hormone, glucocorticoids, fluoroquinolones, vitamin A and vitamin A derivatives such as isotretinoin).

Secondary Intracranial Hypertension. Secondary intracranial hypertension is due to any process that causes excess CSF accumulation resulting in elevated ICP. The culprits include:

1. Anything that results in *blockage of CSF flow* with subsequent CSF accumulation within the ventricles. Venous sinus thrombosis and jugular vein obstruction block venous outflow from the brain, which is the same outflow path utilized by the CSF. Tumors or other mass lesions causing ventricular outflow obstruction (*i.e.*, obstructive hydrocephalus) can also do this.

2. Anything that results in *decreased CSF absorption.* Prior meningitis or subarachnoid hemorrhage can result in scarring and adhesions of the arachnoid granulations that are responsible for CSF resorption.

3. Anything that results in *increased CSF production.* Uncommon but not unheard of, choroid plexus papillomas are tumors that sit within the ventricles and produce excess CSF.

Regardless of cause, the headache associated with intracranial hypertension is positional, but unlike SIH, it is *worsened by lying down and improved by standing up*. Migrainous features are common. Other more specific clinical features that should suggest the diagnosis include:

1. Pulsatile tinnitus

2. Transient visual obscurations, which are brief episodes of vision loss in one or both eyes characteristically precipitated by standing up, and

3. Cranial nerve (CN6) palsy, that is, impaired abduction of the affected eye, a "false localizing sign" (in that it can reflect dysfunction far away from the location suggested by the exam finding); the sixth nerve has the longest intracranial course of all the cranial nerves, and is, therefore, most susceptible to the effects of elevations in ICP. See Chapter 18 for details on the cranial nerves.

Diagnosis requires papilledema on examination (optic nerve swelling due to elevated ICP) and an elevated opening pressure obtained via lumbar puncture (over 25 mm Hg in adults, 28 mm Hg in children). CSF analysis is otherwise normal. An MRI of the brain with and without contrast and an MR venogram (MRV) must be obtained to rule out secondary causes. Classic features of intracranial hypertension on MRI include an empty sella (a saddle-shaped depression in the base of the skull where the pituitary sits), flattening of the posterior globes and torturous-appearing, enhancing optic nerves. The ventricles and brain parenchyma should look normal.

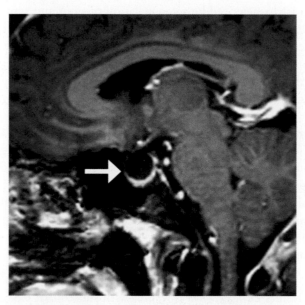

MRI of a patient with intracranial idiopathic hypertension; note the empty sella (*arrow*). (Source: Dr. Daniel T. Ginat, MD.)

Without any intervention, the natural history of pseudotumor cerebri is one of slow symptomatic progression. Treatment is therefore recommended. Conservative management with close observation, weight loss, and other risk factor modifications are first-line treatments in patients without evidence of vision loss. If the headache does not improve or if there is evidence of early vision loss, carbonic-anhydrase inhibitors such as acetazolamide or topiramate are used (these drugs decrease CSF production). If there is progressive vision loss, procedural options include optic nerve sheath fenestration (to relieve pressure on the nerve) and placement of a ventriculoperitoneal shunt (to divert CSF from the brain into the abdomen for better absorption). There is no indication for serial lumbar punctures, which can cause significant discomfort and offer only temporary relief; they may, however, be appropriate as a temporizing measure prior to surgery or in pregnant women who wish to avoid medications during pregnancy.

Posterior Reversible Encephalopathy Syndrome (PRES)

Although the precise incidence of posterior reversible encephalopathy syndrome (PRES) is unknown, it is being increasingly reported in the medical literature. This is one syndrome you really need to know about.

The easiest way to think about PRES is as a constellation of clinical and radiographic features resulting from acute vasogenic edema (*i.e.*, from the extracellular accumulation of intravascular fluid due to disruption of the blood-brain barrier). The name isn't the best, because PRES is not exclusively posterior (*i.e.*, involving the parieto-occipital region), may not be reversible, and does not always cause encephalopathy. So let's go through it carefully.

PRES can be caused by two things:

- The first is *a rapid rise in blood pressure.* The brain is normally able to autoregulate itself such that cerebral blood flow remains stable over a broad range of mean arterial blood pressures. There is an upper limit to this process, however, and when it is exceeded, cerebral blood flow increases. The resulting elevated pressures can cause fluid to extravasate from the cerebral blood vessels into the brain parenchyma, resulting in vasogenic edema.

- The second is *immunosuppressive medication,* such as cyclosporine and tacrolimus. The postulated mechanism here is direct endothelial toxicity caused by the medication itself, resulting in capillary leakage and disruption of the blood-brain barrier, which can occur even after months of exposure to the offending medication. Toxic levels of these medications are not required to cause PRES.

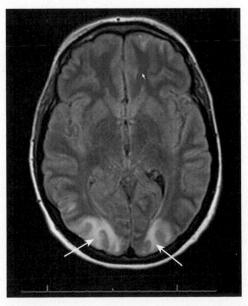

MRI with classic PRES features (symmetric, confluent white matter edema; white arrows). (Modified from Pula JH, Eggenberger E. Posterior reversible encephalopathy syndrome. *Curr Opin Ophthalmol.* 2008;19:479-484.)

Symptoms include headache (often constant and unresponsive to pain medication), visual disturbances (due to preferential posterior cerebral involvement causing visual field cuts, hallucinations, cortical blindness, and so forth), seizures, and encephalopathy (most often lethargy and confusion).

Imaging shows symmetric, confluent white matter edema that often (but not exclusively) involves the posterior parieto-occipital regions. This is best seen on MRI but can be picked up on CT in severe cases. Imaging is essential, because there are no reliable clinical guidelines for diagnosis, and as you might imagine the differential diagnosis of this symptom complex is broad (including stroke syndromes, malignancies, and encephalopathies). An MRI consistent with PRES in the right clinical setting (elevated blood pressure or the use of immunosuppressants) should make you feel confident in the diagnosis.

Treatment is symptomatic, with blood pressure control, seizure control, and, if indicated and feasible, withdrawal or dose reduction of the offending medication. Most patients recover well, but neurologic sequelae (such as motor deficits and epilepsy) and death can occur.

Cardiac Cephalalgia

Cardiac cephalalgia refers to headache due to myocardial ischemia. The headache itself can closely resemble a migraine but is variable in location, intensity, and duration. It can be—but does not have to be—associated with chest pain, but is always exacerbated by exertion and relieved with nitroglycerin or with cardiac stenting and coronary artery bypass graft (CABG) when these interventions are appropriate.

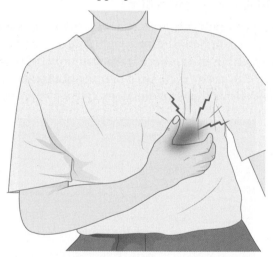

Do not miss the diagnosis of cardiac cephalgia.

This is an uncommon but DO NOT MISS diagnosis and should be considered in older patients with new-onset headache and significant cardiovascular risk factors. It is wise to obtain a resting electrocardiogram (ECG) and a stress test in such patients, particularly prior to prescribing any triptans.

Post-traumatic Headache

If headache onset occurs within 7 days of a head injury, or within 7 days of regaining consciousness following a head injury, the headache is considered to be post-traumatic. Risk factors include younger age, prior headache history, and, paradoxically, *milder* degrees of head trauma (*i.e.*, trauma associated with only transient amnesia and brief if any loss of consciousness).

The headache characteristics are variable and can resemble both migraine and tension type. The key to diagnosis, therefore, is to elicit a history of antecedent trauma. Lightheadedness, mild cognitive slowing, and insomnia are common. Consideration should be given to imaging these patients to rule out an underlying subdural bleed or hemorrhagic contusion.

Treatment is symptomatic. If the headache sounds like a migraine, treat the migraine; if it sounds like a tension-type headache, treat the tension-type headache. Amitriptyline prophylaxis works well for both and is the drug that's been best studied in this patient population. Most patients will fully recover within a few months, although the rare patient may have symptoms that never resolve.

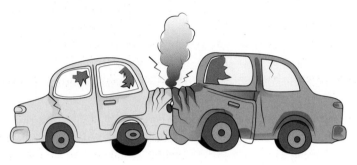

A history of trauma is the key to diagnosing post-traumatic headache.

Box 3.12 Headache in Pregnancy

Headache in pregnancy is a whole different ball game. Pregnancy puts women at risk for a plethora of conditions that can present with headache, some life-threatening, and thus any new or worsening headache that occurs during pregnancy must be taken seriously. It can seem like the diagnostic possibilities are endless, but let's break them down into 5 categories. These are the DO NOT MISS potential causes of headache in pregnant women.

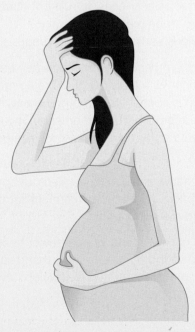

There are many causes of headache in pregnancy and you need to know them all.

(Continued)

Box 3.12 Headache in Pregnancy (Continued)

1. *Cerebrovascular Disorders*: Pregnancy is a hypercoagulable state and thus increases the risk of vascular disorders such as venous sinus thrombosis and acute ischemic or hemorrhagic stroke. The risk of subarachnoid hemorrhage, PRES, and reversible cerebral vasoconstriction syndrome (see Chapter 2) are also increased during pregnancy, especially in the third trimester and postpartum period.

2. *Space-Occupying Lesions*: Previously unrecognized Chiari malformations (see Box 3.11), colloid cysts (see page 400), and other tumors can make themselves known during labor due to increased pressure caused by sustained Valsalva maneuvers. Meningiomas also have a tendency to grow rapidly during pregnancy. The mechanism behind this is unclear, but changes in blood flow dynamics, as well as hormone-mediated cellular proliferation, have been hypothesized.

3. *Disorders Related to High Blood Pressure*: Gestational hypertension can cause both preeclampsia/eclampsia and PRES.

4. *Disorders Related to Changes in Intracranial Pressure*: Idiopathic intracranial hypertension often worsens in pregnancy due to relatively rapid weight gain. Epidural anesthesia also creates a risk for post-dural puncture (low-pressure) headache, as well as pneumocephalus (entry of air into the brain).

5. *Pituitary Apoplexy:* This can present as a sudden and severe headache due to hemorrhage into a preexisting pituitary lesion or enlarged pituitary gland.

The good news is that we can screen for nearly all of these with three imaging studies (none of which require gadolinium, and all of which can be done in just one trip down to the scanner):

- MRI (to look at the brain parenchyma, to rule out PRES, ischemic stroke, bleeds, and underlying structural lesions)
- MRA (to look at the intracranial arteries, to rule out dissection and reversible cerebral vasoconstriction syndrome)
- MRV (to look at the venous sinuses, to rule out venous sinus thrombosis)

All of this said, *not all pregnant patients with headache need to be imaged*. For instance, if a pregnant patient with a history of migraine presents with a slightly more severe headache than is normal for her, but one which is otherwise identical to her normal migraines, you're probably ok not ordering any imaging studies. But the bar to scan pregnant patients is, for obvious reasons, significantly lower than non-pregnant patients, and if you're at all unsure, scan.

Assuming the scans are negative and you have ruled out any potential secondary or dangerous etiologies, options for first-line treatment for headache in pregnancy include acetaminophen and metoclopramide.

Interestingly, patients with migraine tend to have fewer headaches during pregnancy, particularly during the second and third trimesters, than compared to their pre-pregnancy baseline. It is also not uncommon to develop new migraine or even new aura symptoms during pregnancy.

The General Approach to the Headache Patient

We've just gone through a panoply of headache types and it all may seem more than a little overwhelming. But in many instances, the diagnosis will be obvious within minutes of listening to your patient describe his or her symptoms.

No matter what, however, don't be too quick to jump to a diagnosis. In particular, know your red flags—SNOOP2—cold. These are the diagnoses you don't ever want to miss. In addition to your history and examination, there are only a few tools you will need— imaging, CSF analysis, and some laboratory studies. Don't order these indiscriminately. They are expensive, time-consuming, and anxiety-provoking, and with your newfound clinical acumen, frequently unnecessary.

Here are some quick examples that will illustrate the general approach to the patient with headache:

Patient A presents to your office for the first time to establish care. On your review of systems, she reports that she gets "normal headaches" once in a while when she's tired, dehydrated, or stressed out. She usually doesn't have to take any medication but occasionally she'll take an ibuprofen and the pain goes away. Her examination is normal, and you tell her that she has *tension headaches*. Ibuprofen is an appropriate treatment, as long as she restricts its use to less than twice per week.

A quick clinical pearl: if a headache brings a patient to your office or, especially, to the ED, it is in all likelihood *not* a tension headache. These are considered "normal" by most patients who get them and, by definition, are not debilitating. Patient A likely would not have come to see you for her headache; she just happened to mention it (since you asked).

Patient B presents with infrequent but severe headaches for which she's had to miss a day or two of work. Her headaches are usually, but not always, left-sided and associated with nausea and light sensitivity. Her mother gets similar headaches. She feels better when she lies down in a dark room, and ibuprofen or acetaminophen help but often do not fully resolve the pain. Her examination is normal, and you diagnose her with *episodic migraine without aura*. Given her normal examination, family history, and classic migraine history, there is no need for imaging. You prescribe sumatriptan to take at headache onset and tell her she can take it in combination with an NSAID for maximal effect. You ask her to keep a headache diary for you to assess at your next visit and discuss the importance of regular exercise and maintaining a regular sleep schedule.

Patient C comes to the ED after 5 days of excruciating headaches. He tells you that he's had "normal" headaches in the past, but nothing like this. These headaches are right-sided, sharp, and so severe that he tells you he would rather die than continue to experience them. They seem to always come on just after he eats dinner, last about an hour, and are associated with right eye tearing and a droopy eyelid (ptosis). He feels fine right now and his examination is normal. Although his history is consistent with *cluster headache,* obtaining an MRI without contrast while in the ED is reasonable, given the sudden change in headache characteristics and reported focal deficit. His scan is normal, and you discharge him on a steroid taper, with a prescription for subcutaneous sumatriptan and close follow-up in your office.

Patient D comes to your office with a throbbing, right-sided headache that's been going on for 5 days. The pain is noticeably worse at night but never fully goes away. She hasn't had much of an appetite but does report that for the past 2 weeks she has felt a deep ache in her jaw when she chews. She is ill-appearing, but her examination, including her vision, is normal, with the exception of moderate tenderness to palpation over her right temporal artery. You send off an ESR and CRP, both of which return elevated. You tell her you suspect she has *GCA*, start her on empiric steroids and refer her for urgent temporal artery biopsy.

Patient E presents to the ED with a sudden-onset headache that began about 12 hours earlier. She gets headaches frequently but says this one is the worst headache she's ever had and that she's now seeing double whenever she looks to the left. On examination, you immediately note ptosis of her right eye, then discover that her right pupil is dilated and she cannot adduct her right eye across midline. Her head CT, done on arrival to the ED, shows no blood, but this does not reassure you: as you now know (see Chapter 2), the sensitivity of CT for a subarachnoid bleed dramatically decreases more than 6 hours after symptom onset. You tell the ED that she needs an urgent lumbar puncture, which demonstrates significantly elevated red blood cells that don't dilute. Her CT angiogram shows a *ruptured posterior communicating artery aneurysm* (likely compressing her third cranial nerve, causing the focal deficits you found on examination), and she is whisked off to the operating room for endovascular coiling of her aneurysm.

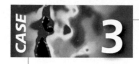

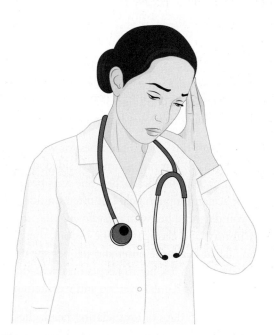

Your Patient's Follow-up: Anna presented with migraine that had transformed from episodic to chronic, likely due to her busy resident's hours and understandable stress. You tailor your "headache hygiene" talk to her unpredictable schedule by suggesting she keep granola bars or almonds in her white coat pockets to avoid long periods without eating, and regularly spend 5 to 10 minutes before bed relaxing with one of the many smartphone meditation apps. You also prescribe sumatriptan to take at the onset of her headaches (although she should do this no more than 2 to 3 times/week), as well as daily candesartan prophylaxis. On her follow-up visit several months later, her headache frequency has improved to one, at most two, headaches per week. Not perfect, but better. You will continue to see her regularly to help as much as possible with her lifestyle habits and titrate her medications as needed.

You now know:

- | Migraines are one of the most common reasons for ED visits worldwide. They are defined not only by their characteristic pain but by specific associated symptoms, genetic risk, and predisposition to other disorders.

- | When patients present with headache, early and accurate diagnosis is crucial, both to distinguish primary from secondary headaches, and to initiate appropriate treatment. The longer a headache disorder goes on, the harder it is to treat.

- | Triptans are commonly prescribed medications for acute migraine. Although evidence is limited, we avoid triptans in patients with significant cardiac and peripheral vascular disease. The newer small molecule CGRP antagonists are another good option for acute migraine, especially in patients who cannot take triptans.

- | Chronic migraine is tough to treat. We have a host of preventive options, all of which work only some of the time. The best treatment approach is often a multifactorial one: medication in conjunction with lifestyle modification, headache hygiene, and other interventions such as botox.

- | The CGRP monoclonal antibodies are the first migraine-specific preventive medications. Although relatively new, they thus far seem to be at least as effective—and with significantly fewer side effects—than the older therapies.

- | The trigeminal autonomic cephalalgias are defined by unilateral trigeminal-distribution pain associated with ipsilateral autonomic features. The different subtypes are best distinguished by the duration of pain and their response to indomethacin.

- | There are many types of secondary headaches, some of which can have serious consequences if they go unrecognized. Each has its own unique presentation, and—when appropriate—prompt imaging and CSF analysis will usually get you the answer you need. Know your SNOOP2 mnemonic!

- | Any headache—and especially any *new* headache—during pregnancy must be taken seriously. The potential differential for underlying etiologies is broad but, when indicated, the combination of MRI, MRA, and MRV can rule out (or in) just about everything.

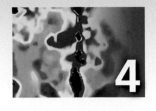

Concussion (aka Mild Traumatic Brain Injury)

4

In this chapter, you will learn:

1 | How to distinguish mild head trauma from more serious trauma that requires imaging and may necessitate inpatient care

2 | What a concussion is and what to expect regarding prognosis

3 | How to guide your patients back to normal activity, with special emphasis on athletes

4 | When to suspect postconcussive syndrome and what to do about it

5 | About chronic traumatic encephalopathy, a devastating complication of repeated head trauma seen most often in athletes involved in contact sports and military personnel

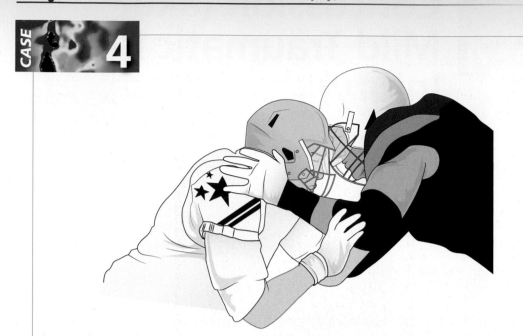

CASE 4

Your Patient: Paul, a 22-year-old college student, is drilled in an (illegal) helmet-to-helmet tackle during his football team's full-contact practice session. He does not lose consciousness but is groggy as he is helped to the sideline. He states that he "saw stars" on impact and is complaining of a severe headache. Within a few minutes, he claims to feel back to normal except for some mild nausea and a slight headache, and he asks to return to the game. Your neurologic assessment, using a standard concussion protocol, is normal. What is your recommendation?

What we don't know about concussion far exceeds what we do know. We are not sure how best to prevent a concussion or how to manage one, and we can't even agree on how precisely to define and diagnose it. Sounds like this might be a short chapter! It will be, but we won't leave you in the lurch. Our knowledge in this field is growing rapidly, in large part because of our belated recognition of the neurologic issues that are troubling many athletes who engage in contact sports and military personnel exposed to severe blast injuries. And we are beginning to know enough to feel some confidence in our ability to evaluate and manage patients with mild traumatic brain injury.

Is It Mild or Severe?

This is the first question you need to ask when you are confronted with a patient with head trauma. Severe trauma can cause an epidural hematoma, subdural hematoma, parenchymal bleed, or acutely increased intracranial pressure, and these potentially life-threatening diagnoses are ones you don't want to miss.

The test of choice in patients with severe head trauma is a CT scan. MRI is less sensitive for acute bleeding and is also more expensive and often not immediately available. But not everyone with head trauma needs a CT. Fortunately, there are reliable guidelines to differentiate those who do from those who can be managed more conservatively. There are many such guidelines, but they tend to converge on a few points that, should you answer "yes" to any of them, necessitate an urgent head CT:

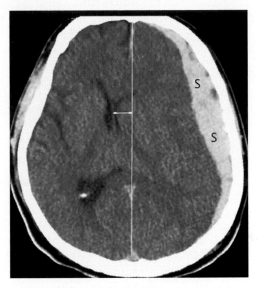

A subdural hematoma (labeled 'S') with mass effect (note the midline shift, indicated by the white arrow) in a patient who suffered acute head trauma. (Modified from Poper TJJr, Harris JHJr. *Harris & Harris' the Radiology of Emergency Medicine.* 5th ed. Wolters Kluwer; 2012.)

- Glasgow Coma Scale (GCS) score < 15 (see Table 4.1).
- A new neurologic deficit (any motor, sensory or cranial nerve deficit, or any alteration in cognition, gait or coordination).
- Two or more episodes of vomiting (this can be a sign of increased intracranial pressure).
- The patient is on anticoagulation or has an underlying bleeding disorder.
- The patient is age 60 years or older (it is important to note that reliance solely on the GCS may underestimate the severity of head injury in the elderly).
- Any evidence of a basilar skull fracture (periorbital bleeding, retroauricular bleeding, hemotympanum (blood in the middle ear cavity), otorrhea or rhinorrhea).
- Evidence suggesting a possible open or depressed skull fracture (*e.g.*, a scalp laceration or hematoma).
- A seizure accompanying or following the trauma.

Table 4.1 The Glasgow Coma Scale (GCS) is the most common scoring system used to help gauge the severity of traumatic brain injury

Domain	Response	Score
Eye opening	Spontaneous	4
	To speech	3
	To pain	2
	None	1
Best verbal response	Oriented	5
	Confused	4
	Inappropriate	3
	Incomprehensible	2
	None	1
Best motor response	Obeying	6
	Localizing	5
	Withdrawal	4
	Flexing	5
	Extending	3
	None	1
Total score	Deep coma or death	3
	Fully alert and oriented	15

Adapted from Institute of Neurological Sciences. *Glasgow Coma Scale*. https://www.glasgowcomascale.org/

Other factors are not as absolute, but if any of these are present, you should have a low threshold for scanning:

- Retrograde amnesia (forgetting memories formed before the traumatic event) of at least 30 minutes.
- Any high-impact injury (such as a motor vehicle accident or a long fall).
- Abnormal behavior (agitation, unusual affect, violent behavior, *etc.*).

These guidelines apply to adults only; there are different protocols for guiding the evaluation of children.

If, using these guidelines, your screen comes up negative but your clinical instinct still tells you that—for whatever reason—there may be more here than meets the eye, get the CT (and don't forget to get an x-ray of the cervical spine if there has been trauma to the neck; you don't want to miss a fracture).

The presence of a fracture or blood on the CT necessitates immediate referral to neurosurgery. If the CT is normal, you should still consider hospital admission for (1) patients with a low GCS score, (2) who present with seizures, or (3) who are on anticoagulation or have a bleeding disorder. Anyone else you can generally feel comfortable sending home.

The critical care management of the patient with severe head trauma causing intracranial hemorrhage and elevated intracranial pressure is discussed in Chapter 14. For the rest of this chapter, we are going to focus solely on those patients who can be managed as outpatients, that is, those with mild traumatic head injury.

 ## So What Is a Concussion?

Definition. You would think there would be a simple answer to this question, but there is considerable disagreement. Probably the simplest definition is to view concussion as *altered mental status, with or without loss of consciousness, caused by head trauma*. Some experts add the term "short-lived" before "altered mental status"; however, there is a difference of opinion as to what "short-lived" actually means, plus this definition is only useful in retrospect (how do you know if the effects of the trauma are short lived until they have resolved or persisted?) and thus of no real utility in practice.

Two important points:

1. Concussion is a *clinical* diagnosis, not one made by either imaging or laboratory testing (although new research on biomarkers that are released by axonal and glial injury is looking promising).

2. This definition—intentionally—does not specify whether or not there is loss of consciousness accompanying the trauma.

Box 4.1 Brain Contusion

The term *contusion* refers to the rupture of blood vessels caused by trauma, and it can occur just about anywhere in the body. A *brain* contusion is a type of intracerebral hemorrhage and is best thought of as a brain bruise. Just like when you bruise your arm or leg and wind up with a "black and blue mark," a cerebral contusion is associated with small microbleeds. The clinical presentation depends on the location and severity of the damage and can include concussion.

Coup–contrecoup is a pattern of injury often associated with brain contusions, in which damage occurs both at the site of impact (often minimal) and at the opposite side of the head (often more severe). The injury at the opposite side of the head— the so-called *contrecoup* injury—occurs when a strong blow to the head causes the brain to strike the side of the skull opposite from the point of impact.

(Continued)

Box 4.1 Brain Contusion (Continued)

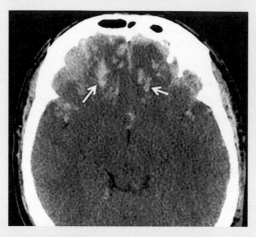

Extensive bifrontal contusions. (Reprinted from Sanelli P, Schaefer P, Loevner L. *Neuroimaging: The Essentials*. Wolters Kluwer; 2015.)

Mechanism. Trauma to the head—from whiplash, for example, or direct injury from a fall, collision, or a blast injury—causes rapid acceleration, deceleration, or rotation of the brain within the cranial vault, resulting in shear strain on the brain parenchyma. Axonal damage and the release of excitatory neurotransmitters appear to play an important role in causing the symptoms of concussion.

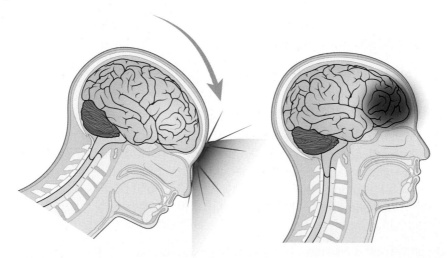

Violent trauma to the head underlies most cases of concussion.

Symptoms and Management. Concussive symptoms may develop immediately or up to several days after the trauma. Symptoms can persist for days to weeks. When they last longer, we refer to the condition as postconcussion syndrome (PCS), which we discuss below.

The most dramatic symptoms of concussion are *loss of consciousness*, *disorientation*, and *amnesia*, but these are *not* the most common symptoms.

Headache is number one. Most concussion-related headaches are migraine-like and can be treated just like other migraines, usually beginning with a nonsteroidal anti-inflammatory drug (NSAID). Tension-type headaches are the second most common headache type. When headache is accompanied by nausea, medications such as prochlorperazine or metoclopramide can be helpful. See the discussion on post-traumatic headache (page 118) for more details.

Dizziness is the second most common symptom. Sometimes it presents as vertigo, but more often patients complain of an ill-defined sense of lightheadedness and disequilibrium. There is no specific therapy, and these symptoms usually resolve with time.

Other symptoms include fatigue, inability to focus or concentrate, slowed reaction times, compromised executive function, emotional lability, sleep disturbances, depression, anxiety, and irritability. These neuropsychiatric symptoms may occur immediately, hours, or even days after the head trauma and tend to last for several weeks before gradually resolving.

Patients who do not require imaging (or who have had a normal CT scan) and do not require inpatient observation can be managed conservatively. Earlier recommendations for a prolonged period of physical and mental rest have been supplanted by more lenient guidelines, but the ideal duration of rest is unknown and should be determined on a case-by-case basis. "Brain rest" is often recommended: limited screens (this includes texting, playing video games, and using a computer) and limited reading. After a short period (typically on the order of 3 to 5 days), patients can gradually resume light cognitive and physical activity as tolerated.

It is important to recognize that it can take weeks for the brain to recover from mild trauma. During this time, the metabolic demands of the recovering brain exceed the available energy supply, and the brain remains at increased risk of further injury.

 ## *Sports-related Concussion*

Athletes who sustain head trauma should be immediately removed from the sports activity. Athletes are often understandably eager to return to the field, but guidelines stress the importance of *objective assessment of neurologic compromise* to determine if there is a concussion or something even more serious.

The most commonly used sideline tests are the *Balance Error Scoring System* and the *Sports Concussion Assessment Tool*. Focus should be directed toward identifying red flags for serious injury, objective signs of neurologic dysfunction (especially gait and balance issues), memory impairment, the GCS score, and a careful cervical spine assessment. However, the accuracy of these tools in predicting serious pathology is still up for debate. Clinical judgment always prevails.

Athletes diagnosed with concussion should not return to play that day and should be totally free of symptoms before beginning a standardized rehabilitation progression that starts with light aerobic exercise and continues for several days.[1] No matter how fast athletes recover, at least 10 days should be allowed before they resume a contact sport; the prolonged recovery of the brain following concussion makes the brain highly susceptible to a second injury, the consequences of which could be much more severe than the first.

---

[1]Some guidelines are a bit more forgiving, allowing very light activity earlier if the athlete's symptoms are mild and improving.

> Important note: The helmets and other protective equipment that are currently available for contact sports such as American football and hockey do not protect against concussion. They do protect against fracture and other head and neck injuries, but not concussion.

 ## *Postconcussion Syndrome*

Patients with mild head trauma should gradually improve over a course of days to a few weeks. However, some patients will have persistent symptoms (i.e., lasting beyond the usual recovery period), a condition referred to as postconcussion syndrome.

For patients with PCS who have already had a normal CT, there is nothing to be gained by repeated imaging *unless they have progressive symptoms, new focal neurologic deficits or their symptoms have become disabling.* The data are clear on this point: other than for those exceptions just mentioned, a repeat CT will in all likelihood add nothing to your management (the chances of detecting a bleed or fracture are virtually nil). If, however, imaging was not done at the time of the trauma, it is appropriate to order it now.

Neuropsychological testing is often recommended for patients with persistent symptoms. However, whereas it may help predict the course of recovery, there is no compelling evidence that it will affect management.

The most common persistent symptom in patients with PCS is *headache* and should be treated more or less as any other headache (see page 118 for details on post-traumatic headache). For patients with persistent dizziness, vestibular rehabilitation may be beneficial. Other symptoms such as depression and anxiety should be addressed in the usual manner. Persistent mental sluggishness and disrupted sleep usually slowly resolve on their own over weeks to months.

Post-concussion syndrome

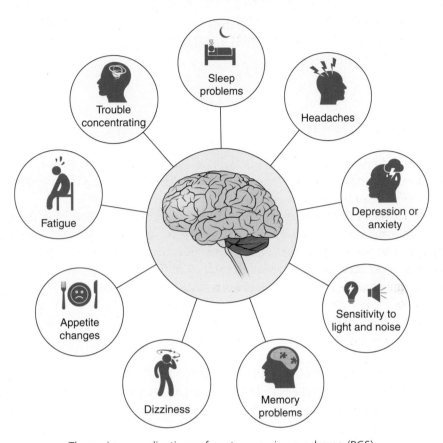

The major complications of postconcussion syndrome (PCS).

Most patients with PCS recover within several months, but as many as one-third may have symptoms that persist for much longer. There is no known intervention that can speed their recovery.

 Chronic Traumatic Encephalopathy

This devastating syndrome appears in patients after multiple repetitive concussions. Athletes and military personnel are the most likely to be affected. Symptoms, which can include depression, anxiety, mental sluggishness, and/or alterations in personality, can be subtle at first, but over time become more pronounced. Suicidal ideation, violence, and aggression are often the most obvious manifestations of the patient's emotional dysregulation. Motor disturbances include ataxia, tremor, parkinsonian symptoms, and motor neuron disease (amyotrophic lateral sclerosis). Symptoms of dementia can appear and progress rapidly.

The precise incidence of chronic traumatic encephalopathy (CTE) is not known. It appears that one or two concussions may not increase the risk, but three or more probably do (it is unlikely this is a hard and fast rule, but it is a useful approximation of risk). Thus, the total number of head impacts, not their severity, may be the best prognosticator. Many young football players sustain thousands of head impacts before their playing days are over. Patients with more than two concussions should, if at all possible, not resume their contact sport (or return to military activity that puts them at risk) even if their recovery from each event has been total.

CTE can only be diagnosed definitively at autopsy. The key finding is the accumulation of tau protein in the brain parenchyma.

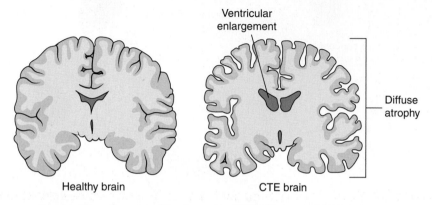

Comparison of a normal brain and a CTE brain at autopsy.

There is no known treatment for CTE.

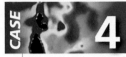

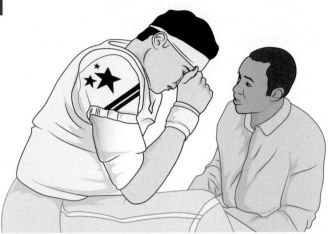

Follow-up on Your Patient: You don't have to be a licensed neurologist to know that Paul should not return to play today. For an athlete engaged in a non-contact sport who is fully recovered, return could be considered. Paul, however, is a football player and is not completely asymptomatic. Most experts would recommend a period of "brain rest," and that he not return to contact sports for at least 10 days, and then only if he remains asymptomatic following a gradual return to full activity protocol.

You now know:

- | The red flags that necessitate urgent evaluation following head trauma
- | How to determine if a patient with mild head trauma requires a CT
- | How to recognize and manage the most common symptoms of concussion
- | The usual arc of recovery following mild traumatic brain injury
- | How to diagnose and manage postconcussion syndrome
- | How to perform a sideline evaluation of athletes suffering head trauma, and how to guide their recovery and return to action
- | The risk factors and often devastating manifestations of chronic traumatic encephalopathy

Dizziness

5

In this chapter, you will learn:

1 | What patients mean when they talk about dizziness

2 | All about vertigo: what it is, when to worry, and how to treat it

3 | How to perform the HINTS exam, which will help you distinguish central from peripheral vertigo

4 | How to think about syncope from a neurologist's point of view

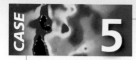

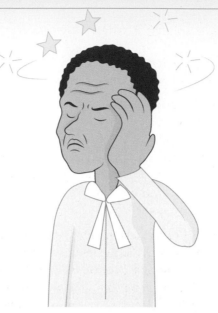

Your Patient: Kyle, a 64-year-old lawyer with a history of hypertension and coronary artery disease, presents to the emergency department with sudden-onset vertigo. He states that he was in his usual state of health until approximately 2 days ago when he began to feel dizzy and off-balance. He initially attributed these symptoms to exhaustion—he'd been working hard on a case and hadn't had much time to eat or sleep—but became worried after he fell this morning on getting out of bed. When you ask him what he means by "dizzy," he tells you that he feels as though the world is spinning around him. The sensation has significantly improved over the past 24 hours, but he still feels unsteady on his feet. He also tells you that he has had "a bit of a headache" and thinks his left hand is weak; he had trouble using it to button his shirt this morning. On examination, you think you detect a few beats of vertical nystagmus when you ask him to look up to the ceiling, but it's hard to tell because he keeps closing his eyes while telling you that your examination is making him dizzy again. His left hand is full strength but dysmetric on finger-nose-finger testing. His examination is otherwise normal. What's the next step in your management?

Dizziness is one of the most common complaints encountered not only by neurologists but by emergency clinicians and primary healthcare providers as well. It is also a highly nonspecific symptom. Dizziness can be the result of an underlying neurologic disease but can also be indicative of cardiac disease, an electrolyte derangement, anemia, infection, and anxiety. Most of the time dizziness is benign, some of the time disabling and—fortunately far less often—life-threatening. How do you tell the difference? That's what we're here for.

A Simple Way to Categorize Dizziness

What do patients mean when they complain of acute dizziness? Despite the many different ways of describing the sensation, there are really only two options:

1. *Lightheadedness.* This is the feeling that you might faint. Some patients will report actual fainting (the formal term for this is *syncope*), and describe lightheadedness as the immediate sensation before losing consciousness; others won't actually syncopize but will report feeling as though they might (*presyncope*). Lightheadedness is incredibly common and most often benign. That said, if the sensation is bothersome enough to bring a patient into the office or the emergency department, or if they have actually experienced syncope or presyncope, it must be taken seriously.

2. *Vertigo.* Most people think of vertigo as a spinning sensation, but that's not always true. The better definition of vertigo is the false sensation of movement or, to put it more simply, *the sensation of movement when nothing is actually moving.* That sensation may be one of spinning—either you yourself or the world around you—but it can also be a feeling of rocking back-and-forth or side-to-side, or even a more vague off-balance, off-kilter sensation.

When patients come to you complaining of acute dizziness, the distinction between lightheadedness and vertigo is the first and most important thing you must determine, because it will drastically alter your diagnostic workup and management. If possible, don't ask your patient specifically about a spinning or lightheaded sensation. Be vague; you don't want to put words into your patients' mouths. '*What do you mean by dizziness?*' is a good place to start. Try to give your patients the opportunity to think about what they're actually experiencing. You might be surprised by how helpful their own words can be in leading you in the right direction.

Box 5.1

Some patients, particularly the elderly, may experience unsteadiness or imbalance when walking or standing, and describe the sensation as one of dizziness. This feeling is referred to as *disequilibrium* and is best thought of as a chronic form of dizziness. Many factors can contribute to this feeling: diminished proprioception, impaired gait, weakness, deconditioning, and even auditory or visual problems. It is important to distinguish disequilibrium from actual dizziness because the therapeutic approaches are different. Treatment of disequilibrium should be directed at specific corrective measures such as hearing aids, new glasses, canes, walkers, or physical therapy.

Vertigo: An Overview

Anatomy

Vertigo is a symptom, not a diagnosis. It can be the result of a disorder of either the central or peripheral nervous system. The differential diagnosis and prognosis are very different for these two anatomic categories. To help you make sense of this distinction, a quick review of the vestibular system is necessary.

The vestibular system is the sensory system that's responsible for the detection of motion, head position, and spatial orientation. The neurologic pathway starts in the inner ear, which contains the cochlea (responsible for sound transduction) and the vestibular labyrinth. The vestibular labyrinth contains two important structures:

1. *The semicircular canals.* These are three tiny, fluid-filled tubes positioned at right angles to one other. They sense *angular acceleration.* When the head is rotated, the fluid (endolymph) within the canal that is situated in the plane of movement flows into an expansion of the canal, called the ampulla. The ampulla contains hair cells, which are the sensory receptors of the vestibular system. Movement of stereocilia attached to these hair cells results in the release of neurotransmitters that relay this information to the brain.

2. *The otolith organs (utricle and saccule).* These detect *linear acceleration*, that is, moving forwards, backwards, and up and down. The utricle detects movement in the horizontal plane, and the saccule detects movement in the vertical plane. These also contain hair cells, which sense movement when gravity-sensing crystals of calcium carbonate (called otoconia), which rest upon a gelatinous membrane that overlies the hair cells, shift in response to motion.

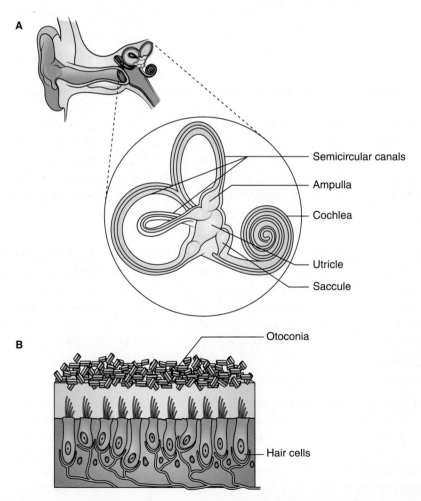

(*A*) The structures of the inner ear. You can see that the vestibular labyrinth is composed of the semicircular canals and otolith organs. (*B*) The hair cells and otoconia within the otolith organs.

The vestibular portion of the eighth cranial nerve receives input from the hair cells and then enters the brainstem to terminate on the vestibular nuclei. These nuclei send projections to the oculomotor cranial nerve nuclei (CN3, CN4, CN6), cerebellum, and spinal cord, among other targets. *Vestibulo-ocular connections* are responsible for stabilization and coordination of eye movements during head motion; *vestibulospinal pathways* help maintain postural equilibrium and balance; *cerebellar connections* modulate these activities.

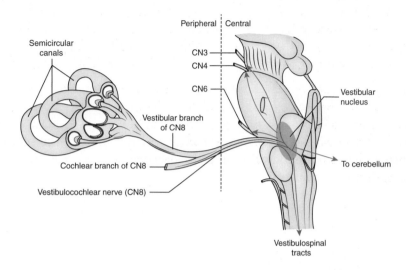

The neurologic pathways from the vestibular labyrinth into the brainstem.

The most important takeaway here is the division between peripheral and central vertigo. When we talk about *peripheral vertigo*, we mean vertigo caused by dysfunction within the inner ear or a process affecting CN8 before it enters the brainstem. *Central vertigo* is due to pathology within the central nervous system itself, typically affecting either the brainstem or the cerebellum. Central vertigo from hemorrhage or infarction in the posterior fossa can be life-threatening.

Peripheral Versus Central Vertigo

So how do we distinguish peripheral from central vertigo? Clinically, peripheral and central vertigo have distinct but overlapping features. Most of the time, your history will give you the answer (benign paroxysmal positional vertigo [BPPV], for instance, is a common cause of peripheral vertigo and is typically relatively straightforward to diagnose just from the patients' descriptions of their symptoms; see page 144). But sometimes, the story isn't so clear. As we've already noted, dizziness can be hard to describe. Your neurologic examination can help, too.

The **HINTS exam** (for **H**ead **I**mpulse test, **N**ystagmus, **T**est of **S**kew) is a screening tool that can help distinguish between central and peripheral vertigo. It has three components:

1. *Head Impulse Test.* This is a test of the vestibulo-ocular reflex (VOR; see Box 5.2). Hold the patient's head in your hands and ask them to fixate their gaze on your nose. Slowly rotate the patient's head side to side and then, abruptly but gently, accelerate the head back to neutral position. If the VOR is intact, the patient will be able to maintain gaze fixation on your nose. If not, you will see a quick corrective saccade (meaning a rapid eye movement that quickly alters the point of fixation) as the eyes "catch up" to the head and quickly re-fixate on your nose. The VOR is a peripherally mediated reflex involving the eighth, sixth, and third cranial nerves (remember, the cranial nerves apart from CN1

and CN2 are part of the *peripheral* nervous system). Therefore, in the appropriate clinical context, that is, in a patient with ongoing vertigo:

- A positive test (the presence of a corrective saccade, indicating a dysfunctional VOR) is suggestive of a peripheral lesion.

- A negative test (the absence of a saccade) is, by default, indicative of a central lesion.

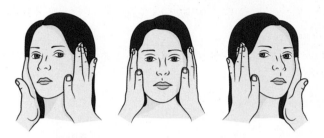

How to do a head impulse test.

2. *Nystagmus.* Nystagmus is an involuntary biphasic oscillation of the eyes characterized by a fast phase in one direction followed by a slow phase in the other. Nystagmus can be horizontal (right- or left-beating), vertical (down- or up-beating), torsional, or mixed.

- Nystagmus due to *peripheral lesions* tends to be either horizontal or horizontal/torsional, not purely torsional or vertical. It is unidirectional (*e.g.*, the fast phase always beats toward the left or toward the right regardless of the direction of gaze), suppressed by visual fixation (*e.g.*, when fixating on a static object), and often most prominent on end-gaze (*e.g.*, the amplitude increases when looking to the extreme left or right).

- Nystagmus due to *central lesions* is often vertical, multidirectional (*e.g.*, right-beating on right gaze, left-beating on left gaze), and does not suppress with visual fixation.

Horizontal

Vertical

Torsional

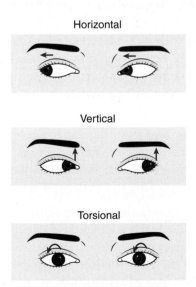

Different types of nystagmus. Note that nystagmus is named for the fast phase: if the fast phase is to the left and the slow phase to the right, we refer to it as left-beating nystagmus.

3. ***Test of Skew.*** This is a test of vertical ocular alignment. Cover one of the patient's eyes with your hand and ask him or her to fixate on your nose, then move your hand back and forth, from eye to eye. As you do so, look for any vertical movement—either up or down—of the uncovered eye, as though the eye is trying to re-focus on your nose. Skew deviation, or vertical misalignment of the eyes, is thought to be caused by supranuclear (higher in the chain of command than the oculomotor nuclei; these pathways project to the nuclei of CN3, 4, and 6, and—unlike CN3, 4, and 6—are part of the central nervous system [CNS]) oculomotor damage. Therefore:

- The presence of any vertical misalignment (*i.e.*, skew deviation) suggests *central etiology*.

- The absence of any vertical misalignment suggests *peripheral etiology*.

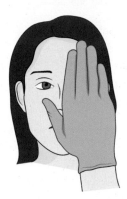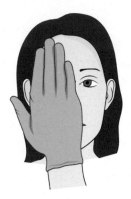

Testing for skew.

If any one of these three clinical signs is concerning for central vertigo, an MRI of the brain should be done in order to exclude a central cause. That said, do not be falsely reassured by a normal HINTS examination. The findings are subtle and, as you can imagine, the tests aren't always the easiest to reliably perform. Therefore, in the absence of a convincing clinical history that favors a peripheral etiology, maintaining a low threshold to scan—regardless of the HINTS examination—is important.

The HINTS Exam to Distinguish Between Peripheral and Central Vertigo

	Head Impulse Test	Nystagmus	Test of Skew
Peripheral vertigo	Positive (+corrective saccade)	Horizontal, unidirectional, suppressed by fixation	Negative (no skew)
Central vertigo	Negative (no corrective saccade)	Vertical, multidirectional, not suppressed by fixation	Positive (+skew)

Box 5.2 The Vestibulo-Ocular Reflex (VOR)

The purpose of the VOR is to stabilize vision during head movement. Look in a mirror while shaking your head side-to-side. See how your eyes move opposite your head, allowing you to remain fixated on your image? That's the VOR. The vestibular system by way of CN8 and the vestibular nuclei comprises the afferent limb of the reflex (it detects head motion), and the oculomotor system by way of CN6 and CN3 comprises the efferent limb (it enables eye movement in the opposite direction).

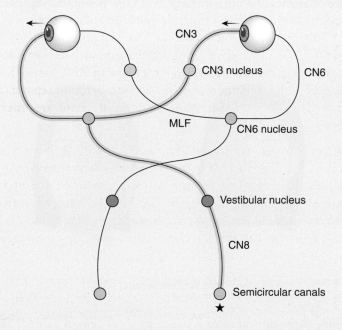

The vestibulo-ocular reflex (VOR). Activation of the right horizontal semicircular canal from a rapid head turn to the right results in excitation of the left CN6 nucleus and right CN3 nucleus (via the medial longitudinal fasiculus [MLF]; see page 232), driving the eyes to the left and thereby stabilizing the gaze.

Peripheral Vertigo

The majority of patients with vertigo (approximately 80%) have peripheral vertigo. Benign paroxysmal positional vertigo (BPPV), vestibular neuritis and Meniere disease are three of the most common causes.

1. **BPPV** is caused by displacement of the otoconia within either the left or right inner ear. For whatever reason (aging, trauma, and inner ear disease are all

risk factors, but sometimes it's just bad luck), the crystals get displaced from their normal location within the otolith organs and float into the fluid-filled semicircular canals. This abnormal, asymmetric stimulation results in the false sensation of head rotation whenever the head moves even the slightest bit in specific directions.

Most of what you need to remember about BPPV is in the name. It's benign—it typically self-resolves over a period of days to weeks; paroxysmal—it presents with very brief episodes of vertigo; and positional—these episodes are predictably provoked by movement. Patients will report sudden-onset seconds-long episodes of severe vertigo that occurs whenever they sit up or turn their head to one side or the other. Associated nausea and vomiting are common. The diagnosis is suggested by the clinical history and confirmed with the Dix-Hallpike maneuver (see Box 5.3). Treatment is with canalith repositioning maneuvers, such as the Epley (Box 5.3). Pharmacologic therapy is often given to patients with BPPV as well, but it is not curative. However, antihistamines (*e.g.*, meclizine), benzodiazepines, and antiemetics can be used for symptomatic relief while awaiting successful treatment with the Epley maneuver.

Unfortunately, despite substantial evidence supporting the use of the Epley maneuver (one study cites an 80% cure rate at 24 hours), patients are far more likely to be prescribed medication such as meclizine or to undergo expensive and often unnecessary neuroimaging tests. BPPV is "benign" in that it will eventually spontaneously resolve, but patients are miserable in the meantime. So be proactive and try the Epley—there's little harm and potentially significant benefit.

2. **Meniere disease** is a heterogeneous condition of unknown cause[1] that presents with episodic inner ear dysfunction, characterized by tinnitus, fluctuating low-frequency hearing loss, and vertigo associated with ear fullness. Autoimmune disease, a genetic predisposition, and migraine potentially contribute to its pathogenesis. Episodes of vertigo last (by definition) 20 minutes to 12 hours, but hearing impairment and nausea can persist for several days. The diagnosis is suggested by history and confirmed by formal hearing evaluation, which will show low-frequency sensorineural hearing loss on audiometry. There is no proven treatment. Supportive measures include avoidance of triggers (alcohol, caffeine, nicotine, and high-salt foods are common triggers) and vestibular rehabilitation. There is no clinical evidence to support the use of diuretics or steroids.

3. **Vestibular neuritis** is thought to be a viral or postviral disease affecting the vestibular portion of CN8. Classically, vestibular neuritis is characterized by severe and

---

[1]Meniere disease was previously believed to be the result of excess endolymph within the semicircular canals, but the current consensus is that so-called endolymphatic hydrops is more likely a marker for disease in some patients rather than the cause; it isn't evident in all patients, and many patients with hydrops do not have clinical evidence of Meniere disease.

persistent vertigo that is associated with unidirectional horizontal nystagmus due to the sudden asymmetry in vestibular input. Nausea, vomiting, and gait instability are also common. If hearing is affected as well, the disorder is called vestibular labyrinthitis. Acute symptoms last for hours to days, often with residual oscillopsia (the sensation that the world is unstable and in motion) and imbalance lasting for days to weeks or even longer. The diagnosis is based on history and examination (a positive head impulse test is crucial; the HINTS test was initially developed to distinguish vestibular neuritis from central causes). Treatment is supportive, typically with antiemetics and vestibular rehabilitation. In severe cases, there is some evidence that corticosteroids may hasten recovery.

Box 5.3 Dix-Hallpike and Epley Maneuvers

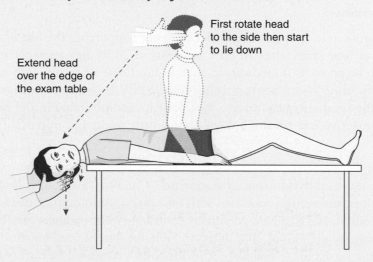

First rotate head to the side then start to lie down

Extend head over the edge of the exam table

The Dix-Hallpike maneuver (remember, the Dix-Hallpike is diagnostic; **D**ix = **D**iagnostic!). To perform this maneuver, position the patient sitting upon an examination table. Turn the head 45° to one side (you'll need to do this twice, once with the head turned left and once right; typically, only one side will be symptomatic), then quickly lower them backwards, so the head is extended about 20° over the back of the table. Remember to support the patient's neck when you do this. Then observe the patient's eyes closely; if the patient has BPPV you should see nystagmus appear within about 30 seconds. It's not a perfect test (the sensitivity is about 80%), but if the history seems to fit the diagnosis, a positive Dix-Hallpike maneuver can be very useful as confirmation. Remember to warn the patient beforehand: if they do have BPPV, you are effectively provoking an episode, and they will likely find the experience unpleasant to say the least.

Box 5.3 Dix-Hallpike and Epley Maneuvers (Continued)

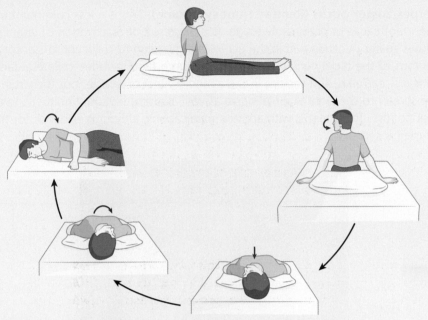

The Epley maneuver is the most well-established treatment for BPPV. Put simply, the idea is to knock the crystals back into their correct position. The Epley begins with the Dix-Hallpike maneuver (which will help you determine laterality), followed by rolling the patient onto the opposite shoulder before sitting up. You can and should perform this on the patient in the office (the patient's symptoms may entirely resolve!), but—especially for those with residual symptoms or a history of recurrence and because the Epley often takes several attempts to work—you should also send the patient home with instructions on how to do it themselves. You can also refer them to a physical therapist with expertise in vestibular disorders.

Key Features of Peripheral Vertigo

	Duration	Other Distinguishing Features	Diagnosis	Treatment
BPPV	Episodic (seconds)	Positional	Positional testing	Epley maneuver
Meniere	Episodic (minutes-hours)	Unilateral hearing loss, tinnitus, ear fullness	Audiogram	Supportive
Vestibular Neuritis	Persistent (hours-days)	Preceded by a viral infection, rarely recurs	Head impulse test (+audiogram, if hearing changes are present)	Supportive

Box 5.4 Other Causes of Peripheral Vertigo

- **Herpes zoster oticus (Ramsay Hunt syndrome).** This is a less common but important cause of peripheral vertigo. It is the result of reactivation of latent herpes zoster infection within the geniculate ganglion (a collection of sensory neurons of the facial nerve). The classic symptom triad includes ipsilateral facial paralysis, ear pain, and vesicles in the auditory canal or auricle, but the virus can spread to the eighth cranial nerve as well, causing vertigo, tinnitus, and/or hearing loss. Treatment is with antiviral medications, although evidence for their efficacy is sparse.

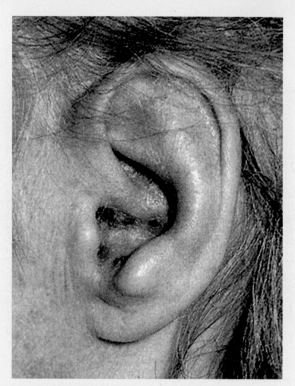

Vesicles seen in Ramsay Hunt syndrome.

(Reprinted from Campbell WW. *DeJong's the Neurologic Examination*. 7th ed. Wolters Kluwer; 2012.)

Box 5.4 Other Causes of Peripheral Vertigo   (Continued)

- **Vestibular schwannoma** (acoustic neuroma). Schwann cells myelinate peripheral nerves. It makes sense, then, that schwannomas—relatively common, benign tumors—grow along peripheral nerves. Any cranial nerve besides CN1 and CN2 can be affected (CN1 and CN2 are technically part of the CNS; they are myelinated by oligodendrocytes, not Schwann cells); when CN8 is affected, the tumor is called a vestibular schwannoma. Because these tumors are slow-growing, the CNS is able to compensate for subtle vestibular imbalances, and severe vertigo is relatively uncommon. More often patients experience gradual-onset unilateral hearing loss and tinnitus, along with a vague sense of imbalance or gait instability. When vestibular schwannomas are associated with neurofibromatosis type 2, they are often bilateral (see Chapter 17). An MRI of the internal auditory canal (IAC) is diagnostic.

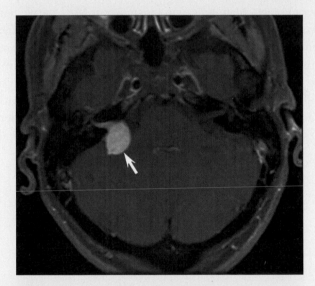

An MRI showing a vestibular schwannoma (white arrow) located at the cerebellopontine angle, where the eighth cranial nerve enters the brainstem.

(Modified from Johnson J. *Bailey's Head and Neck Surgery*. 5th ed. Wolters Kluwer; 2013.)

- **Aminoglycoside toxicity.** Many aminoglycoside antibiotics are both vestibulotoxic and ototoxic and can therefore cause peripheral vestibular damage and permanent hearing loss.

Central Vertigo

Central vertigo is caused by lesions within the central nervous system.

Infarction (ischemic or hemorrhagic) and *multiple sclerosis* affecting the brainstem and cerebellar vestibular pathways are common causes, but any lesions located in these areas (including tumors, abscesses, etc) can cause central vertigo. Because there are so many cells and axons packed into these areas, vertigo is usually not isolated but is associated with other signs and symptoms. Therefore, when vertigo presents with these so-called "neighborhood" signs and symptoms—that is, signs and symptoms attributable to damage of nearby neuronal pathways—red flags should go up for a potential central etiology. Common "neighborhood" symptoms that localize to the brainstem include diplopia, dysarthria, and dysphagia (if you add dizziness, you've got the classic "4 Ds" of brainstem lesions). Ataxia, truncal instability, and limb incoordination are more indicative of a cerebellar lesion. The presence of any of these associated symptoms, when a patient presents with new-onset vertigo, is an indication for an urgent MRI to rule out a central etiology.

Migraine is becoming increasingly recognized as a cause of vertigo. *Migraine with brainstem aura* is considered a subclass of migraine with aura, defined as migraine associated with an aura consisting of classic brainstem symptoms such as vertigo, diplopia, and dysarthria. *Vestibular migraine* is characterized by frequent vertiginous episodes lasting from 5 minutes to 72 hours, at least half of which are temporally associated with migraine. Both of these diagnoses remain incompletely understood but are worth considering in patients for whom your workup of other central causes has been unrevealing.[2]

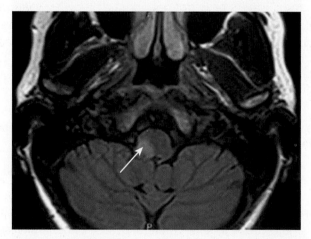

Lateral medullary syndrome (or Wallenberg syndrome), caused by posterior inferior cerebellar artery (PICA) occlusion, classically presents with vertigo as well as a host of other neighborhood signs and symptoms including hoarseness, dysphagia, nystagmus, Horner syndrome, and hemisensory loss (see page 68). White arrow is pointing to the lateral medullary infarct. (Courtesy of Carlos Torres, MD.)

---

[2]It is thought that migrainous vertigo is a type of central vertigo predominantly because evaluation for peripheral causes (*i.e.*, ear or nerve dysfunction) comes up negative.

Box 5.5

When neurologists hear a patient describe their symptoms as "acute onset," the first thing that comes to mind is vascular pathology: ischemic or hemorrhagic stroke. This is an absolutely appropriate response, but it is certainly worth pointing out that "acute-onset" vertigo should not sway you inexorably toward a central etiology. Both peripheral and central vertigo can (and often do) present acutely.

Box 5.6 Disembarkment Syndrome (mal de debarquement)

Have you ever had a transient sense of imbalance—like you are still floating up-and-down on the waves—when you step off a boat onto dry land? That unpleasant sense of disequilibrium may occur with your first step onshore or several minutes to hours after abandoning the high seas. This sensation is normal if it is brief (lasting minutes to hours), but if it becomes persistent it is referred to as disembarkment syndrome. Formal diagnostic criteria include persistent, non-spinning vertigo (patients often describe a sensation of swaying or rocking) lasting more than 48 hours, with onset less than 48 hours from exposure. Re-exposure to passive motion should transiently relieve symptoms. Disembarkment syndrome can last weeks to years. Disabling fatigue and cognitive difficulties can also occur. The etiology is unknown, and treatment is difficult. Scopolamine, meclizine, anticonvulsants, and diuretics have not been found to be reliably effective. Some patients may experience some benefit from a benzodiazepine or selective serotonin reuptake inhibitor. Vestibular rehabilitation has not been found to be consistently beneficial.

 A Brief Word on Syncope

Syncope is the transient loss of consciousness due to inadequate blood flow to the brain. Patients present with a loss of muscle tone and subsequent collapse, followed by a relatively quick return to baseline. Preceding lightheadedness is common. Brief tonic or myoclonic movements can also occur; this is known as *convulsive syncope* and is a common and benign syncopal variant (see page 165). Presyncope should be evaluated the same as true syncope, as the causes—both benign and serious—are the same.

There are, for our purposes, three major types of syncope:

1. **Reflex syncope** is very common. It is caused by a sudden drop in blood pressure or heart rate due to alterations in autonomic activation, either increased parasympathetic or decreased sympathetic tone. *Vasovagal syncope* is the most common type of reflex syncope and classically presents with prodromal

lightheadedness, diaphoresis, pallor, palpitations, nausea, and/or blurring or darkening of vision prior to the loss of consciousness. If you suspect vasovagal syncope but, for whatever reason, are not certain, tilt table testing can be helpful to confirm the diagnosis. ***Situational syncope*** is another type of reflex syncope and refers to syncope due to an identifiable trigger such as urination (referred to as micturition syncope) or coughing.

2. **Syncope due to cardiopulmonary disease.** Since this is a book about neurology, we won't expound on this topic. Causes include arrhythmias and structural cardiopulmonary diseases, such as aortic stenosis or hypertrophic cardiomyopathy with significant left ventricular outflow obstruction. From a neurologic perspective, it is important to have a low threshold to refer to cardiology when patients present with otherwise unexplained syncope. Concurrent neurologic and cardiac evaluations are often ideal.

3. **Orthostatic Syncope.** Orthostatic hypotension is defined as a decrease in systolic blood pressure of at least 20 mm Hg or a decrease in diastolic blood pressure of at least 10 mm Hg within 3 minutes of standing. There are three main causes:

• *Volume depletion.* Significant volume depletion can be due to vomiting, bleeding, or just dehydration, among many other potential causes.

• *Medications.* This list is a long one and includes medications that cause vasodilation, volume depletion, and autonomic dysregulation.

• *Autonomic failure.* Autonomic failure can be due to neurodegenerative diseases (such as Parkinson disease or Multiple System Atrophy; see Chapter 13) or autonomic neuropathy (caused most often by diabetes, but don't forget to consider the many other potential etiologies including amyloidosis, connective tissue diseases, vitamin deficiencies, and various infections; see Chapter 11).

Are you wondering why transient ischemic attacks (TIAs) are not on this list of causes of syncope? It's a common misperception that TIAs frequently present with syncope. Vertebrobasilar TIAs can cause loss of consciousness if thalamic structures are involved, but for this to occur in isolation, without any other neurologic deficits, is very rare. The American Academy of Neurology recommends against carotid artery imaging for syncope without the presence of other neurologic symptoms; occlusive carotid artery disease results in ischemia of brain tissue supplied by the ophthalmic, anterior and middle cerebral arteries, as we discussed in Chapter 2, and causes focal deficits such as weakness, numbness, and visual field cuts, but it does not cause syncope.

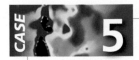

CASE 5

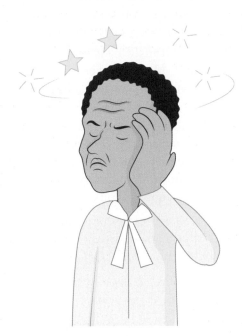

Your Patient's Follow-up: Although Kyle's vertigo is improving, you order an MRI because you've found convincing focality on his examination. The nystagmus is hard to see—this is not unusual!—but you think it's there, and you are confident about the left upper extremity dysmetria. Now that you know about the HINTS test, you've also noted a negative head impulse test and positive test of skew, both concerning for a central etiology. His symptoms are all but resolved by the time the MRI is completed, but the scan is notable for a small acute infarct in the left cerebellum. You admit him for a stroke evaluation and, on reviewing his telemetry the following morning, note about 30 minutes of atrial fibrillation. He's soon discharged on anticoagulation and is grateful for your help.

You now know:

- | That acute dizziness can mean either lightheadedness or vertigo. Lightheadedness is most often not a primarily neurologic complaint; it is more often the result of dehydration or, less commonly but importantly, underlying cardiac disease. Vertigo is a neurologic symptom and requires a careful history and examination to appropriately manage and treat. Disequilibrium is another type of vertigo—chronic, as opposed to acute—that's most often seen in the elderly.

- | Vertigo does not always mean spinning! Vertigo is defined as the false sensation of movement, or *the sensation of movement when nothing is actually moving.*

- | BPPV, Meniere disease, and vestibular neuritis are common causes of peripheral vertigo. If the history is straightforward and the examination consistent, an MRI is not needed. But if you are unsure, or if your examination is concerning for central etiology, get an MRI.

- | Central vertigo is most often caused by ischemic or hemorrhagic stroke within the brainstem or cerebellum. Multiple sclerosis lesions in the same regions can also present with vertigo. Suspect central vertigo when "neighborhood" signs or symptoms are present.

- | Syncope can be divided into reflex syncope, syncope due to cardiopulmonary disease, and orthostatic syncope. TIAs rarely cause syncope. If they do, it is the posterior circulation (*i.e.*, vertebrobasilar system) that is responsible and not the anterior circulation. Carotid dopplers are not recommended for patients who present with simple syncope without other associated neurologic findings.

Seizures

6

In this chapter, you will learn:

1 | How to classify and distinguish among different types of seizures

2 | How to manage a first-time seizure in an urgent setting

3 | How to sort through and make sense of the antiepileptic medications

4 | How to define, classify, and treat status epilepticus

5 | How to diagnose and manage psychogenic nonepileptic seizures (PNES)

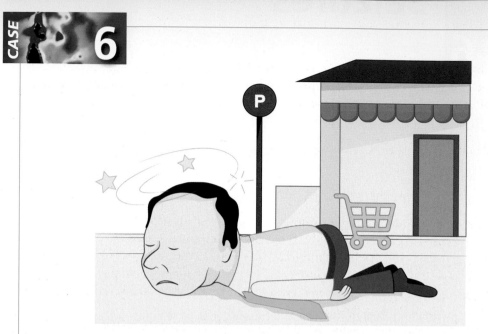

Your Patient: Carlton, a 58-year-old accountant with no known medical history, is brought into the emergency department (ED) by emergency medical services (EMS) after he was found on the ground in a supermarket parking lot. EMS tells you that a witness at the scene saw several minutes of full-body shaking, but this had resolved by the time EMS arrived. The patient's vitals are stable and his fingerstick glucose is within normal limits. He appears sleepy, but when he opens his eyes, you notice that he's looking preferentially to the left. You don't notice any abnormal shaking movements. He won't follow commands but seems to withdraw his right arm and leg less briskly than his left to noxious stimuli. What is the first step in your management?

Seizures are sudden bursts of abnormal electrical activity occurring within the cerebral cortex. Because they can happen in any area of the cortex, seizures can cause almost any neurologic manifestation you can imagine, from dramatic motor events with loss of consciousness to subtle sensory or behavioral abnormalities. Sometimes you can even find electrical activity on an electroencephalogram (EEG) indicative of a seizure without any associated clinical manifestations at all. Seizures are among the most common and treatable conditions in all of neurology.

Epilepsy

Not everyone who has a seizure has epilepsy. As many as 1 in 20 people will have a single seizure in their lifetime, but only approximately 1 in 50 will be diagnosed with epilepsy. The diagnosis of epilepsy requires:

- At least *two unprovoked seizures* occurring more than 24 hours apart

OR

- One unprovoked seizure, *plus* the probability of further seizures must be similar to the risk of recurrence after two unprovoked seizures (at least 60%)—don't worry, we will explain this in just a moment

OR

- The diagnosis of a specific epilepsy syndrome (see page 170)

Provoked Versus Unprovoked Seizures

According to the International League Against Epilepsy (ILAE) guidelines, a *"provoked"* seizure is a seizure that is directly caused by an *acute, symptomatic*[1] condition. Sepsis, hypo- or hyperglycemia, and alcohol withdrawal are common causes of provoked seizures. Other conditions—stroke, traumatic brain injury, intracranial surgery, and postanoxic encephalopathy—are considered *acute, symptomatic* conditions only if the seizure occurs within the first 7 days following the insult.

An *"unprovoked"* seizure is a seizure of unknown etiology or a seizure related to a preexisting brain lesion or preexisting disorder (*i.e.*, a *"remote, symptomatic"* condition[2]). Such lesions—an old stroke, for instance, or a brain tumor—can act as seizure "niduses" in that they can create irritable brain tissue that is prone to seize. But why, for example, does a patient with a stroke that occurred many years ago seize for the first time today? The answer is often elusive; thus, in the absence of an *acute, symptomatic* condition, that seizure is considered unprovoked.

What Conditions Increase the Risk of Recurrence After a Single Seizure?

Let's go back to that second definition of epilepsy for a moment: *one unprovoked seizure, plus the probability of further seizures similar to the general recurrence risk after two unprovoked seizures.* The chance of seizure recurrence is low following a single seizure but increases significantly after a second seizure. So, what factors increase this risk after just a single seizure such that the risk is high enough to potentially warrant the diagnosis of epilepsy? There are only a handful of things:

- *An abnormal EEG.* An EEG that is "irritable" or "epileptiform" shows a brain that is not actively seizing but has the potential to seize. It is therefore not surprising that specific "irritable" features on an EEG (the details of this are beyond the scope of this book) are associated with a significantly increased risk of further seizures.

---

[1]The term "symptomatic" here simply means that the condition has caused a seizure, hence it is "symptomatic."
[2]Note the distinction between acute, symptomatic conditions and remote, symptomatic conditions.

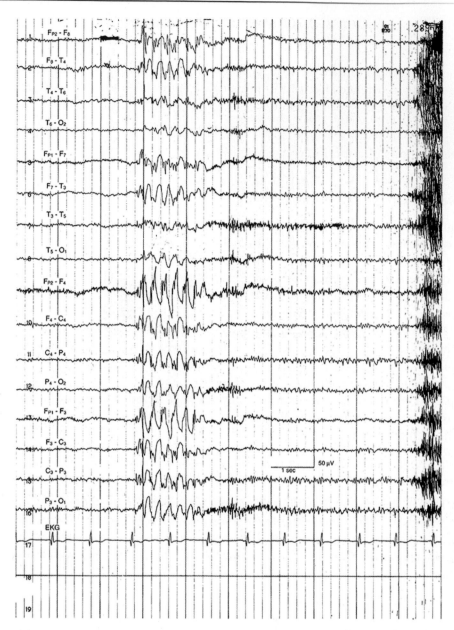

An abnormal EEG showing high-amplitude generalized fast 4-to-6 Hz and slow waves in a teenager with myoclonic and generalized tonic-clonic seizures upon awakening, characteristic of juvenile myoclonic epilepsy (see page 173). (Reprinted from Wyllie E, Cascino GD, Gidal BE, Goodkin HP. *Wyllie's Treatment of Epilepsy.* 5th ed. Wolters Kluwer; 2012.)

- *Remote, symptomatic seizures.* Although an old stroke or known brain tumor does not "count" as an acute, provoking factor, these lesions can represent a locus of irritable brain tissue. Patients with these lesions have an increased risk for further seizures.

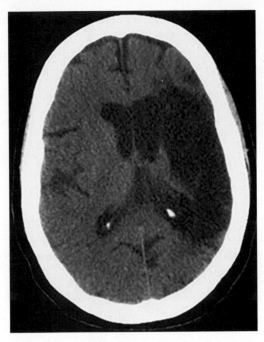

A chronic left middle cerebral artery (MCA) distribution infarct on CT that could serve as the source of seizure activity. (Reprinted from Weiner WJ, Goetz CG, Shin RK, Lewis SL. *Neurology for the Non-Neurologist.* 6th ed. Wolters Kluwer; 2010.)

- *Nocturnal seizures (i.e., seizures that happen during sleep).* There is no known, satisfying explanation for this one. We think of this as a risk for recurrence because seizures that occur during sleep strip away many of the potential "seizure mimics," and therefore reflect actual, ongoing seizure activity. For example, nonepileptic seizures, vasovagal syncope, and convulsive syncope are not risk factors for seizure recurrence and do not wake a patient from sleep.

Thus, if a patient presents with a single unprovoked seizure and has any of the three items listed above—an abnormal EEG, a relevant brain lesion identified on imaging, or a seizure during sleep—that patient can be diagnosed with epilepsy.[3]

First-Time Seizure

Seizures account for approximately 2% of all ED visits. Approximately 25% of these will be for first-time events. Such visits can be scary, both for the patient and for the healthcare provider, but there is a simple algorithm to help you manage these patients.

---

[3]There are caveats to this rule. For example, a patient with a prior stroke can have nonepileptic seizures. And an abnormal EEG—assuming it isn't performed during the event—does not necessarily mean the event itself was a true seizure. Don't worry if all this doesn't make perfect sense to you now; it will by the end of the chapter. The point is that, as with any diagnosis, don't forget to use your clinical judgment!

Start with the basics. *First, take a good history.* There are several "seizure risk factor" questions to ask every patient who presents with a first-time seizure, including a history of developmental delay, febrile seizures during infancy, a history of significant head trauma with loss of consciousness, prior central nervous system (CNS) infections such as encephalitis or meningitis, and a family history of seizures.

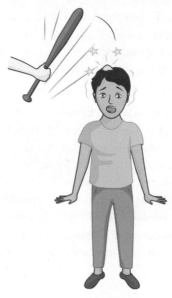

A thorough history for seizure risk factors, including head trauma, is essential when you see a patient for a first-time seizure.

Next, perform a complete neurologic examination. Patients may be entirely back to their baseline or (as is often the case) very sleepy, because:

1. they are *postictal* (this term refers to the altered state of consciousness that is present immediately post-seizure) and/or

2. they have been given benzodiazepines by EMS or ED providers to treat the seizure.

Although sleepiness is not unexpected, focality is a red flag that should prompt concern for an underlying neurologic lesion such as an intracranial mass or bleed. Note that, although the postictal state is most often associated with lethargy and confusion, it can be associated with agitation and psychosis as well.

Check labs. You want basic studies (including a STAT fingerstick glucose and a metabolic panel, as both hypo- and hyperglycemia and various electrolyte abnormalities can cause seizures), as well as a serum alcohol level and urine toxicology screen. Notably, if the seizure semiology[4] was reported to be several minutes of generalized, full-body shaking, you should not be surprised to see a mild-to-moderate leukocytosis, an elevated creatine kinase (CK),

---

[4]No, you are not suddenly reading a thriller by Dan Brown, and yes, this is really the term used by neurologists to mean the signs or manifestations of a seizure.

and an elevated lactate; in fact, if you do *not* see these things, you may want to dig a bit deeper into the history and consider diagnoses other than a seizure.

Finally, a noncontrast CT of the head should always be performed to rule out any obvious underlying pathology.

At this point you now have two big decisions to make:

1. *Does the patient require admission?* If the above workup is unrevealing (as it often is), the neurologic examination is non-focal, and your patient has returned to his or her clinical baseline, admission is often not necessary. If the laboratory work or imaging is abnormal and requires further evaluation, if the patient remains lethargic or agitated for an extended period of time, or if there are focal neurologic abnormalities on examination, then admission is indicated.

2. *Should you start the patient on an antiepileptic medication?* Immediate treatment with an antiepileptic drug (AED) has been shown to reduce the risk of seizure recurrence within the first 2 years following the initial event but has *not* been shown to improve prognosis (defined as sustained seizure remission) in the long term. Further, as already discussed, the risk of seizure recurrence after a single event is not that high. Thus, we need to weigh the benefits of starting an AED against the possible side effects and risks. Common practice is to defer AED initiation following a first-time event, but there are three exceptions. You should recognize these from the discussion above, and they make sense: these are the factors that significantly increase the risk of seizure recurrence.

   a. Nocturnal seizure

   b. Remote, symptomatic seizure (*e.g.*, if there is a relevant finding on imaging, such as encephalomalacia [softening or loss of brain tissue] from an old stroke or calcifications from prior neurocysticercosis; other lesions, such as a small arachnoid cyst or an incidentally found pituitary lesion, are likely incidental and do not warrant AED initiation)

   c. An abnormal EEG (the caveat here is that EEGs are not routinely performed in most EDs; if the patient has returned to his or her baseline, it is fine to defer the EEG to the outpatient setting).

Although this algorithm works nearly all of the time, we want to emphasize that these decisions should be individualized and, when possible, made in conjunction with the patient. And there are exceptions. If a patient works in construction, for instance, and spends his or her days climbing ladders, it may be reasonable to start an AED at least temporarily to avoid potentially significant injury should a second seizure occur while at work.

If the plan is for discharge, it is imperative to ensure close outpatient follow-up. An EEG and MRI of the brain (ordered with a "seizure protocol," which specifies thin cuts through the temporal lobes; you'll understand why shortly) should ideally be scheduled prior to the first outpatient visit so the results can be reviewed and the patient appropriately treated at that time. An MRI of the brain *with gadolinium* is often indicated if you suspect neoplastic, infectious, or inflammatory etiologies.

Seizure Types

What exactly is a seizure? To build on the simplified definition we used at the beginning of this chapter, we can say that a seizure is a *sudden, paroxysmal* event caused by *synchronous hyperactivity* of neurons in the *cerebral cortex* (in simpler words, a whole bunch of neurons in the brain start firing pretty much all at once). There are two main types of seizures, generalized and focal.

1. *Generalized seizures.* The onset of generalized seizures involves both hemispheres of the brain simultaneously. There are several types.

   a. *Generalized tonic-clonic* (GTC) *seizures.* Previously known as grand mal seizures, these are the most common type of generalized seizure. They can be broken down into four phases:

      i. The *onset,* classically characterized by the abrupt loss of consciousness, often accompanied by a loud moan (also known as an "ictal cry" due to strong muscle contractions that rapidly push air out of the lungs).

      ii. The *tonic (stiffening) phase,* during which the muscles of all four extremities, chest, and back become stiff. This can last anywhere from several seconds to approximately 1 minute.

      iii. The *clonic (jerking) phase,* during which there is *generalized, rhythmic, nonsuppressible* jerking of all extremities. This typically lasts another 1 to 2 minutes

      iv. The *postictal period.* As mentioned earlier (see page 160), this is most often characterized by sleepiness and confusion but can also be associated with agitation and psychosis. This can take anywhere from several minutes to several hours to fully resolve.

Box 6.1

It is very common for patients' family members (or anyone who witnesses a generalized tonic-clonic seizure) to report that the episode of shaking went on for 5, 10, or even 20 minutes. Most often, this is not because the patient was in true status epilepticus (see page 177), but because the family members were scared and their sense of time became understandably distorted.

During the seizure, family members or other witnesses should:

1. turn the patient on his or her side to decrease the risk of aspiration;
2. NOT stick a spoon or anything else in the patient's mouth (this is not only unhelpful but can actually be dangerous);
3. time the event and, if possible, take a video (this can be extremely helpful diagnostically for the healthcare provider who will eventually care for the patient); and
4. call 911 if the seizure lasts longer than 5 minutes, if there are recurrent seizures without return to baseline, if the patient's skin color turns blue, or if there is evidence of serious head injury or laceration.

b. *Tonic seizures*: These consist of abrupt muscle stiffening, often associated with loss of consciousness and falling.

c. *Clonic seizures*: Characterized by repetitive jerking movements usually involving the face and arms.

d. *Myoclonic seizures*: Sudden, brief muscle contractions that can affect any muscle group (most often the arms); these can occur as a single event or a cluster of events. Consciousness is almost always preserved.

Box 6.2 Myoclonus

Myoclonus has many different etiologies. In this chapter, we are talking specifically about epileptic myoclonus, meaning myoclonus that originates from abnormal epileptic activity in the cerebral cortex. *Physiologic myoclonus* is a normal phenomenon that occurs in healthy people: common examples include *hypnic myoclonus* (those sudden jerks that occur when you're falling asleep) and *diaphragmatic myoclonus* (hiccups!). *Essential myoclonus* is myoclonus of no clear cause, or is suspected to be due to genetic causes. For more details, see Chapter 13.

---

e. *Atonic seizures*: Colloquially known as "drop attacks," these are effectively the opposite of tonic seizures in that they cause a sudden loss of muscle tone resulting in abrupt collapse to the ground. Patients who experience recurrent atonic seizures often need to wear helmets to protect themselves.

f. *Absence seizures*: Absence seizures are brief staring spells typically lasting 5 to 10 seconds, accompanied by behavioral arrest and impaired consciousness. They can be associated with stereotyped automatisms (repetitive, purposeless movements) such as eyelid fluttering, lip-smacking, or picking at buttons, and are almost exclusively seen in children.

2. **Focal seizures.** Unlike generalized seizures, which begin in both hemispheres simultaneously, the onset of focal seizures is limited to a single, focal region of brain tissue. Although they begin this way, they can "secondarily generalize" such that the neuronal hyperexcitability spreads to involve both hemispheres; clinically, the patient is observed to progress to a generalized tonic-clonic seizure. Most first-time unprovoked seizures in adults are focal-onset seizures that have secondarily generalized.

a. *Focal Aware Seizures* (FAS; previously called simple partial seizures). The patient is awake and aware that something abnormal is happening. The symptoms depend entirely on the part of the cortex that is involved. Examples include flashing lights (due to involvement of the occipital cortex) and rhythmic, jerking movements of an arm or leg (due to involvement of the motor cortex). When these movements begin in one body part (let's say the fingertips) and gradually spread to another (up the wrist and into the arm), we call this a **"Jacksonian March,"** and it's typical for this type of seizure. You can picture the wave of hyperexcitability spreading up the homunculus of the motor cortex, causing the propagation of these symptoms.

b. *Focal Impaired Awareness Seizures* (FIASs; previously called complex partial seizures). These are the most common type of seizures in adults with epilepsy. Patients will appear to be awake but are unresponsive and minimally reactive with their environment. They may stare straight ahead or demonstrate automatisms such as chewing movements, lip smacking, grimacing, or word repetition. These typically last several minutes and are followed by a postictal period. Patients are typically amnestic for the event but are often aware of their preceding aura, if one exists (see Box 6.3).

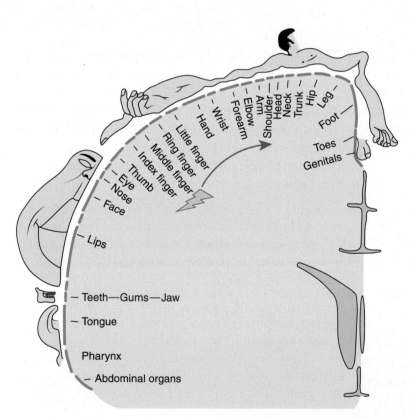

You can imagine a focal seizure affecting the motor cortex that begins in the hand and then spreads upward into the arm.

Box 6.3 Absence Seizures versus Focal Seizures With Impaired Awareness

After reading these definitions, it may seem tricky to distinguish between absence seizures and focal seizures with impaired awareness, but it's usually quite straightforward. First, absence seizures are almost exclusively seen in childhood. Second, absence seizures are very brief (lasting only seconds), never begin with an aura, and do not have a postictal phase, whereas focal seizures with impaired awareness usually persist for several minutes, often begin with an aura, and are typically followed by a postictal phase.

Box 6.4 Auras

Many patients will tell you that they know when they are about to seize. What they are describing are their auras, which are relatively brief, focal seizures that occur at the onset of a seizure episode and are substantial enough to cause symptoms but not so large as to interfere with consciousness. Common examples include a "rising" sensation in the stomach, a metallic taste in the mouth and pleasant or unpleasant smells, but auras can really be just about anything. A sudden sensation of familiarity (*deja vu*), unfamiliarity (*jamais vu*), euphoria, or word-finding difficulty are other common examples. Visual auras are also common; those that originate from the occipital lobe are un-formed elementary hallucinations (think flashing white or colored lights), whereas those that originate from the temporal lobe can be more complex (images of letters, animals, and even people).

A Quick Note on the Differential Diagnosis of Seizures

As you now know, seizures can present in many different ways and can therefore—at times—be difficult to diagnose. Two of the most common, and arguably the most important, alternative diagnoses to consider are syncope and stroke.

Seizure Versus Syncope. Syncope is the loss of consciousness due to a sudden drop in blood pressure. It can look a lot like a seizure. Syncope is most often the result of an underlying cardiac or neurocardiogenic (vasovagal) etiology (see page 151), the treatment of which is distinctly different from the management of a seizure. Both seizures and syncope can be associated with loss of consciousness and incontinence. Convulsive syncope—a common variant of syncope that is associated with brief tonic or myoclonic activity—can look for all the world like a seizure. So how do we distinguish between them? Certain features can help:

- The period of confusion after a seizure can last minutes to hours, whereas with syncope it lasts at most a minute or two.
- Whereas premonitory symptoms can occur with both, with syncope they tend to be cardiac (palpitations, diaphoresis, lightheadedness) or visual (tunnel vision,

"blacking out"), and with seizures are more often an aura (glittering lights, a funny smell, a gastric rising sensation, a sense of deja vu).

- Tongue biting occurs almost exclusively with seizures.

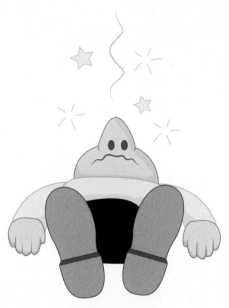

The distinction between syncope and a seizure can be challenging.

Seizure Versus Stroke. This one's a little harder, but it comes up all the time in the ED and can be challenging—sometimes even impossible—to sort out.

Let's return to our patient at the beginning of this chapter, Carlton. He presented to the ED with a left gaze preference and right-sided weakness after being found down in a parking lot, with several minutes of full-body shaking reported by a bystander. Although the shaking should absolutely prompt you to think he has had a seizure, the first step in his management is to activate a stroke code. Why? Carlton is presenting with the acute onset of focal neurologic deficits (left gaze preference and right-sided weakness), so stroke (which can occasionally present with seizure at the time of onset) has to be at the top of your differential because—as discussed in Chapter 2—strokes are treated in a highly time-sensitive manner. So do everything you can to first rule a stroke in or out, and then consider the rest of your differential.

A common feature of seizures that can be confused with stroke is **Todd paralysis,** a transient postictal weakness involving the part of the body that was actively seizing. Let's assume that Carlton's seizure began in his left cerebral hemisphere (and then generalized, consistent with the description of full-body shaking). His right arm and leg must have been initially involved. Once he stopped actively seizing, he could be disproportionately weak on the right side of his body due to Todd paralysis, lasting anywhere from minutes to several hours. Why? The neurons that were firing away are now exhausted and can take some time to recover. You can imagine that this kind of focal weakness can initially be difficult if not impossible to distinguish from weakness caused by a stroke.

Box 6.5

Todd paralysis is named after Robert Bentley Todd, an Irish-born physician who first described the phenomenon. He was also known to prescribe wine and brandy for fevers, and some attribute one of our better-known cocktails—the hot toddy—to him as well. Whereas its medicinal value is debatable, it might be just what you need to get you through the rest of this chapter!

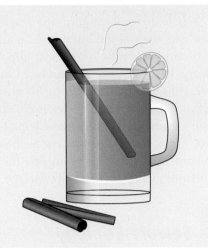

Box 6.6 Gaze Preference During and After a Seizure

Gaze preference must also be considered. Patients typically look "toward their stroke" and "away from their seizure" (see page 62). If we think Carlton's seizure began in his left hemisphere, he should be looking to the right *if he is actively seizing*. But we don't think he is actively seizing; instead, we suspect that he is postictal. Just as a Todd paralysis causes weakness due to "burned out" neurons, gaze preference often reverses sides postictally due to "burned out" frontal eye fields. The eye fields were initially pushing the eyes to look away from the seizure focus but are now exhausted, and thus the eyes drift back in the opposite direction—in Carlton's case, to the left—which is the same direction you would expect if he'd had a left hemispheric stroke.

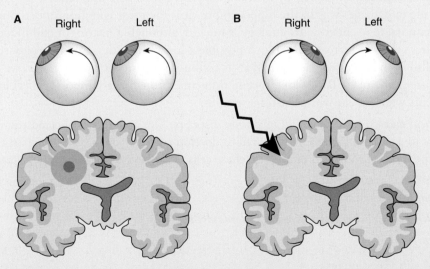

(A) Ablation (due to stroke or the postictal state after a seizure) of the frontal eye fields, and *(B)* stimulation (from a seizure) of the frontal eye fields.

So how do we distinguish the postictal state from stroke? There is no easy answer. We must take the whole clinical picture into account: what we find on examination, what we see on imaging and—often most important—what we are able to obtain from a careful history. If, for instance, we contact Carlton's spouse who tells us that he has a known seizure disorder and ran out of his medications several days ago, we likely have our answer. Perfusion imaging studies can also help to determine if there is decreased blood flow to the brain suggestive of stroke (see Chapter 2). But sometimes we just can't be certain, and in those cases, we treat the patient as if he or she has had a stroke even if we suspect seizure. The potential downside of missing the opportunity to treat a stroke is often far worse than that from giving thrombolytic therapy to a postictal patient.

 ## Seizure Etiology

Seizures can be due to lots of things, but we can simplify it to four:

1. An epileptogenic lesion

2. Toxic-metabolic derangements

3. Medications and other substances

4. An epilepsy syndrome

Epileptogenic Lesions

Epileptogenic lesions are lesions in the brain that act as seizure foci. They can be present from birth or acquired later in life. Some common examples include:

- *Mesial temporal sclerosis* (MTS). This is a pathologic diagnosis (although often detectable on MRI) defined by neuronal loss and gliosis (the proliferation of glial cells at a site of damage) within the hippocampus. It is the most common underlying cause of temporal lobe epilepsy. Its etiology is unclear, although a history of childhood febrile seizures seems to increase the risk. A possible association with human herpesvirus 6 has also been suggested. Because MTS is common in patients with seizures, we order "seizure protocol" MRIs (which specify thin cuts through the temporal lobes) in patients who present with first-time seizures.

- *Cortical dysplasia and neuronal migration disorders.* This rather complicated terminology refers to a situation when neurons fail to develop correctly or to reach the parts of the brain they were meant to end up in; these cells often have a high propensity to cause seizures.

- *Prenatal or perinatal cerebral injury*

- *Poststroke or post-traumatic encephalomalacia*

- *Brain tumors*

- *Brain abscesses*

- *Vascular anomalies* (such as arteriovenous or cavernous malformations)

Acute intracerebral hemorrhage and ischemic stroke can also present with seizure.

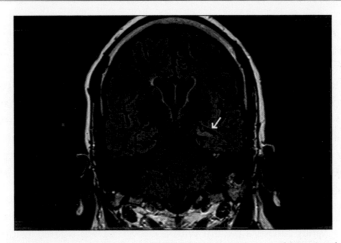

Mesial temporal sclerosis on MRI, characterized by volume loss and increased signal of the hippocampus (*arrow*). It can be bilateral but is often asymmetric. (Reprinted from Yamada T, Meng E. *Practical Guide for Clinical Neurophysiologic Testing.* Wolters Kluwer; 2011.)

Toxic-Metabolic Derangements

This category is a catchall for seizures caused by metabolic and other systemic processes. Common examples include:

- Hypoglycemia
- Hyperglycemia
- Hyponatremia
- Hypocalcemia
- Hypomagnesemia
- Uremia

Seizures due to any of these metabolic derangements would be considered provoked seizures. There are no definitive guidelines regarding the use of antiepileptic medications in these situations. Most often, if the toxic-metabolic derangement is severe, you should start medication and continue it through hospital discharge. If the toxic-metabolic derangement is corrected and the patient remains clinically stable for several weeks, you can consider tapering the medication as an outpatient.

Medications and Other Substances

Many medications and illicit drugs decrease the seizure threshold in patients who are already prone to seize. These agents typically do not in and of themselves cause seizures but in certain situations—in the setting of overdose, for instance, or with severe liver or renal impairment—they can cause seizures in patients who do not have any other reason to seize. Common examples include pain medications (such as tramadol), several antibiotics (the carbapenems, cephalosporins, and fluoroquinolones are highest risk) and psychiatric medications (most often bupropion at high doses). Alcohol and benzodiazepine withdrawal are other common causes of seizures.

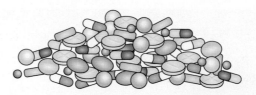

Many medications and other substances can cause seizures.

Box 6.7 Seizure Triggers

In contrast to the above categories, which alone can predispose to seizures, seizure triggers are things that provoke seizures in patients who are already predisposed. In other words, what causes a patient with a known epileptogenic lesion to seize *today*? We often don't know, but there are a host of things we ask about when trying to find an explanation. These most commonly include:

- Infection (systemic or neurologic)
- Severe stress or anxiety
- Lack of sleep
- Missed antiepileptic medications
- Use of seizure-threshold lowering medications
- Menstrual periods (when seizures consistently occur at specific times during the menstrual cycle, it is called *catamenial epilepsy*)

If a patient with a previously well-controlled seizure disorder presents to your office with a breakthrough seizure, it is crucial to ask about each of these items as it will help determine your management. If, for example, your patient had a breakthrough seizure in the setting of pulling an all-nighter while studying for a midterm, you may not need to change that patient's medications; a conversation regarding the importance of consistent sleep might suffice. However, if none of these triggers are present, the patient likely needs medication adjustment.

Epilepsy Syndromes

Epilepsy syndromes are disorders defined by specific features that usually occur conjointly. These features can include particular seizure types and EEG patterns, age at seizure onset, and the characteristic presence or absence of other associated features such as developmental delay and motor regression. There are hundreds of epilepsy syndromes; here are a few you should be familiar with. All but the last have their onset very early in life.

West Syndrome
- Etiology: Approximately 70% of patients have underlying brain lesions (such as lesions associated with tuberous sclerosis or neurofibromatosis; see Chapter 17). Thirty percent are considered cryptogenic (*i.e.*, of uncertain etiology).
- Age at onset: Typically <1 year old.
- Clinical features:

- Infantile spasms (symmetric, brief muscle contractions usually involving the trunk, neck, and/or extremities, followed by several seconds of tonic stiffening; often occur in clusters, often in the morning)

- Arrest of psychomotor development

- EEG:

  - ***Hypsarrhythmia*** (an electrographic pattern characterized by high-voltage, irregular and diffuse slow waves and multifocal spikes seen predominantly interictally, *i.e.*, between seizures; disappears during REM sleep)

- Treatment:

  - Hormonal therapy (corticotropin/ACTH)

  - Vigabatrin (a gamma-aminobutyric acid [GABA] analog that increases GABA activity; can cause peripheral visual field defects and thus requires regular ophthalmologic monitoring)

- Prognosis: Poor, with significantly increased morbidity and mortality; associated with the development of Lennox-Gastaut syndrome (see page 172).

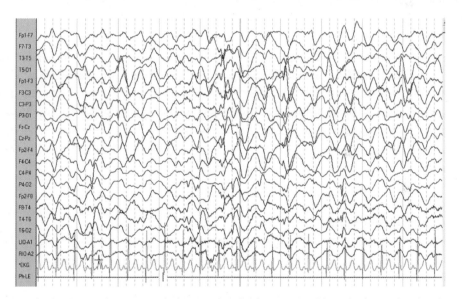

Hypsarrhythmia on electroencephalogram (EEG), characterized by a high-amplitude, chaotic interictal background with multifocal spikes. (Reprinted from Greenfield LJ, Carney PR, Geyer JD. *Reading EEGs: A Practical Approach.* 2nd ed. Wolters Kluwer; 2020.)

Childhood Absence Epilepsy

- Etiology: Presumed to be genetic (but no clear gene defect yet identified)
- Age at onset: Childhood (usually 5 to 10 years old)
- Clinical features:
  - Absence seizures (can be hundreds per day, often provoked by hyperventilation)
  - Generalized tonic-clonic seizures (can occur, but rarely before puberty)

- EEG: 3 Hz spike-and-wave discharges (seen during seizures, with abrupt onset and offset); usually normal between seizures
- Treatment: Ethosuximide (first line in most children), valproate, lamotrigine
- Prognosis: Most children grow out of this. You can usually wean AEDs if the patient is seizure-free for 1 to 2 years.

Dravet Syndrome

- Etiology: Genetic (70% to 80% of cases are due to mutations in the voltage-gated sodium channel known as SCN1A; most mutations are de novo)
- Age at onset: Around 6 months
- Clinical features:
  - Drug-resistant epilepsy with multiple seizure types (often generalized and focal, often provoked by fever and bright lights)
  - Cognitive and motor delay (development is usually normal prior to first seizure)
- EEG: Evolves over time; typically normal up to 1 year of age, with progressive slowing, poor organization, and nonspecific and variable epileptiform abnormalities
- Treatment: First line is typically valproate, often with adjunctive clobazam. Other options include levetiracetam and topiramate. Avoid sodium channel blocking agents (such as lamotrigine). Because seizures are often drug-resistant, ketogenic diet and various epilepsy surgeries should be considered as other therapeutic options.
- Prognosis: Poor, with significantly increased morbidity and mortality. These patients have a high risk of sudden unexpected death in epilepsy (SUDEP; see page 176).

Lennox-Gastaut Syndrome

- Etiology: Approximately 60% have underlying secondary etiologies (including tuberous sclerosis, tumors, cortical malformations, and genetic syndromes). Forty percent of cases are considered cryptogenic.
- Age at onset: Childhood (usually 3 to 5 years old)
- Clinical features:
  - Drug-resistant epilepsy with multiple seizure types (most often tonic and atypical absence, but myoclonic and focal impaired awareness seizures are seen as well)
  - Intellectual disability (development is usually normal prior to first seizure)
- EEG: Slow 1–2 Hz spike-and-wave pattern (interictally)
- Treatment: Broad-spectrum, or generalized, agents (often required in combination; see AED discussion beginning on page 173). Narrow-spectrum agents are often added, given the high prevalence of mixed (generalized and focal) seizure types. As with Dravet Syndrome, nonpharmacologic measures are often indicated as well.
- Prognosis: Poor, with significantly increased morbidity and mortality.

Juvenile Myoclonic Epilepsy

- Etiology: Presumed to be genetic (suspected polygenic or multifactorial mechanisms in most cases)

- Age at onset: Adolescence (usually seen in otherwise healthy teenagers)

- Clinical features:

  - Triad of seizure types (from most to least common: myoclonic, generalized tonic-clonic, and absence). Seizures often occur in the morning, and can be triggered by sleep deprivation and alcohol use.

- EEG: 4–6 Hz polyspike-and-wave pattern (interictally)

- Treatment: valproate is first line (but often avoided in teenage girls given teratogenicity); levetiracetam, lamotrigine, and topiramate are also often used

- Prognosis: Most patients achieve excellent seizure control with a single agent but often require life-long treatment.

Anti-Epileptic Drugs (AEDs)

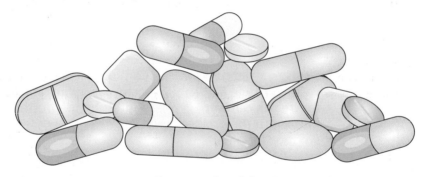

There are a lot of them!

Learning the AEDs can feel a little like wading through alphabet soup. There are, happily for our patients, a lot of them, but their varying mechanisms of action, pharmacologic properties and side effect profiles can be overwhelming to master. But there is no need to despair. There are just four main principles you need to know:

1. Although some AEDs may work better than others for specific seizure types or epilepsy syndromes, there is little evidence to indicate any significant differences in general efficacy among them. Medication decisions are typically made based on age and sex of the patient, side effect profile and relevant drug–drug interactions.

2. All of these medications work by suppressing neuronal activity. They do this by blocking sodium or calcium channels, inhibiting glutamatergic (excitatory) or increasing GABAergic (inhibitory) neurotransmission, or—most often—some combination of the above.

3. We can divide these medications into broad-spectrum agents (those that work for both generalized and focal-onset seizures) and narrow-spectrum, or partial agents (which work for focal-onset seizures only). Because it can be difficult to distinguish between generalized and focal-onset seizures when patients are first diagnosed with epilepsy, we often start with broad-spectrum agents, and afterward (once we have more data, typically in the form of an EEG and MRI) narrow the treatment to partial agents, if indicated.

4. Approximately 50% of patients will achieve complete or near-complete seizure control with a single AED. An additional 15% or so will do so with a second AED. The percent who will significantly improve with a third AED, however, drops to 3%–4%. This is why the definition of drug-resistant epilepsy is failure to respond to two or more AEDs.

Listed below are some of the most commonly used AEDs. These tables are by no means comprehensive but are a concise summary of some of the most important and relevant information for each drug.

BROAD SPECTRUM AGENTS

AED	Mechanism of Action	Adverse Effects
Valproate	• GABA agonist • Sodium and calcium channel antagonist	**Common:** weight gain, tremor, hair loss, gastrointestinal (GI) upset **Rare but serious:** hepatotoxicity (can be fatal in children <2 years old), pancreatitis, thrombocytopenia, hyperammonemia, teratogenic (causes neural tube defects)
Levetiracetam	• Binds to synaptic vesicle protein SV2A (decreases calcium influx into the pre-synaptic terminal)	**Common:** sedation, mood disturbance (irritability, aggression, depression)
Topiramate	• Sodium channel antagonist • Carbonic anhydrase inhibitor	**Common:** paresthesias, weight loss, mental slowing and word-finding difficulty **Rare but serious:** nephrolithiasis, acute glaucoma, metabolic acidosis, hypohidrosis/heat stroke
Zonisamide	• Sodium and calcium channel antagonist • Carbonic anhydrase inhibitor	Similar to topiramate
Lamotrigine	• Sodium channel antagonist • Inhibits glutamate release	**Common:** dizziness, sedation, headache **Rare but serious:** Stevens-Johnson syndrome
Clobazam	• A benzodiazepine: binds postsynaptic receptors on GABAa neurons and increases the frequency of receptor opening	**Common:** sedation, hyposalivation/dry mouth, constipation **Rare but serious:** respiratory depression, Stevens-Johnson syndrome

COMMON NARROW SPECTRUM AGENTS

AED	Mechanism of Action	Adverse Effects
Phenytoin	Sodium channel blocker	**When given IV:** cardiac arrhythmias, hypotension, purple glove syndrome (infusion site phlebitis) **Long-term:** loss of bone density, cerebellar atrophy, gingival hyperplasia, coarse facial features, generalized lymphadenopathy **Acute overdose:** ataxia, diplopia, vertigo
Carbamazepine	Sodium channel blocker	**Common:** dizziness, fatigue, nausea **Rare but serious:** hyponatremia (most often in patients >65 years old), aplastic anemia, agranulocytosis, hepatitis, Stevens-Johnson syndrome
Oxcarbazepine	Sodium channel blocker	Similar to carbamazepine (typically better tolerated, but has a higher risk of hyponatremia)
Eslicarbazepine	Sodium channel blocker	Similar to carbamazepine (but lower risk of hyponatremia)
Lacosamide	Sodium channel blocker	**Common:** dizziness, nausea **Rare but serious:** PR prolongation, bradyarrhythmias, hypotension, syncopal episodes
Gabapentin	Modulates calcium channel activity	**Common:** sedation, dizziness **Less common:** tremor/abnormal movements, peripheral edema, weight gain
Pregabalin	Modulates calcium channel activity	**Common:** sedation, weight gain, peripheral edema **Less common:** tremor/abnormal movements

Box 6.8 Drug-Resistant Epilepsy

Patients are diagnosed with drug-resistant epilepsy if they have failed two or more appropriately chosen antiepileptic medications. Approximately one-third of epilepsy patients are drug-resistant. Although it is often reasonable to continue to try different combinations of AEDs, there are other nonpharmacologic interventions that should be seriously considered as well.

- *Epilepsy surgery.* When feasible, epilepsy surgery can be the patient's best chance at better seizure control and, for some, seizure freedom. There are two options:
  - *Resective surgery.* The idea here is to resect the seizure focus. Candidacy requires an identifiable seizure focus in a nonessential (or so-called "noneloquent") and safely-resectable area of the brain.
  - *Neuromodulation devices.* These include the *responsive neurostimulation device (RNS),* which is implanted in the skull and can respond almost instantaneously to abnormal electrical activity (similar to a heart pacemaker), ideally stopping seizures before they even begin; and the *vagal nerve stimulation device (VNS),* which is implanted underneath the skin in the chest with a wire wound around the vagus nerve. The mechanism of action of the VNS is unknown.
- *Dietary modification.* The classic ketogenic diet is a high-fat, low-carbohydrate (in an approximately 4:1 ratio) diet that can be effective for some patients (for reasons that remain largely unclear) regardless of their age or seizure type. But it can be difficult to adhere to, given the significant side effects associated with such a drastic nutritional change, including GI upset, dyslipidemia, and hypoglycemia. The modified Atkins diet and low–glycemic index treatment are newer and slightly less stringent alternatives.

Box 6.9 Sudden Unexpected Death in Epilepsy (SUDEP)

SUDEP is said to occur when a person with epilepsy dies suddenly without any obvious cause. It can be witnessed or unwitnessed (the majority of cases are unwitnessed), and with or without any evidence of seizure. Seizure-induced respiratory changes and cardiac arrhythmias have been proposed as potential mechanisms, but the etiology remains unknown. The most significant risk factors for SUDEP are the presence and frequency of generalized tonic-clonic seizures, but younger age (SUDEP is most often reported in children and young adults) and specific genetic variants also increase risk. SUDEP is, unfortunately, not uncommon; it is thought to be responsible for approximately 10% to 15% of all deaths in patients with epilepsy. Optimizing antiepileptic treatment as best as possible, instructing patients (or patient's parents, if the patient is an infant) to try to sleep in a prone position, and informing patients and patients' families about this risk, are—for now—the best we can do. Ongoing studies will hopefully continue to shed light onto the mechanisms of SUDEP and lead to better prevention strategies.

Status Epilepticus

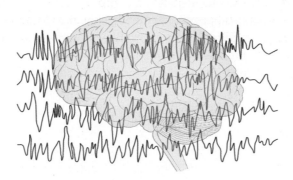

Status epilepticus can be (but is not always) a true neurologic emergency that requires immediate evaluation and management. It can be scary to see but is often easy to diagnose and relatively straightforward to treat. There are two main types of status: convulsive and nonconvulsive.

1. ***Convulsive status epilepticus*** was historically defined as a single, convulsive seizure lasting at least 30 minutes, or a series of convulsive seizures lasting at least a total of 30 minutes without interictal (or "between seizure") return to baseline. However, because of the now-recognized urgency to treat generalized convulsive status, these definitions have been updated and now include:

   a. 5 or more minutes of continuous seizure activity OR

   b. 2 or more back-to-back seizures without return to baseline in between.

   Although it is generally believed that it takes approximately 30 minutes for ongoing generalized convulsive seizure activity to pose significant risk of long-term brain damage, it is highly unlikely that seizure activity will spontaneously cease once it has persisted for 5 minutes, and thus—at the 5-minute mark—it is necessary to diagnose status and treat it.

2. ***Nonconvulsive status epilepticus*** (NCSE). NCSE is just what it sounds like: prolonged seizure activity (in this case, the threshold is at least 10 minutes) *without* prominent (or any) associated motor activity. This is most often seen in critically ill patients—patients with severe sepsis, acute neurologic insults, or patients who are post-cardiac arrest—and should always be considered when these very sick patients are "not waking up" despite adequate medical management. The diagnosis, as you can imagine, relies almost exclusively on EEG, but neither diagnosing nor treating NCSE is straightforward. It is therefore important to know that NCSE exists and to have a low threshold for EEG monitoring when persistently poor or fluctuating mental status is otherwise unexplained.

> ## Box 6.10 Generalized Versus Focal Convulsive Status Epilepticus
>
> When people talk about convulsive status epilepticus, what they typically mean is *generalized* convulsive status epilepticus, that is, shaking of the entire body. But convulsive status can also be focal—for example, prolonged shaking of one arm or one leg. Focal motor status without impaired consciousness (also known as **Epilepsia Partialis Continua**) is nearly always due to an underlying focal brain lesion. It is not an emergency in the same way that generalized convulsive status is: it can, in fact, last for days, months, or even years without any evidence of brain damage. It can also be notoriously difficult to treat, and often requires a balance between symptom management (reducing the shaking to a tolerable level) and medication side effects (primarily avoiding over-sedation caused by too many AEDs).

The treatment algorithm for generalized convulsive status epilepticus is straightforward and effective. Memorize this. It is easy to panic when confronted with a patient in convulsive status, but if you know this algorithm, you won't hesitate before jumping into action.

1. *First line:* Benzodiazepines. Options include IV lorazepam, midazolam, and diazepam. These act rapidly but can cause significant respiratory depression and can therefore only be given up to certain doses in order to avoid intubation.

2. *Second line:* You have several options, all of which are equally efficacious. Decide which way to go based on side effect profile.

    a. IV levetiracetam. The dose has to be adjusted to the patient's renal function, but otherwise, levetiracetam has no significant, immediate adverse effects that you need to worry about.

    b. IV valproate. Avoid in pregnant patients, or in patients with known thrombocytopenia or liver dysfunction.

    c. IV phenytoin. Avoid in patients with known cardiac arrhythmias, or who are currently hemodynamically unstable. If it is available, you should give IV fosphenytoin instead of phenytoin: it is a prodrug of phenytoin and can be infused up to 3x faster with less risk of thrombophlebitis or cardiac arrhythmias.

    d. IV lacosamide. Lacosimide is a newer agent and has less supporting evidence than the medications above. Thus far, however, it seems to be equally as effective and is another second-line option. Avoid this drug in patients with known cardiac arrhythmias.

3. *Third line:* Choose a second option from the above list. If you've given levetiracetam without response, for instance, try valproate.

4. *Fourth line:* Sedate and intubate. At this point, you are essentially attempting to temporarily shut down—and hopefully reset—the brain. Midazolam and propofol drips are the most commonly used therapies. Pentobarbital and ketamine are other options.

Box 6.11

You might wonder why phenytoin—a narrow-spectrum antiepileptic medication—is used to treat generalized status. Just as most first-time unprovoked seizures in adults are focal-onset seizures that have secondarily generalized, most cases of status in adults are also focal-onset seizures with secondary generalization.

Box 6.12 Imaging Changes Associated With Status Epilepticus

Aside from identifying underlying structural lesions, an MRI can reveal abnormalities due to ongoing seizure activity itself. Leptomeningeal enhancement as well as areas of T2 hyperintensity on fluid-attenuated inversion recovery (FLAIR) sequences and diffusion restriction on diffusion-weighted imaging (DWI) sequences are common (most often seen in cortical, thalamic, and deep limbic structures such as the hippocampus) and are believed to be related to seizure-induced cellular edema.

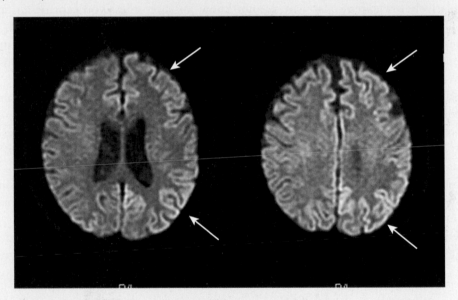

An example of post-status changes on diffusion-weighted MRI, showing predominantly left-sided hyperintensity (arrows) along the cortical rim (referred to colloquially as the cortical ribbon) that comprises the outermost layer of the brain.

Modified from Biller J, Espay A. *Practical Neurology Visual Review*. 2nd ed. Wolters Kluwer; 2013.

Box 6.13 Refractory and Super-Refractory Status Epilepticus

Refractory status epilepticus is defined as ongoing seizure activity despite first-line and second-line treatment. Super-refractory status epilepticus is status epilepticus that has not responded to anesthetic therapy.

Psychogenic Nonepileptic Seizures (PNES)

Previously called pseudoseizures, PNES are paroxysmal events that clinically resemble epileptic seizures but have no EEG correlate; that is to say, if a person experiences a psychogenic seizure while hooked up to an EEG, the EEG will be normal without any epileptiform activity.

Clinically, PNES may sometimes closely resemble true seizure activity (*i.e.*, relatively brief, rhythmic, nonsuppressible stereotyped movements) or sometimes not (lasting much longer—often 15 to 20 minutes—nonrhythmic, nonstereotyped, and suppressible). PNES tend to be characterized by asynchronous, erratic movements that start and stop; associated back arching and crying are common. No matter how many epileptic and nonepileptic seizures you have seen, however, it is important to remain humble. True epileptic seizures originating in the frontal lobe, for instance, can appear "psychogenic" with bizarre bicycling of the legs or other hypermotor behaviors, and can easily be mistaken for psychogenic events. You may suspect nonepileptic seizures, but—with relatively few exceptions—you cannot know for sure unless you capture an episode on EEG.

Patients with PNES often have a relative or close friend with epilepsy. Many patients experience both epileptic and nonepileptic seizures. A history of sexual abuse is common, as are other comorbid psychiatric conditions.

Explaining this diagnosis to the patient can be challenging but is critically important. The longer patients believe they have—and are treated for—true epilepsy, the worse their prognosis for recovery from PNES. Emphasizing the seriousness of this diagnosis is often helpful. Although these events may not be epileptic in nature, they are just as "real" as epileptic seizures, and can have serious and debilitating consequences (*e.g.*, leading to multiple hospital admissions, even unnecessary intubations, as well as causing understandable anxiety and exacerbating other mental health disorders) if not appropriately managed.

Referral to psychotherapy and—if needed—gradually peeling off previously started antiepileptic medications, are the mainstays of treatment. If diagnosed early, the prognosis is good.

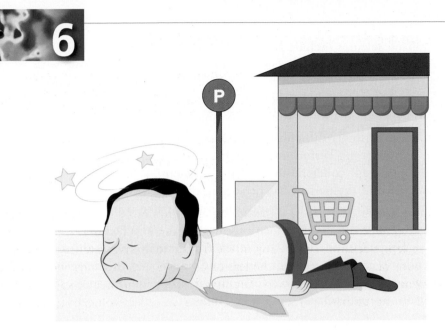

Your Patient's Follow-up: Carlton presented with a left gaze preference and right-sided weakness after being found down on the ground by EMS, with reported full-body shaking prior to EMS arrival. Shortly after his arrival to the ED, you activate a stroke code. CT of the head and CT angiogram are both unremarkable. As you are trying to gather information regarding his history and potential candidacy for thrombolytic therapy with tPA—because you cannot yet rule out a stroke—you are able to reach his wife on the phone, who tells you that he has had seizures since he was a child. She does not know what antiepileptic medication he takes or if he has been taking it but does tell you that he has been sick for the past few days with high fevers and chills. On re-examination, you note that his gaze preference has resolved. He still seems to be slightly weaker on the right than the left, but he is gradually waking up, and after some prompting is able to tell you his name and his birthday.

Although you still cannot know for sure that he has not had an ischemic event, his examination is rapidly improving; besides the subtle weakness of his right arm, his examination is now non-focal and thus you decide, appropriately, to defer tPA. An MRI performed several hours later is normal, without evidence of acute ischemia. The patient, now fully awake, is able to tell you that he normally takes levetiracetam twice a day but missed 2 doses in the last 2 days because he was feeling so ill. You counsel him on the importance of medication adherence, load him with levetiracetam to bump up his level and discharge him home, with strict precautions to return to the hospital if he has another seizure.

You now know:

- | Generalized seizures include generalized tonic-clonic, tonic, clonic, myoclonic, atonic, and absence seizures. Focal seizures are divided into those with impaired awareness and those with retained awareness. Focal seizures with impaired awareness (previously known as complex partial seizures) are the most common type of seizure in adults with epilepsy.

- | It can be surprisingly difficult to distinguish the postictal state from stroke in the acute setting. Performing a careful neurologic examination and quickly obtaining relevant collateral information is essential. Sometimes, if you still are not sure and the patient has persistent and significant neurologic deficits, treating that patient as if he or she is having a stroke is imperative.

- | There are many antiepileptic medications, no one of which has been shown to be significantly superior to any other. Approximately one-third of patients with epilepsy are drug-resistant and should be referred to comprehensive epilepsy centers and considered for nonpharmacologic therapies, such as diet modifications and epilepsy surgery.

- | Not all types of status epilepticus are true emergencies. Generalized convulsive status is an emergency and must be rapidly recognized and treated. Focal convulsive status, also known as Epilepsia Partialis Continua, is not an emergency and can go on for days, months, and even years without significant brain damage.

- | Nonconvulsive status is most frequently seen and diagnosed in critically ill patients with persistently poor or fluctuating mental status. Rapid diagnosis (via EEG) and treatment can often help with patient prognostication.

- | Psychogenic nonepileptic seizures are common, particularly among patients with close friends or family with epilepsy, and those with a history of other comorbid psychiatric conditions or sexual abuse. PNES can be difficult to distinguish from epileptic seizures; diagnosis often requires prolonged monitoring to capture an episode while the patient is hooked up to an EEG. With early diagnosis and appropriate management, the prognosis is good.

7 Neurocognitive Disorders and Dementia

In this chapter, you will learn:

1 | How to distinguish the cognitive changes of normal aging from those of mild cognitive impairment (MCI) and dementia

2 | To distinguish among the most common types of dementia, including Alzheimer disease (AD), vascular dementia, and dementia with Lewy bodies (DLB), among others

3 | How to screen for reversible causes of dementia

4 | What treatments are available to help our patients with dementia

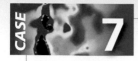

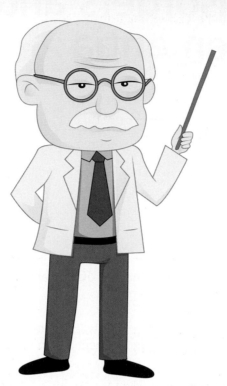

Your Patient: Aaron, a 65-year-old physics professor, comes to see you because of concerns about his memory. Work is going fine, but on a couple of occasions he has forgotten where he parked his car and more than once during a lecture he has forgotten the name of one of his students. One other time he forgot the name of the engineer who was the founder of the science of thermodynamics (Sadi Carnot, for those of you who are interested). He is on no medications and denies that he is depressed. His father was diagnosed with Alzheimer dementia in his seventies, and Aaron is afraid he is showing the first signs of dementia. Should he be evaluated, and if so, how?

 Cognitive Impairment

There is a broad spectrum of cognitive function that we regard as normal. Our abilities in the many different modalities of intelligence vary from person to person, and thank goodness for that; after all, a world of all lawyers or accountants or even healthcare providers would be a very limited and boring place indeed.

There is also a spectrum of normal cognitive decline as we age: memory, executive function, processing speed, and word-finding typically all decline, varying in how much and how fast each modality regresses from individual to individual (the good news: other cognitive functions, such as reading and verbal reasoning, often improve with age). With normal aging, most of these changes are slow and subtle and do not impact our work or social interactions. At the other extreme, there is dementia—*not* a part of normal aging—in which daily activities become significantly impaired. Between normal aging and dementia, there is something called mild cognitive impairment (MCI).

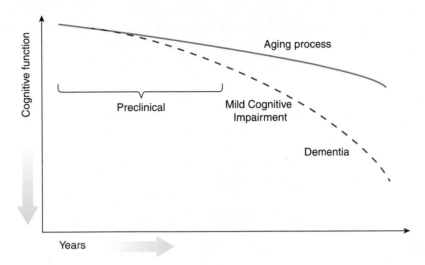

One simplified view of how cognition declines with aging.

Before we dive into the details of the multiple types of dementia, here are some useful definitions to help you keep things straight.

Dementia. So what exactly do we mean when we use the term *dementia*? When cognitive decline impairs a patient's ability to function independently, that patient has crossed over the vague, ill-defined gray line that separates MCI (see the next page) from dementia[1]. It is a line that is crossed too often: about one in seven individuals over the age of 70 carries the diagnosis of dementia, and by age 90 that number is greater than one in three. Dementia is one of the leading causes of death and disability worldwide, and because of our steadily aging population, its prevalence is expected to increase as much as threefold by 2050.

Patients with dementia will show a decline in at least one of the following domains:

- Memory and learning
- Executive functioning (organizational skills such as planning and problem-solving, self-control and moral reasoning)
- Language (word finding, fluency and comprehension)
- Social cognition (socially-appropriate insight and emotions)
- Complex attention (the ability to maintain and manipulate information, and the ability to stay on task despite distraction)
- Perceptual motor function (ability to use one's sensory and motor skills to interact with the environment)

---

[1]The Diagnostic and Statistical Manual of Mental Disorders (DSM) IV and V use the term *major neurocognitive disorder* to refer to what is more colloquially known as dementia.

> ## Box 7.1 Dementia Versus Delirium
>
> Dementia tends to present insidiously and is both progressive and irreversible, whereas delirium presents acutely, with a waxing-and-waning course and often reversible etiology. For a comprehensive discussion of delirium and encephalopathy, see Chapter 15.

Alzheimer dementia (AD), vascular dementia, dementia with Lewy bodies (DLB), frontotemporal dementia (FTD), and prion disease (such as Creutzfeldt-Jakob disease) are all important types of dementia that will be discussed in depth later in this chapter.

Mild Cognitive Impairment (MCI). Estimates vary, but MCI affects as many as one in ten people up to age 69, and nearly two in ten up to age 74. Fifteen percent of patients with MCI over the age of 65 will go on to develop overt dementia within 2 years; this statistic can unnerve even the most stoical among your patients, so remember to emphasize to them that this means that 85% of people with MCI will *not* progress to dementia during that period.

The simplest definition of MCI is *cognitive impairment that does not fully meet the diagnostic criteria for dementia;* in other words, cognitive impairment that does not significantly impair activities of daily living. Everyone's baseline is different, so it is important not to make the diagnosis of MCI unless there is a decline from the patient's own particular baseline.

Distinguishing MCI from the cognitive changes that accompany normal aging is largely based on clinical judgment, relying in no small part on the patient's own (and the patient's family's, friends', and colleagues') assessment. Symptoms that suggest something more than normal aging is going on include:

- Getting lost in familiar places
- Forgetting recent events
- Demonstrating a declining ability to comprehend things that previously were within the patient's grasp
- Exhibiting a decline in executive functions such as planning and organizing
- Experiencing behavioral changes, ranging from apathy to aggression

Should You Screen for Cognitive Impairment?. Routine screening of the older population is not recommended by most (although not all) current guidelines, primarily because there is no evidence that it improves meaningful clinical outcomes. We currently do not have much in the way of evidence-based methods to slow cognitive decline beyond the same lifestyle recommendations—healthy diet, exercise, *etc*—we would make to any patient. The data on physical exercise, however, are starting to get interesting, with preliminary evidence showing that it can delay the progression from MCI to dementia.

How to Assess Cognitive Impairment. Testing is appropriate if and when you suspect your patient may be cognitively impaired, and various tools for cognitive assessment are available. Some, which can be done in your office, are quick and easy, whereas others require referral to a specialty center and are more involved (often requiring a whole day's session of cognitive testing done by a neuropsychologist). The utility of testing lies more in providing "objective" evidence of the diagnosis and the trajectory of the illness to concerned patients and family members than in guiding therapy and improving clinical outcomes. The validated in-office tests each take only a few minutes to perform and include the Mini-Mental State examination, the Mini-Cog, the Montreal Cognitive Assessment, and the 8-Item Ascertain Dementia.

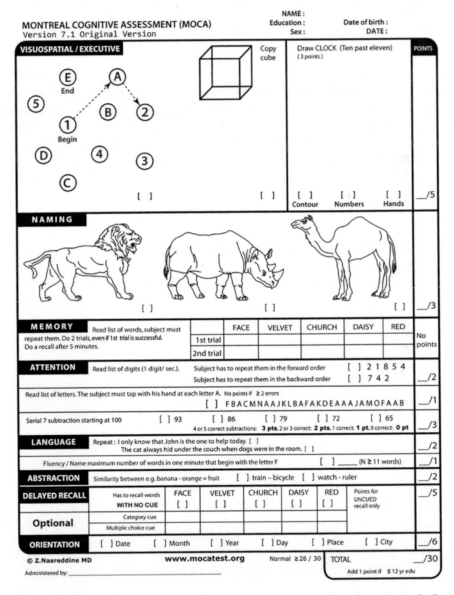

The Montreal Cognitive Assessment (MOCA) tests multiple cognitive domains, including visuospatial function (*i.e.*, the patient must copy the cube), naming (name the animals), and memory (remember a list of 5 words). (Copyright Z. Nasreddine, MD. Reproduced with permission. http://www.mocatest.org)

When Testing Is Abnormal. When your clinical assessment leads you to suspect the diagnosis of MCI or dementia, you need to rule out other confounding disorders as well as any reversible factors that may be contributing to the patient's decline. In particular, you want to consider:

- Depression
- Sleep disorders
- Alcohol and substance abuse
- The contribution of prescription medications
- Reversible disorders, such as vitamin B12 deficiency and hypothyroidism
- Normal pressure hydrocephalus (NPH)

The recommended laboratory tests for a basic dementia work-up include a complete blood count, basic metabolic panel, vitamin B12, and thyroid-stimulating hormone (TSH). A rapid plasma reagin (RPR) and HIV test can also be considered in specific high-risk patient populations. All patients should undergo depression screening. A brain MRI is also often appropriate to rule out any underlying structural pathology and assess the burden of vascular disease. Additional testing such as cerebrospinal fluid (CSF) analysis and positron-emission tomography (PET) scanning maybe valuable depending on the clinical presentation but are not indicated in the routine workup of dementia.

Dementia (aka Major Neurocognitive Disorder)

As previously stated, patients with dementia will show a decline in at least one of the following domains: memory and learning, executive functioning, language, social cognition, complex attention, and perceptual motor function. When this decline impairs the patient's ability to function independently, that patient is diagnosed with dementia.

Important types of dementia include:

- Alzheimer disease
- Vascular dementia
- Dementia with Lewy bodies
- Frontotemporal dementia
- Prion diseases (including Creutzfeldt-Jakob disease)

Alzheimer Disease (AD)

The lifetime prevalence of AD is over 11% among men and over 21% among women. Most of these patients will have *late-onset AD* (65 years of age and older). *Early-onset AD* is far less common. AD is the most common cause of dementia worldwide.

Genetics. Late-onset (*i.e.*, sporadic) AD has been most closely linked genetically to the genes that code for apolipoprotein E, in particular the apolipoprotein E epsilon 4 allele (APOE4), which is present in 14% of the general population. Heterozygotes have a

Box 7.2 Early-Onset Alzheimer Disease

Presenting in patients younger than 65, early-onset AD can occur sporadically, but more often there is an identifiable genetic component with a strong autosomal pattern of inheritance associated with mutations in several genes. Most common is a mutation in presenilin 1 on chromosome 14, a protein that is involved in the conversion of amyloid precursor protein (APP) into beta-amyloid, and less often mutations in presenilin 2 (on chromosome 1) and APP itself (on chromosome 21). Early-onset AD is far less common than late-onset AD. It tends to pursue a more aggressive course, and memory impairment can be overshadowed by other cognitive deficits.

3-fold increased risk of AD, whereas homozygotes have an 8- to 12-fold increased risk. However, 30% to 60% of patients with AD do *not* carry this allele. Using APOE4 as a screening tool is not recommended, both because it is not specific and because there are no preventive or therapeutic interventions that we can offer based on the test results. For patients who want to proceed with testing, referral to a genetic counselor should be considered.

Just as a side note, the impact of the APOE4 allele is not limited to increasing the risk of AD; it also increases the risk of dementia with Lewy bodies. In addition, APOE4 carriers are less able to maintain neuronal health following a stroke or head trauma. Data suggest that APOE2, on the other hand, can be protective against AD, and is associated with increased lifespan in both patients with and without AD.

Risk Factors. Aging, female sex, and the APOE4 allele are well-established non-modifiable risk factors. Potentially preventable or reversible risk factors include:

- The same factors that raise the risk of cardiovascular disease (*e.g.*, hypertension, metabolic syndrome, and hyperglycemia)
- A history of traumatic brain injury
- Sleep disorders
- Some drugs with anticholinergic activity (*e.g.*, antidepressants, antipsychotics, and anti-Parkinson drugs)
- A low level of both physical and cognitive activity throughout one's lifetime

Histology. The pathologic hallmarks of AD are neurofibrillary tangles (composed of *intracellular* flame-shaped aggregates of hyperphosphorylated tau protein, a microtubule-associated protein), and senile neuritic plaques (*extracellular* aggregates of amyloid-beta). Accumulation of these substances in brain tissue is associated with neuronal degeneration, cell death, and cerebral angiopathy. Are tau and amyloid-beta the causes of AD? We still don't know for certain, but the smart money says yes—stay tuned.

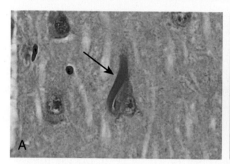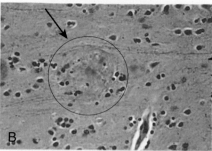

(*A*) Neurofibrillary tangles, and (*B*) neuritic plaques in hematoxylin and eosin (H&E)-stained brain sections. (Modified from Mills SE. *Histology for Pathologists*. 4th ed. Wolters Kluwer; 2012.)

Clinical Presentation and Diagnosis. AD typically presents with the insidious progression of memory deficits. Problems with short-term memory—difficulty recalling recent events as opposed to remote events—are usually the first to appear. Over time other cognitive deficits will appear, often fluctuating from day to day, and may include impaired intellectual, executive and visuospatial functioning along with language deficits and changes in personality and behavior. Patients may exhibit impaired judgment, confusion, disorientation, depression, anxiety, and—ultimately—delusions and hallucinations. Some patients may develop profound apathy, others agitation, and still others alternating periods of one with the other. Except when AD is in its earliest stages—when intellectual function is still to some extent preserved—patients are unaware of what is happening to them. Eventually, patients become bed-bound, unable to walk independently, and develop bladder and bowel incontinence.

With the exception of the mental status examination, neurologic examination is typically normal until the very late stages of the disease. The presence of focal neurologic signs or parkinsonian features should prompt an evaluation for other causes.

The differential diagnosis of AD is broad, and it is important to rule out other causes of dementia, particularly reversible causes (see page 199). Laboratory testing, as outlined above, should be ordered. Detection of tau proteins in the blood is a new test, not yet commercially available, that may eventually offer an expedited means of making the diagnosis of AD.

An MRI is recommended to rule out structural causes of dementia. Classic features that suggest AD on a brain MRI include cortical atrophy with ventricular enlargement along with atrophy of the hippocampus and medial temporal lobes. These changes are not specific to AD but highly suggestive of the diagnosis in the right clinical context. PET scanning, while not routinely done, can demonstrate hypometabolism in the posterior temporoparietal lobes.

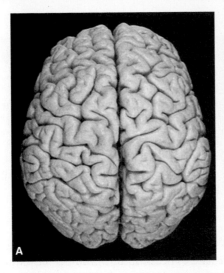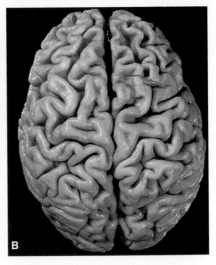

A healthy brain (*A*) compared with the brain of a patient with Alzheimer disease (*B*). Note the significant cortical atrophy, characterized by widened sulci and thinned gyri. (Courtesy of Dr. F. Stephen Vogel, Duke University.)

CSF biomarkers are still mostly used for research protocols, but the finding of elevated tau protein and low levels of amyloid-beta are reasonably sensitive and specific for AD.

Treatment. There is unfortunately no cure for AD. The available medications do not reverse existing symptoms and may at best only slightly slow a patient's decline.

Disease-Directed Therapies. Both cholinergic and glutaminergic pathways appear to be important in cortical function, and these are targeted by current therapies. Acetylcholinesterase inhibitors (*e.g.,* donepezil) may show some modest benefit in slowing disease progression for patients with mild to severe AD, and memantine, an NMDA (*N*-methyl-D-aspartate) receptor antagonist, may benefit some patients with moderate to severe disease. A combination of memantine and an acetylcholinesterase inhibitor may be slightly more efficacious than either alone.

Aducanumab, a recombinant monoclonal antibody, is the first drug that specifically targets the amyloid-beta protein. It has been shown to reduce amyloid accumulation in the brain, but evidence of clinical benefit has been at best very modest. Its approval by the FDA has been controversial, but as of this writing it can be considered for patients with mild memory or cognitive issues.

Supportive Therapies. Social support systems (for both the patient and the patient's caregivers) are paramount. Antipsychotics (often quetiapine) and antidepressants (selective serotonin reuptake inhibitors [SSRIs] and serotonin and norepinephrine reuptake inhibitors [SNRIs]) can be used to help manage behavioral symptoms. No complementary or alternative therapies have been found to offer any significant benefit. In particular, ginkgo biloba, a popular over-the-counter "memory enhancer," has not been found to slow cognitive decline in older adults.

Never forget that the toll AD takes on the patient's caregivers can be overwhelming, and they may benefit from counseling and support.

Table 7.1 Drugs for Alzheimer Disease

Medication	Mechanism of Action	Indications
Memantine	NMDA Receptor Antagonist	For moderate to severe dementia; usually well tolerated although worsening confusion, hallucinations, and dizziness have been reported
Donepezil, Rivastigmine, Galantamine	Acetylcholinesterase Inhibitors	For mild to severe dementia; GI side effects are common (including nausea and diarrhea), especially when starting therapy
Aducanumab	Monoclonal antibody targeting amyloid-beta	For mild dementia; appears to be well tolerated

GI, gastrointestinal; NMDA, *N*-methyl-ᴅ-aspartate.

Prevention. No single intervention appears to make a meaningful difference in reducing the risk of AD, but there is evidence that a multimodal approach can be helpful: blood pressure should be controlled, physical and mental activity encouraged, and a healthy diet (such as the Mediterranean diet) consumed. No supplements or medications have been shown to reduce the risk of developing AD.

Vascular Dementia

This is the other dementia you will see most frequently. Sometimes referred to as "multi-infarct dementia," vascular dementia is responsible for approximately 8% to 15% of cases of cognitive impairment. Many patients have elements of both AD and vascular dementia, hardly surprising because (1) they are both common, and (2) they share many of the same risk factors.

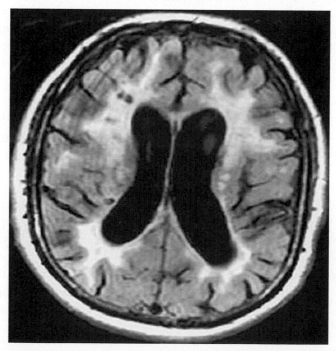

MRI of a patient with vascular dementia. Note the significant burden of microvascular ischemic disease, characterized by extensive white matter and periventricular fluid-attenuated inversion recovery (FLAIR) hyperintense lesions. (Reprinted from Guermazi A, Miaux Y, Rovira-Cañellas A, et al. Neuroradiological findings in vascular dementia. *Neuroradiology*. 2007; 49(1):1-22.)

Vascular dementia is the result of cerebrovascular disease, a result of the cumulative burden of years of uncontrolled hypertension, hyperlipidemia, diabetes, and obesity on the brain. Smoking also significantly increases the risk.

Clinical Features and Diagnosis. Vascular dementia should be suspected in any patient with cognitive dysfunction who also has risk factors for cerebrovascular and cardiovascular disease. Unlike AD, which progresses slowly and steadily, vascular dementia can evolve in a stepwise fashion; new cognitive deficits may appear suddenly, presumably the result of new cerebral infarctions. Compared with AD, the physical examination is more often abnormal, notable for focal deficits resulting from the accumulating stroke burden. MRI will show evidence of microvascular disease (see figure above) and often, more discrete and larger areas of infarction.

Treatment. Cardiovascular risk factors should be controlled. Antihypertensives, cholesterol-lowering agents (usually statins), and medications to ensure tight glycemic control are recommended as indicated to prevent progression—which, taking a step back and remembering the global burden of dementia worldwide—is critical. The cholinesterase inhibitors that are used for AD may be of some small benefit for some of these patients as well.

Box 7.3 The Role of Stroke in Vascular Dementia

Recall that the definition of stroke—*the acute onset of focal neurologic deficits*—is a clinical one. Patients with vascular dementia often have a history of stroke, but it is not necessary for the diagnosis of vascular dementia. Although the MRI will show significant microvascular ischemic disease sufficient to cause progressive cognitive decline, we would not diagnose them as having a history of stroke in the absence of a history of sudden focal neurologic deficits.

Dementia With Lewy Bodies (DLB)

When you see a patient with cognitive impairment and at least one parkinsonian[2] feature, such as bradykinesia (i.e. slowness of movement), rigidity or postural instability, consider the diagnosis of DLB.

What is the difference between this entity and Parkinson disease with overlapping dementia? The distinction is not an easy one to make, and the two disorders may represent two ends of a single spectrum; there is considerable clinical and pathologic overlap between the two. The diagnosis of DLB should only be made if dementia and parkinsonism appear within 1 year of each other. Tremor also tends to be less prominent in DLB.

Lewy bodies, the pathologic hallmark of DLB, are inclusions of alpha-synuclein within neurons and can only be recognized at autopsy.

---

[2]See Chapter 13 for a comprehensive review of Parkinson disease.

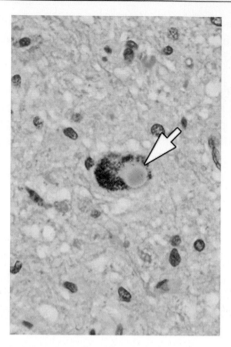

Lewy bodies are concentric intraneuronal hyaline inclusions. (Reprinted from Jankovic J, Tolosa E. *Parkinson's Disease and Movement Disorders*. 6th ed. Wolters Kluwer; 2015.)

There are several hallmark features of DLB that can make it easy to recognize and that distinguish it from other forms of dementia:

- Features of parkinsonism, as just discussed.
- Fluctuating level of cognition. Patients often display varying levels of attention and alertness over the course of the day. But unfortunately, as with the other dementias, the natural history of DLB is ultimately one of relentless progression.
- Early and prominent visual hallucinations. *Lilliputian hallucinations*—in which patients see non-threatening tiny people and animals—are classic for DLB, but more abstract hallucinations can occur as well. Visual hallucinations in AD are rare.

Anxiety is also common, and new onset of anxiety (often fluctuating as well) later in life should prompt consideration of DLB.

Treatment. Treatment is symptomatic; as with the other dementias, no treatment has been shown to modify the course of the disease. Patients with DLB are deficient in both cholinergic and dopaminergic activity. Therefore, anticholinesterase inhibitors are often used with some modest success, and levodopa can be helpful for the parkinsonian features (although it is often less effective than with idiopathic Parkinson disease). Antipsychotic medications can be considered in patients with severe psychosis, but keep in mind that these medications act as dopamine antagonists and can therefore worsen parkinsonian symptoms. Interestingly, levodopa—when titrated carefully—is usually well tolerated and does not seem to significantly exacerbate psychotic features.

Life expectancy is less than half that of patients with AD.

Frontotemporal Dementia (FTD)

This is actually a group of dementias, the most serious and common form being *behavioral variant frontotemporal dementia (bvFTD)*. BvFTD is one of the most common causes of early-onset dementia, with a prevalence similar to that of AD in patients younger than 65. It is most often sporadic, although there are familial forms.

Clinical Presentation. BvFTD affects a younger population than AD, with a mean age of onset in the 50s. Because the clinical picture is dominated by behavioral and personality changes, it can be confused with a primary psychiatric illness. The first signs, such as poor performance at work, marital problems, social disinhibition, apathy, and a lack of empathy, may be dismissed and falsely attributed to the normal stressors of life. Repetitive and compulsive behaviors are common, as are changes in eating behavior (overeating and a strong predilection for sweets are common, but these dietary behaviors hardly distinguish these patients from the general population!). Less common variants of FTD include progressive nonfluent aphasia and progressive fluent aphasia, characterized by prominent word-finding difficulty and impaired language comprehension, respectively. Memory impairment eventually occurs with all variants but is often not the most salient feature.

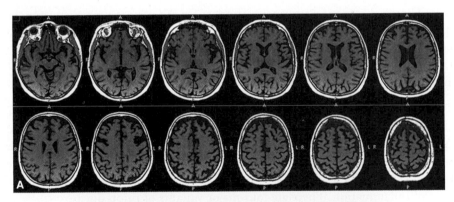

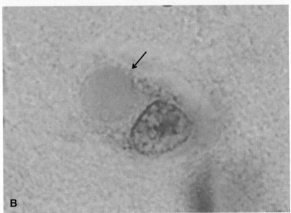

(*A*) An MRI of a patient with frontotemporal dementia (FTD), showing extensive atrophy most pronounced in the frontal cortex. (*B*) A microscopic section of a large Pick body just beside the nucleus. (*A*, reprinted from von Schulthess GK. *Molecular Anatomic Imaging*. 3rd ed. Wolters Kluwer; 2015; and *B*, reprinted from Rubin R, Strayer DS. *Rubin's Pathology*. 5th ed. Wolters Kluwer; 2007.)

> ## Box 7.4 FTD and Amyotrophic Lateral Sclerosis (ALS)
>
> In 2011, a specific gene mutation was identified that could cause both FTD and amyotrophic lateral sclerosis (ALS). Several other mutations that can cause both diseases have since been discovered. Although FTD is thought of as a purely cognitive dementia and ALS as a movement disorder, there actually can be considerable clinical overlap between the two (approximately 50% of patients with ALS, for example, ultimately exhibit some degree of cognitive impairment). The precise genetics and clinical features that characterize the *FTD-ALS spectrum* remain an area of active research. See Chapter 11 for a review of ALS.

Histology. Pick bodies, which are round intracellular aggregates of tau protein, are found in approximately half of all cases of FTD.

Diagnosis. Depending on the specific form of FTD, the diagnosis is primarily a clinical one, which can be supported by neuroimaging (CT or MRI will show frontal and/or temporal atrophy) and histopathological analysis (to provide a definitive diagnosis, although rarely necessary).

Treatment. There is no specific treatment. Support for the patient's caregivers may be the most important intervention, as the behavioral changes can be a source of terrible distress to the patient's family. Genetic counseling should also be offered.

Prion Diseases and Creutzfeldt-Jakob Disease

Prion diseases are neurodegenerative diseases caused by the accumulation in the brain of insoluble and infectious prion protein, a misfolded variant (PrP^{SC}) that replaces the normal prion protein (PrP^c) (see Box 7.5). Histologically, these diseases are characterized by intraneuronal cytoplasmic vacuoles that give the brain tissue a spongiform appearance (*spongiform encephalopathy* is another term for these diseases), along with neuronal loss and the absence of inflammation. There are four major variants of prion disease:

- Creutzfeldt-Jakob Disease (CJD)
- Fatal Familial Insomnia
- Gerstmann-Straussler-Scheinker syndrome
- Kuru

Creutzfeldt-Jakob Disease. We will focus on CJD because—although rare (approximately 1 new case of sporadic CJD occurs per 1,000,000 people per year worldwide)—it is the most common of the prion diseases. CJD is always fatal, with 90% of patients dying within 1 year of diagnosis. The patient's course is dominated by rapid cognitive, motor, and behavioral decline. The rapidity of progression distinguishes CJD from the other dementias we have discussed. Psychiatric symptoms (including anxiety and apathy) and cognitive symptoms (memory loss, aphasia, apraxia) often dominate the clinical picture early in the course, followed by myoclonus (present in ~90% of patients), ataxia, and weakness. Patients eventually lapse into coma, and death most often is the result of a superimposed respiratory infection.

CJD can be inherited as an autosomal dominant trait, but in the majority of cases it arises sporadically. It can also be transmitted and acquired in various other ways—via

Box 7.5 Prions

Prions are protein particles that arise from mutations of the PRNP gene on the short arm of chromosome 20. The precise function of the PRNP gene is not understood; it is expressed throughout the body but predominantly in the brain, suggesting that it probably has some neurologic function. The disease progresses so rapidly because the prions can use normal PrP^C protein as a template to replicate, bypassing the more complex mechanics of replication via cellular DNA.

contaminated neurosurgical instruments and cadaveric material (*e.g.*, corneal transplants, dura mater transplants) and contaminated pituitary derived growth hormone. Rarely, it can be caused by exposure to bovine spongiform encephalopathy (this is referred to as *new variant CJD*, or, colloquially, as Mad Cow Disease).

The diagnosis is usually made by a combination of the clinical picture, MRI findings (see below), EEG abnormalities (showing generalized periodic sharp wave complexes; these are *not* seen in the new variant form), and CSF analysis for the 14-3-3 protein (a neuronal protein present in the CSF indicative of neuronal injury; elevated levels, however, are not specific to CJD). A newer test (known as real-time quaking-induced conversion, or RT-QuIC), which detects misfolded prion proteins within the CSF, looks promising. However, at present definitive diagnosis can be made only by means of neuropathologic analysis performed at autopsy. Treatment is purely supportive.

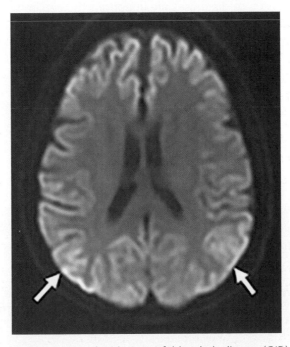

MRI findings that can be associated with Creutzfeldt-Jakob disease (CJD) include diffuse cortical gyral hyperintensities (*arrows*; this is referred to as "cortical ribboning" and can also be seen in the context of status epilepticus) as well as signal hyperintensities in the bilateral basal ganglia and thalami (not pictured). (Reprinted from Louis ED, Mayer SA, Noble JM. *Merritt's Neurology*. 14th ed. Wolters Kluwer; 2021.)

Fatal Familial Insomnia is inherited as an autosomal dominant disease (sporadic cases have been reported, but these are rare) and is characterized by severe insomnia associated with an exaggerated startle response and sympathetic hyperactivity. Like CJD, progression is rapid, and death usually occurs within 1 year of diagnosis.

Gerstman-Straussler-Scheinker Syndrome is also inherited in an autosomal dominant fashion. Cerebellar symptoms such as ataxia and gait incoordination dominate the clinical picture, followed by weakness and varying degrees of memory loss. The course is a bit more gradual, with most patients surviving for 4 to 5 years after diagnosis.

Kuru was the first prion disease to be identified and was endemic among the Fore tribes in Papua New Guinea in the early-to-mid 1900s. Kuru is acquired via cannibalism (*i.e.*, eating brain tissue of an infected human; deceased family members were traditionally eaten in order to help free their spirits). It was thought that it had been eradicated decades ago with the cessation of cannibalism, but a handful of cases have since been reported. Symptoms include early and prominent tremors (the word kuru derives from a Fore word meaning "to shake"), ataxia, and myoclonus, followed by dementia and death usually within 1 to 2 years of diagnosis.

Box 7.6 Differential Diagnosis of Rapidly Progressive Dementias

There is a long list of diseases and substances that can cause rapidly progressive dementia, but all of these, like CJD, only rarely present as rapidly advancing dementia in this way. These diagnoses are important to keep in mind, however, because unlike CJD, most are potentially reversible:

- Infections (HIV, Lyme disease, herpes simplex virus, neurosyphilis)
- Toxins (alcohol, drugs, heavy metals)
- Paraneoplastic syndromes
- Autoimmune diseases (systemic lupus erythematosus [SLE], Sjogrens, Hashimotos)
- Granulomatous diseases (Behcets, sarcoidosis)
- Vasculitis

Table 7.2 What You've Learned so Far, Pared Down to the Basics

Type of Dementia	Most Characteristic Features
Alzheimer dementia	Memory deficit is predominant
Vascular dementia	Progresses stepwise
Dementia with Lewy Bodies	Parkinsonian features, visual hallucinations, fluctuating cognitive function
Frontotemporal dementia	Behavior changes
Creutzfeldt-Jakob disease	Very rapid progression, myoclonus

Reversible Dementias

There are several reversible dementias that, because they can be treated, are important diagnoses not to miss.

Psychiatric disorders. Various psychiatric disorders, such as *major depression*, can masquerade as dementia. When dementia occurs as a consequence of mental illness, it is referred to as dementia syndrome of depression, previously pseudodementia. Treatment with antidepressants will usually resolve the cognitive symptoms.

Metabolic Disorders. Cognitive impairment associated with *Hashimoto thyroiditis* can evolve acutely or subacutely. Vitamin B12 deficiency (which can be a cause of peripheral neuropathy [page 281] or subacute combined degeneration of the spinal cord [page 269]) can also cause reversible mild cognitive impairment and dementia. Long-standing alcohol abuse resulting in *Wernicke-Korsakoff syndrome* (page 380) is another example.

Normal Pressure Hydrocephalus (NPH). This disorder is discussed far more often than it is seen; NPH is rare. It classically presents with the triad of cognitive decline, gait disturbance, and urinary incontinence ('wet, wobbly and wacky' is a common way to remember this). You can understand, therefore, why it comes up so often in discussion, since all three of these features are common in the elderly.

Most cases of NPH are idiopathic, the result of an imbalance between the production and absorption of CSF. The CSF pressure is normal or only slightly elevated. Secondary causes include infections, inflammatory conditions, and hemorrhagic strokes that impair CSF absorption. The increased CSF volume in both idiopathic and secondary NPH leads to ventricular enlargement and compression of adjacent brain tissue.

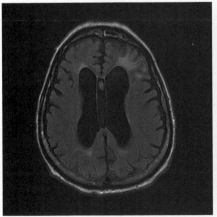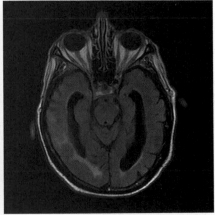

An MRI of a patient affected by normal pressure hydrocephalus (NPH), with ventriculomegaly out of proportion to the degree of generalized brain atrophy. However, keep in mind that NPH is first and foremost a clinical diagnosis. You will often see radiology reports that comment on ventriculomegaly (often followed by *"may be consistent with NPH"*) but you need to *"correlate clinically;"* if the patient does not present with features consistent with NPH, the diagnosis is not NPH, regardless of the imaging findings. (Reprinted from Louis ED, Mayer SA, Noble JM. *Merritt's Neurology.* 14th ed. Wolters Kluwer; 2021.)

NPH progresses slowly. The patient's cognitive impairment can take almost any form and can mimic Alzheimer Disease. Urinary incontinence is the least common of the three classic features (about 50% of patients). The typical gait disturbance is often described as shuffling, and can closely mimic the shuffling gait associated with Parkinson disease.

Suspect NPH in any patient with dementia and a gait disturbance with or without urinary incontinence. The first diagnostic test is an MRI or CT scan, and if this shows enlarged ventricles *out of proportion to the degree of generalized brain atrophy*, proceed with a lumbar puncture, which has both diagnostic and therapeutic implications. If removal of a small amount of CSF leads to an improvement in the patient's symptoms, then the patient may be a candidate for a shunt. Gait should improve quickly, within minutes of CSF removal, but some patients may improve as long as 24 hours later. CSF drainage is not a perfect test; it has a relatively low sensitivity for predicting who will benefit from a shunt, so some patients who might benefit will be missed.

The most common shunt used today is a ventriculoperitoneal shunt, and an adjustable valve allows for careful titration of the CSF pressure. Complications from shunt placement requiring neurosurgical intervention occur in approximately 25% of patients and include subdural hematomas and the need for shunt revision. Most patients with the classic presentation of NPH who show improvement with CSF removal will improve with shunting; gait shows the most improvement; cognitive function is less likely to improve.

Transient Global Amnesia (TGA). A favorite of books, television and movies, amnesia may be a great plot device but can be a terrifying reality. Transient global amnesia (TGA) is not a dementia at all—neither is it a neurodegenerative disorder—but we want to discuss it here because of its sudden, dramatic memory deficit.

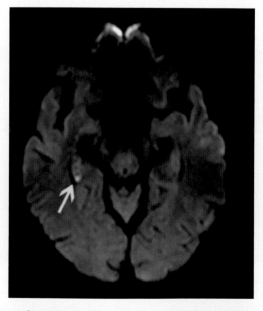

MRI with a small focus of restricted diffusion in the right hippocampus in a patient with transient global amnesia. (Reprinted from Cuello Oderiz C, Miñarro D, Dardik D, et al. Teaching NeuroImages: hippocampal foci of restricted diffusion in transient global amnesia. *Neurology.* 2015; 85(20):e145.)

TGA is a reversible amnesia. The neurologic examination is normal except for the sudden development of the inability to create new memories. Patients will keep asking the same questions over and over again: Where am I? Who are you? and so on. They will, however, remain oriented to self and be fully capable of carrying out complex cognitive tasks. The degree of retrograde amnesia—the inability to remember things prior to the event—is variable.

Symptoms typically last 1 to 24 hours, although some patients may experience very mild residual memory impairment that persists for weeks.

TGA occurs most often in patients 50 to 70 years of age and can affect both men and women. The cause is not known. Patients with TGA do not appear to have an increased risk of stroke or seizure, or of developing dementia later in life.

Patients with TGA should be observed until they return to baseline mental status. An MRI is often obtained to rule out stroke or an underlying seizure focus and can show incidental small diffusion-restricting lesions in the hippocampi (see image on page 200). If any neurologic abnormalities are present, or if the memory deficit persists beyond 24 hours, then imaging as well as an EEG are definitely indicated.

No treatment is required beyond reassurance. Recurrence is rare but can occur, and for unclear reasons is more common in patients with a personal or family history of migraine.

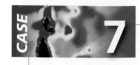

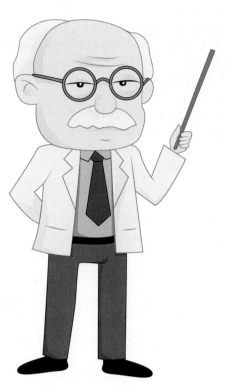

Follow-up on Your Patient: Although Aaron's presentation did not ring any immediate alarm bells, you use one of the quick in-office mental status evaluations and discover he appears to have mild cognitive impairment. You assure him he does not have dementia. You let him know that there is no medication currently available to reduce his risk of progression, but he readily agrees to your recommendations for a healthy lifestyle—daily exercise in particular. He will come back to see you regularly to monitor his cognitive status.

You now know:

- | There is a fine line that separates the cognitive changes of normal aging with those of mild cognitive impairment; mental status testing can be helpful to distinguish between the two.

- | Important types of dementia include Alzheimer disease (profound memory loss), vascular dementia (progresses in stepwise fashion), dementia with Lewy bodies (parkinsonism and often visual hallucinations), frontotemporal dementia (behavioral and personality changes) and Creutzfeldt-Jakob disease (rapid progression).

- | Always rule out reversible causes of dementia, such as depression, alcoholism, Hashimoto thyroiditis, vitamin B12 deficiency, and normal pressure hydrocephalus.

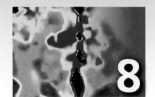

8 Meningitis, Encephalitis, and Other Infectious Diseases of the Nervous System

In this chapter, you will learn:

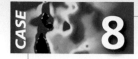

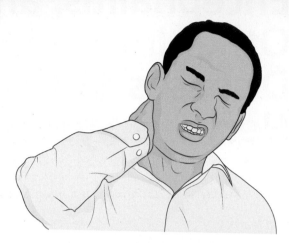

Your Patient: Amir, a 33-year-old management consultant, comes to see you with a severe headache that began just a few hours ago, associated with photophobia and chills. He has a history of migraine headaches, but this headache is far more severe than his usual migraines. You measure a temperature of 103.2 °F and demonstrate marked nuchal rigidity (a stiff neck) on his examination. There is no obvious rash. There are no focal neurologic abnormalities. He is lethargic but not disoriented. What is your immediate next step in his management: do you order a CT or MRI, perform a lumbar puncture for CSF analysis, or start him on empiric antimicrobial therapy right away?

Encephalitis refers to inflammation of the brain parenchyma. *Meningitis* refers to inflammation of the meninges. They are traditionally distinguished from each other by the presence of neurologic impairment (encephalitis) or the preservation of normal neurologic function (meningitis).

Because encephalitis, unlike meningitis, affects the brain parenchyma, it can cause focal neurologic deficits, including altered mental status (most commonly), hemiparesis, hemisensory loss, and language impairment.

On the other hand, although meningitis can cause altered mental status, most often this is a secondary phenomenon that can be attributed to a combination of lethargy and pain (remember that, unlike the brain parenchyma, the meninges are pain sensitive). Cerebral function is otherwise normal. The classic syndrome associated with meningitis is the result of meningeal irritation and is termed, aptly enough, *meningismus*: a combination of stiff neck, headache, and photophobia.

It is not uncommon for meningitis and encephalitis to coexist to some degree (meningoencephalitis). Meningitis, for instance, can present with focal neurologic deficits as a result of involvement of the nearby brain cortex and spinal cord. However, for purposes of clarity in sorting out the differential diagnoses, it is a good idea to maintain the following distinction:

- Fever + focal neurologic deficits = encephalitis
- Fever + meningismus + no focal neurologic deficits = meningitis

Warning: we are going to poke several holes in this categorization as we make our way through this chapter. But thinking about meningitis and encephalitis in this way provides a solid framework for understanding infectious diseases of the central nervous system.

 ## *Meningitis*

In the United States, the majority of adult cases of meningitis (and encephalitis, too) are caused by viruses. Viral meningitis is relatively benign. Although these viral infections are often very unpleasant and can be debilitating, the vast majority of patients make a complete recovery. Fewer than 1 in 5 cases of meningitis are caused by bacteria, but these can be so deadly so quickly that it is appropriate that we first turn our attention to them.

Bacterial Meningitis

Bacterial meningitis is a medical emergency. Although there are other causes of meningitis besides bacterial infection (we've just mentioned that viral meningitis is more common, and, as you will shortly see, there are numerous other infectious and noninfectious etiologies), patients who present like Amir with fever, headache, nuchal rigidity, photophobia, and/or confusion have bacterial meningitis until proven otherwise. Your first step is to start treatment immediately, before you proceed with any further evaluation.

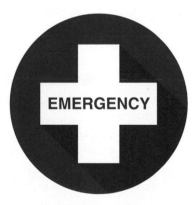

Suspected bacterial meningitis should be treated as a medical emergency.

Clinical Presentation. Most patients with bacterial meningitis look very sick. The classic presentation consists of fever, nuchal rigidity, photophobia, and altered mental status. Patients who do not have at least one of these classic symptoms almost certainly do *not* have bacterial meningitis. On the other hand, fewer than half of patients with bacterial meningitis present with the full symptom complex. Especially in infants,[1] the elderly and immunosuppressed patients, one or more of these symptoms is often muted or absent altogether. Headache is actually the most common presenting symptom of bacterial meningitis (reported by approximately 80% of patients), followed by fever and nuchal rigidity. The quality and location of the headache pain are variable and cannot be used to help guide diagnosis.

Box 8.1 Brudzinski and Kernig Signs

Nuchal rigidity reflects underlying inflammation of the pain-sensitive pia and arachnoid meninges around the spinal roots and nerves. Movement of the neck is very painful, so patients attempt to hold their neck as still as possible. If during your examination you try to force neck flexion, patients will flex their knees and hips; this is called the *Brudzinski sign*. Forcing patients to extend one knee with the thigh at a right angle to the trunk will cause pain in the back and hamstrings, a finding termed the *Kernig sign*. When positive in the right clinical setting, these tests are highly specific for meningitis. However, they are not sensitive, that is, their absence cannot be used to rule out the diagnosis.

A Brudzinski sign

Elicits hip and knee flexion

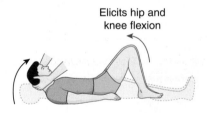

1. Passive flexion of neck

B Kernig sign

Elicits pain or limited extension

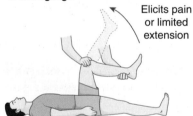

1. Knee is flexed to 90 degrees
2. Hip is flexed to 90 degrees
3. Extension of the knee is painful or limited in extension

Eliciting the Brudzinski and Kernig signs.

Other features of bacterial meningitis can include:

- Nausea and vomiting
- Seizures
- Coma

---

[1]Manifestations of bacterial meningitis in infants can be particularly nonspecific and can include both hyper- and hypothermia, poor feeding, seizures, and a bulging fontanelle; neck stiffness is uncommon.

- Focal neurologic signs (we're poking holes in the standard definition already)—most commonly these are cranial nerve abnormalities due to inflammatory exudate that crosses the pial barrier and compresses the nerves

- Rash—meningococcal meningitis, which carries a particularly poor prognosis, is often accompanied by a transient and rapidly progressive maculopapular rash

Causes of Bacterial Meningitis. Bacteria can find their way into the subarachnoid space either by hematogenous spread (bacteremia) or by direct extension from a local site of infection, such as acute sinusitis or otitis media. Different age groups are affected by different organisms (see table), but in adults the most common causes of bacterial meningitis are:

1. *Streptococcus pneumoniae* (aka pneumococcus)

2. *Neisseria meningitidis* (aka meningococcus)

The Most Common Pathogens and Their Treatment, by Age Group

Age	Most Common Pathogens	Empiric Treatment
<1 month	*Group B Streptococcus (GBS), E. coli (+ other enteric gram-negative rods), listeria*	Ampicillin + cefotaxime
1–23 months	*GBS, E. coli, S. pneumoniae, N. meningitidis, H. flu*	Vancomycin + ceftriaxone
2–50 years	*S. pneumoniae, N. meningitidis*	Vancomycin + ceftriaxone
>50 years	*S. pneumoniae, N. meningitidis, listeria, aerobic gram-negative rods (pseudomonas)*	Vancomycin + ceftriaxone + ampicillin

GBS, group B streptococcus.

Box 8.2 Meningococcal and Pneumococcal Vaccines

Routine vaccination against the A and C meningococcal serogroups has led to a marked decline in meningococcal infection, and vaccination against the B serogroup is now available as well. Pneumococcal vaccination is now recommended routinely for adults 65 years and older as well as for those at risk of invasive disease, that is, those with a cochlear implant, CSF leak, or a prior history of invasive pneumococcal disease, and has decreased the incidence of invasive pneumococcal infection.

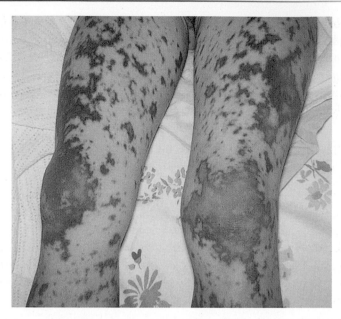

Fulminant rash in a patient with meningococcemia. (Reprinted from Scheld MW, Whitley RJ, Marra CM. *Infections of the Central Nervous System*. 4th ed. Lippincott Williams & Wilkens; 2004.)

S. pneumoniae, a gram-positive diplococcus, is the most common cause of bacterial meningitis in adults. This bacterial infection more commonly causes pneumonia (hence its name), and many patients with meningitis also have evidence of pneumonia. Of importance, however, the absence of pneumonia does not preclude the diagnosis of *S. pneumoniae* meningitis.

N. meningitidis, a gram-negative diplococcus, is the second most common cause. Meningitis caused by *N. meningitidis* is unique in that it often presents with devastating suddenness, progressing rapidly over just a few hours. It should be suspected immediately in a patient who presents with the classic nonblanching maculopapular rash (see above), which can be seen in about 50% of patients at the time of presentation. Complications can include shock, which can cause adrenal infarction and adrenal insufficiency (known as Waterhouse-Friderichsen syndrome); disseminated intravascular coagulation; heart failure; and purpura fulminans (diffuse cutaneous bleeding and necrosis).

The incidence of meningitis caused by ***Haemophilus influenzae,*** a gram-negative rod, has declined dramatically in the United States and other developed nations since the early 1990s because of widespread childhood vaccination against *H. flu* type b (known as Hib, the most virulent strain and, of the typeable strains, the most likely to cause invasive disease). Worldwide, however, *H. flu* remains one of the most common causes of meningitis. Children less than 5 years of age are most likely to be affected.

Listeria monocytogenes, a gram-positive rod, causes about 5% to 8% of cases of bacterial meningitis and occurs mostly in neonates, pregnant women, adults over 50 years and immunocompromised patients. It is primarily a foodborne illness (most often acquired from contaminated and unpasteurized milk or cheese). Meningoencephalitis is actually more common than meningitis alone, and the course can range from mild (fever with subtle mental status changes) to fulminant, resulting in coma or death.

Less common bacterial causes include *streptococci* (group A streptococcal infection can be seen following basilar skull fracture; group B streptococcal infection predominantly affects neonates and infants), as well as *staphylococci* and *aerobic gram-negative bacteria* (*S. aureus* and *pseudomonas* can be associated with penetrating skull trauma or neurosurgery; immunocompromised patients are at increased risk of *pseudomonas* meningitis). *Escherichia coli* most often affects neonates as a result of exposure during vaginal delivery.

Diagnosis. Patients with suspected bacterial meningitis should have a complete blood count and blood cultures drawn immediately. If possible, blood cultures should be obtained before initiating antibiotic therapy; they are positive in a majority of cases of bacterial meningitis. However, the key to diagnosis is a lumbar puncture for cerebrospinal fluid (CSF) analysis. If the lumbar puncture is, for whatever reason, contraindicated or delayed, antibiotic therapy should not be delayed, because any delay in treatment can be fatal.

CSF analysis allows you to (1) quickly distinguish bacterial from viral and other causes of meningitis, (2) immediately identify the organism if the Gram stain is positive,[2] and (3) send off definitive tests to pin down the precise etiology and antibiotic susceptibility of the causative organism.

CSF Findings Associated With Meningitis

	Opening Pressure	Predominant Cell Type	Protein	Glucose
Bacterial	↑	Polymorphonuclear leukocytes	↑	↓
Fungal	↑	Lymphocytes	↑	↓
Viral	↑ or normal	Lymphocytes	↑ or normal	normal

The essential CSF tests to order include:

- a cell count and differential
- glucose and protein levels
- a Gram stain
- cultures (bacterial, viral and, if the patient is immunocompromised or has other risk factors, fungal) and polymerase chain reaction (PCR) testing (both viral and bacterial)

A CT of the head is indicated before performing a lumbar puncture only if there is concern for increased intracranial pressure, which could lead to herniation when CSF is withdrawn during the lumbar puncture. Suspect increased intracranial pressure if:

1. there are any neurologic abnormalities on examination (papilledema specifically is indicative of elevated intracranial pressure, but any focality on examination is potentially concerning for a concomitant or alternative diagnosis, including intracranial abscess or other mass lesion);

2. the patient experienced a seizure; or

3. the patient is immunocompromised.

---

[2]Negative Gram stains are common in patients with bacterial meningitis who have already been on antibiotic therapy and in those with listeriosis or gram-negative bacterial infection.

Treatment. One more time: *if you suspect bacterial meningitis, do not delay treatment to pursue your diagnostic evaluation.* Empiric antibiotic therapy in adults usually consists of a third-generation cephalosporin (ceftriaxone) combined with vancomycin (see Table on page 207). Ampicillin should be added in older or immunocompromised patients to provide coverage for listeria. Therapy can be adjusted once the actual pathogen has been identified and antibiotic resistance patterns have been assessed.

Intravenous (IV) dexamethasone should also be given for suspected or proven pneumococcal meningitis (no benefit has been found for other causes of bacterial meningitis) and continued only if gram-positive diplococci (*i.e.*, pneumococci) are confirmed on Gram stain. Although it is unclear if corticosteroids decrease mortality in patients with pneumococcal meningitis, they do appear to improve neurologic outcomes and reduce the risk of hearing loss. IV hydration may also reduce neurologic sequelae.

IV acyclovir is also often added empirically because of the overlap in the clinical presentation of herpes simplex virus (HSV) meningitis/encephalitis (see below, and page 216) and bacterial meningitis. Once HSV infection is ruled out, acyclovir can be stopped.

Prognosis. Despite modern techniques of diagnosis and today's powerful antibiotics, about 25% of patients hospitalized with bacterial meningitis still die, and many who survive have residual hearing loss, seizures, cognitive impairment, or other focal neurologic deficits. One important risk factor for mortality that we should be able to keep improving is delay in initiating antibiotic therapy.

Other Causes of Meningitis

We can group the many other causes of meningitis into those that are infectious and those that are not. In either case, routine bacterial cultures in CSF will be negative. The resulting CSF profile is often termed *aseptic meningitis* (*i.e.*, culture-negative meningitis).

Infectious (Viral) Causes. Viral meningitis is the leading cause of aseptic meningitis. Symptoms tend to be far less severe than those seen with bacterial meningitis. The most common viral causes include:

- *Enteroviruses* (including echovirus, coxsackie virus, and other nonpolio enteroviruses). In the United States, these infections usually occur in the summer months. Patients almost always recover completely, although symptoms such as headache and fatigue can persist for months.

- *Herpesviruses.* Unlike herpes encephalitis (see page 216), which is almost always caused by HSV-1, meningitis is most often caused by HSV-2. Genital lesions are often present. Patients are treated with IV acyclovir, although the benefit remains unclear. HSV-1, varicella-zoster virus (VZV) and cytomegalovirus can also cause meningitis, usually in immunocompromised patients.

- *HIV.* HIV meningitis tends to present at the time of initial seroconversion and typically resolves without treatment.

- *Mosquito-borne infections.* In recent years a number of mosquito-borne infections have surfaced in the United States. Chief among them is West Nile virus. This particular virus can also cause encephalitis or acute flaccid paralysis (see page 217).

- *Mumps.* Before the MMR vaccine was introduced, mumps was one of the most common causes of aseptic meningitis. Today, because of the increasing numbers of children who are not being vaccinated, the incidence is again rising. Meningitis remains the most frequent extrasalivary, extratesticular complication of mumps.

Infectious (Non-viral) Causes. Other infectious causes of aseptic meningitis include spirochetal infections, fungal infections, tuberculosis (TB), and parasitic infections. Note that, although spirochetes and tuberculosis are bacteria, routine bacterial cultures will be negative and thus these infections are, in this setting, considered *aseptic*.

- Spirochetal infections include Lyme disease, syphilis, and leptospirosis.

  - *Borrelia burgdorferi*, which causes Lyme disease, produces a lymphocytic meningitis that is typically seen several weeks after the appearance of the initial rash of erythema migrans (see page 223 for more information about the neurologic manifestations of Lyme disease).

  - Syphilitic meningitis, caused by *Treponema pallidum*, tends to occur in the setting of secondary syphilis and is often associated with a disseminated rash (see page 220 for more information about syphilis).

  - Leptospirosis, caused by *Leptospira* spirochetes that prefer warm climates, is acquired through exposure to contaminated water or soil. It tends to present with the abrupt onset of fever, myalgias, and headache; meningitis is observed in over 50% of those infected.

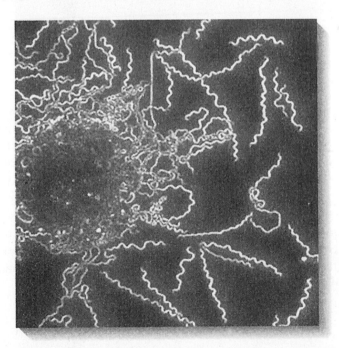

The corkscrew-appearing *Borrelia burgdorferi*, as seen by darkfield microscopy. (Reprinted from Strohl WA, Rouse H, Fisher BD. *Lippincott's Illustrated Reviews: Microbiology.* Lippincott Williams & Wilkins; 2001.)

- Among the fungi, the major culprits are cryptococcus and coccidioides.

  - *Cryptococcus*, an encapsulated budding yeast, is a leading cause of meningitis among patients with HIV and those who are for any reason severely immunocompromised. Infection presents indolently, evolving over a period of several weeks, often with signs and symptoms of elevated intracranial pressure (the fungal capsules can clog up the ventricular system, preventing normal CSF outflow). CSF analysis is notable for an elevated opening pressure and a positive cryptococcal antigen. A mild lymphocytosis and elevated protein are common but not always present; the basic CSF profile can be normal. Initial treatment is with amphotericin and flucytosine. Repeated lumbar punctures may be necessary to remove excess CSF and thereby prevent elevated intracranial pressure. Fluconazole is usually used for long-term maintenance.

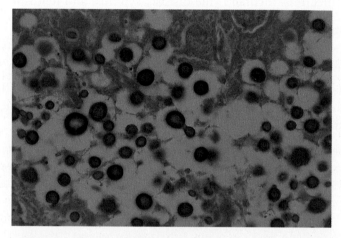

Cryptococcus appear as budding yeast surrounded by mucoid capsules. (Reprinted from McClatchey KD. *Clinical Laboratory Medicine*. 2nd ed. Lippincott Williams & Wilkins; 2002.)

  - *Coccidioides* is endemic in the southwestern United States as well as in Central and South America (although with climate change, cases are being seen farther north as well). Most patients who have been exposed either remain asymptomatic or have only mild flu-like symptoms. Severe disease, when it occurs, most often manifests as pneumonia, but the organism can disseminate and cause osteomyelitis, septic arthritis, and meningitis. Unlike cryptococcus, coccidioides can affect both immunocompetent and immunosuppressed patients. Patients at risk for severe disease include pregnant women, diabetic patients, cigarette smokers, and the elderly, as well as patients who are immunosuppressed. Lifelong antifungal treatment (typically with fluconazole) is necessary; if left untreated, coccidioides meningitis is universally fatal.

Box 8.3 Other Fungi That Can Attack the Central Nervous System

Certain fungi that can attack the central nervous system do so without actually causing meningitis. However, it's worth taking a brief look at them here within the context of CNS fungal disease.

Aspergillus can cause both parenchymal disease (including abscesses and granulomas) and disease due to vascular invasion (multifocal ischemic and/or hemorrhagic infarcts). Immunosuppressed patients are at greatest risk, particularly those that are neutropenic or on chronic glucocorticoid therapy. A combination of positive blood cultures, serum biomarkers (galactomannan and beta-D-glucan assays), bronchoalveolar lavage, and neuroimaging is often necessary for diagnosis. Voriconazole, often in combination with caspofungin, is first-line treatment.

Mucormycosis is a mold that most often affects patients with diabetes (particularly those in diabetic ketoacidosis), hematologic malignancies, or other immunocompromised states (post transplant, HIV/AIDS). It is inhaled and attacks the paranasal sinuses and vasculature. The infection typically presents as an acute sinusitis, with fever, purulent nasal discharge, headache, and sinus pain. But this is not your everyday sinus infection. It can spread with devastating speed to cause pulmonary disease, orbital complications (resulting in proptosis and eventual blindness), and cerebral manifestations (often due to spread from the sphenoid sinus into the cavernous sinus, causing multiple cranial neuropathies). Suspect mucormycosis in a patient, particularly one at risk, who presents with fever, acute sinusitis, and associated neurologic symptoms. A black eschar, the result of tissue necrosis, may be visible within the nasal passages or elsewhere in the oropharynx or around the orbits. Diagnosis is difficult and usually requires both nasal endoscopy and neuroimaging. Treatment includes surgical debridement and antifungal therapy with amphotericin B. Despite aggressive therapy, mortality is high, ranging in some studies above 60%.

- *Tuberculosis* causes a subacute basilar meningitis (meaning it affects the base of the brain). The onset is usually gradual with headache, vomiting, and lethargy. Cranial nerve deficits result from inflammation that is concentrated in and around the brainstem. Diagnosis can be difficult, because the CSF acid-fast bacilli smear is often negative and the culture can take weeks to grow. CSF adenosine deaminase can be a useful adjunctive test, but a positive result is not specific to TB and can be seen with other bacterial infections. In most cases, multiple lumbar punctures with repeated CSF samples are needed to conclusively make the diagnosis. Additional testing—positive findings on skin testing (purified protein derivative [PPD]) or an interferon-gamma release assay along with a chest x-ray consistent with tuberculosis—strongly support the diagnosis. Treatment should be started empirically on the basis of clinical suspicion and not be delayed for diagnostic confirmation. Initial four-drug therapy (typically with rifampin, isoniazid, pyrazinamide, and ethambutol) is given for 2 months; rifampin and isoniazid are then continued for an additional 7 to 10 months.

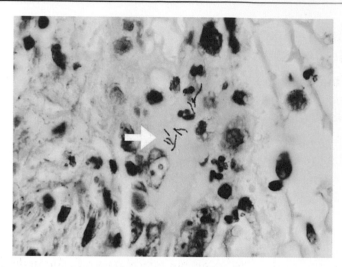

AFB stain for TB. (Reprinted from Shields JA, Shields CL. *Eyelid, Conjunctival, and Orbital Tumors: An Atlas and Textbook*. 3rd ed. Wolters Kluwer; 2015.)

Box 8.4 Other Neurologic Complications of Tuberculosis

A *tuberculoma* is a collection of tubercles (hard nodules formed by TB) that clump together into a firm mass. Tuberculomas can occur in both the brain and the spinal cord and, when symptomatic, present like a tumor or other mass lesion with headache, seizure, and/or focal deficits, depending on the location. They appear as ring-enhancing lesions on MRI. Treatment is largely the same as for tuberculous meningitis.

When TB affects the joints and bones, it is referred to as skeletal TB. Osteomyelitis and arthritis can occur; spondylitis (inflammation of the vertebrae, also known as *Pott disease*) is another manifestation. The thoracic and lumbar vertebrae are most often affected, causing progressive back pain and gait instability. Treatment involves antimicrobial therapy and, in certain advanced cases, surgical debridement, decompression, and/or drainage.

- Finally, a number of *parasites*, most notoriously Naegleria, can cause a meningoencephalitis that can be fatal.

Noninfectious Causes. Leukemia, lymphoma, and metastatic carcinoma can all seed the meninges, causing what is known as *leptomeningeal carcinomatosis*. CSF analysis will show no infection, but cytology may be positive for malignant cells (see Chapter 16 for details). Various medications can also cause aseptic meningitis, including nonsteroidal anti-inflammatory drugs (NSAIDs), the antibiotic trimethoprim-sulfamethoxazole, and IV immunoglobulin (IVIG).

Causes of Aseptic Meningitis

Viral meningitis

Spirochetal infections

Fungal infections

Tuberculosis

Malignancy

Medication-induced

Chronic Meningitis

Yes, there is such a thing. It is defined as the presence of inflammation in the CSF (*i.e.*, a CSF pleocytosis, another word for an increased white blood cell count in a body fluid, in this case the CSF) persisting for at least 1 month without resolution. The typical patient presents with several weeks of headache, nausea, one or several cranial neuropathies and polyradiculopathy.

Chronic meningitis can be caused by infections (including viral, bacterial, fungal, and parasitic infections), as well as by a variety of noninfectious conditions including malignancy, autoimmune diseases (such as systemic lupus erythematosus and sarcoid), vasculitis (Behcet syndrome and granulomatosis with polyangiitis), and medications (NSAIDs, intravenous immunoglobulin [IVIG], and intrathecal agents).

Empiric antibiotic therapy is not recommended, because the diagnostic possibilities are so diverse and difficult to sort out. Small cases studies have shown that some patients with idiopathic chronic meningitis may respond to antituberculosis therapy and some to glucocorticoids, but these therapies, particularly the latter, are not benign and only should be considered after extensive evaluation and consultation with specialists from all pertinent fields.

The overall prognosis for patients with chronic meningitis is good if a cause can be diagnosed and treated. For those with idiopathic disease, most patients also do well; their symptoms either improve or stabilize over a period of 1 to several years.

 ## Encephalitis

An Overview

Almost all cases of infectious[3] encephalitis are viral. Most viruses can cause either meningitis or encephalitis, but the majority are more likely to cause one rather than the other. HSV-1, for instance, is most likely to cause encephalitis but can cause meningitis; HSV-2, as previously discussed, is much more likely to cause meningitis and is less likely to cause encephalitis. In most cases, however, the specific cause of encephalitis is never found. Patients with viral encephalitis tend to have a benign and self-limited course, but there are exceptions (see below).

---

[3]Like meningitis, encephalitis does have non-infectious etiologies, including autoimmmune encephalitis (see page 248), which will be discussed later on.

Here is a list of some of the more common viruses that can cause encephalitis:

Herpesviruses (HSV-1 > HSV-2, VZV, EBV, HHV-6)

Arboviruses (West Nile, Japanese, St. Louis, Eastern and Western equine)

Enteroviruses (echo, coxsackie, polio)

HIV

Rabies

Measles

Influenza

HSV-1, herpes simplex virus 1; HSV-2, herpes simplex virus 2; VZV, varicella zoster virus; EBV, epstein barr virus; HHV-6, human herpesvirus 6.

Encephalitis presents most commonly with fever and altered mental status, ranging from subtle confusion to obtundation. Signs of meningeal irritation, including neck stiffness and photophobia, are usually absent. Seizures are common. Focal neurologic deficits, such as hemiparesis or aphasia, can occur. A typical viral prodrome (fevers, chills, myalgias) usually precedes the brain involvement.

As with meningitis, CSF analysis is critical. Since most cases are viral in origin, an aseptic profile predominates (*i.e.*, lymphocytic pleocytosis with a normal to mildly elevated protein and a normal glucose). PCR testing is available for many of the viral causes, including herpes viruses, enteroviruses, and West Nile virus.

Herpes Encephalitis

This is the one you don't want to miss, because treatment is available and early intervention can be lifesaving. HSV-1 causes most cases, and encephalitis can occur with primary infection or reactivation. Patients present with the typical features of encephalitis described above; more than half will experience seizures. The CSF profile is notable for an elevated protein, a lymphocytic predominance of cells and, unlike most viral encephalitides, although certainly not pathognomonic, an elevated red blood cell count. CSF PCR testing for HSV-1 has a high diagnostic sensitivity and specificity. MRI of the brain will often reveal *edema or hemorrhage within the temporal lobes,* and an EEG will classically show *periodic sharp waves arising from one or both temporal lobes.* Treatment is IV acyclovir,[4] which should be given empirically if there is any clinical suspicion. Mortality used to be exceedingly high (over 70%), but early treatment has reduced this substantially. However, many patients will suffer residual neurologic deficits that may include cognitive deficits, memory impairment, and behavioral abnormalities.

---

[4]Remember to give IV acyclovir with IV fluids to prevent acyclovir-induced renal injury from crystal formation.

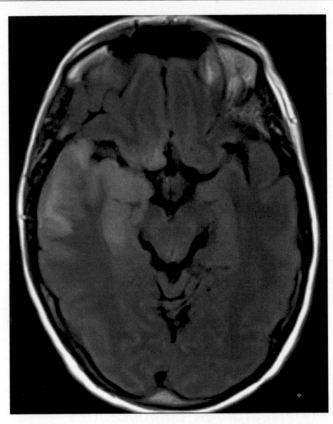

An MRI of a patient with HSV-1 encephalitis showing marked edema of the right temporal lobe. (Reprinted from Louis ED, Mayer SA, Rowland LP. *Merritt's Neurology*. 13th ed. Wolters Kluwer; 2015.)

Arthropod-Borne Encephalitis

Insects can carry a number of pathogens that can cause encephalitis. Among the ones you've probably heard of are West Nile virus, Japanese encephalitis, St. Louis encephalitis, Eastern and Western equine encephalitis, dengue fever, and Lyme disease. The patient's geographic location and history of possible exposure (often via travel) can be helpful, but patients must undergo CSF analysis to rule out other treatable causes. Serology and nucleic acid testing can aid in the diagnosis. Only supportive treatment is available for the viral etiologies. Doxycycline is the recommended therapy for Lyme disease.

West Nile virus (WNV) is a single-stranded RNA virus that first appeared in the United States in 1999. Although the majority of cases are asymptomatic, neuroinvasive disease can occur and is associated with a high mortality. In adults, WNV encephalitis is often associated with extrapyramidal symptoms such as tremor, parkinsonism, and myoclonus. In children, meningitis is the more common presentation and looks just like other viral meningitides. WNV can also cause an acute myelitis similar to poliomyelitis, characterized by an asymmetric flaccid paralysis, hyporeflexia, and autonomic dysfunction. The diagnosis of WNV infection is made by serum (antibody) and CSF (antibody and PCR) testing. There is no known treatment, although some studies have shown a potential benefit of IVIG, particularly in immunocompromised patients.

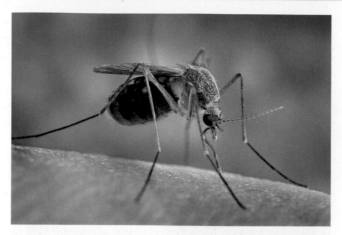

West Nile virus is most commonly spread in the summer by the bite of an infected mosquito. (Gathany J. *Public Health Images Library*. Centers for Disease Control and Prevention; 2014. http://phil.cdc.gov)

Now that you are well versed in both meningitis and encephalitis, we need to spend some time on several specific infections, many of which we have already briefly discussed, that can have important neurologic consequences. These include HIV, syphilis, Lyme disease, neurocysticercosis, leprosy, poliomyelitis, and COVID-19.

HIV Infection: Neurologic Complications

Before the advent of modern antiretroviral therapy, CNS opportunistic infections were common in HIV-positive patients. Fortunately, these infections are significantly less common today.

- *HIV meningitis* is technically not an opportunistic infection but rather a manifestation of acute HIV infection. It presents as a typical aseptic meningitis that tends to self-resolve within 2 to 4 weeks. *Guillain-Barre syndrome* can also occur in association with acute HIV infection, although it usually appears several weeks later.

- *Progressive multifocal leukoencephalopathy* (PML), the result of infection with the JC virus, is much less common today in patients with HIV thanks to the widespread use of antiretroviral therapy. PML is a disease of the white matter (white matter, *leuko*, in the brain, *encephalo*, is damaged, *pathy*) that typically presents with subacute neurologic deficits; the symptoms depend on the location of the white matter lesions. Seizures, a manifestation of cortical disease, are also common, presumably due to lesions that lie adjacent to the cortex. Various medications, including natalizumab and ocrelizumab (used to treat multiple sclerosis), can also increase the risk of PML (see page 246).

- *Toxoplasmosis*, caused by the intracellular protozoan parasite *Toxoplasma gondii*, is the most common CNS infection in patients with untreated or inadequately treated HIV. Toxoplasmosis in immunocompetent patients is nearly always asymptomatic, but when CD4 counts fall below 100 cells/μL, the parasite can reactivate and cause both CNS and systemic disease. Encephalitis is the most common neurologic manifestation. A presumptive diagnosis is made by brain imaging (see below, and Box 8.5) and serologic testing in the appropriate clinical context; although often unnecessary, biopsy is required for definitive diagnosis. Acute treatment is with pyrimethamine and sulfadiazine. Leukovorin is given as well, to prevent pyrimethamine-induced hematologic toxicity. Trimethoprim-sulfamethoxazole is used for prophylaxis in HIV-positive patients with CD4 counts below 100 cells/μL.

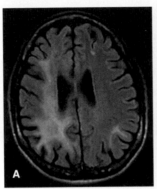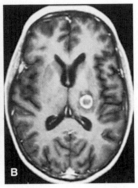

(*A*) Fluid-attenuated inversion recovery (FLAIR) MRI of a patient with PML, showing the characteristic nonenhancing, asymmetric, and confluent white matter lesions.
(*B*) Postcontrast T1-weighted MRI of a patient with toxoplasmosis, showing the classic ring-enhancing lesion. Toxoplasmosis can be indistinguishable from CNS lymphoma on imaging; clinical context is key, but brain biopsy may be required to differentiate the two diseases. (Reprinted from Atlas SW. *Magnetic Resonance Imaging of the Brain and Spine.* 5th ed. Wolters Kluwer; 2016.)

- *Other infectious complications* include cytomegalovirus encephalitis and, as mentioned earlier, cryptococcal meningitis.

Noninfectious neurologic complications of chronic HIV infection include:

- a *distal symmetric polyneuropathy* (either from the infection itself or as a side effect of antiretroviral therapy)
- *chronic inflammatory demyelinating polyneuropathy* (see page 287)
- *immune reconstitution syndrome* (IRIS). IRIS can occur when patients with low CD4 counts start antiretroviral therapy. Symptoms range from headache and dizziness to delirium and coma
- *HIV-associated neurocognitive disorder,* or HAND. This is a form of dementia that can present with varying types and degrees of cognitive deficits. It is the result of ongoing inflammation that persists despite viral suppression. Although the prevalence and severity have decreased in recent years, mild forms of cognitive dysfunction still develop in as many as 20% of HIV-positive individuals.

One final neurologic complication of HIV infection is *primary CNS lymphoma,* which can occur in both immunocompetent and immunocompromised patients, and is discussed in detail in Chapter 16.

Box 8.5 Cerebral Ring-Enhancing Lesions

This descriptor, "ring-enhancing," comes up frequently in neurology—we just mentioned it in our discussion of toxoplasmosis (take a look again at the MRI on page 219)—so we thought it deserved a short paragraph. What does it mean? A ring-enhancing lesion is an abnormal radiographic finding that can be seen on a contrast-enhanced CT or MRI that is characterized by a region of hypo- or isodensity (on CT) or hypo- or isointensity (on MRI) surrounded by a rim of brightly enhancing contrast. The diagnostic differential is long, but some of the more common etiologies include:

- *Infections* (bacterial or fungal abscess, tuberculoma, toxoplasmosis, neurocysticercosis)
- *Neoplastic disorders* (CNS lymphoma, glioblastoma, metastasis)
- *Inflammatory disorders* (sarcoid and a rare form of multiple sclerosis (MS) called tumefactive MS that appears like a tumor on imaging)
- *Vascular disorders* (subacute infarct, resolving hematoma)

The ability to differentiate among these potential causes relies heavily on clinical context. However, further evaluation, with a lumbar puncture or brain biopsy, is sometimes necessary.

Neurosyphilis

Syphilis, caused by the spirochete *Treponema palladum*, has experienced a resurgence in recent years. Because most patients are treated early in the primary phase when the disease is still localized, the neurologic complications of syphilis, which are associated with untreated disease, are only rarely encountered. Nevertheless, neurosyphilis has not vanished from the population. It is especially prevalent in the HIV-positive population. Because the long-term complications of neurosyphilis can be devastating and treatment with penicillin is curative, this is another diagnosis you don't want to miss.

The clinical manifestations of neurosyphilis are typically divided into early (occurring within months to a few years of the initial infection) and late (occuring 10 or more years after the initial infection) phases.

Early Neurosyphilis. Primary syphilis presents as a painless genital ulcer. During the secondary phase of infection, the spirochete, if untreated, disseminates throughout the body causing a diffuse rash and can seed multiple organs, including the meninges.

- *Meningeal involvement* may remain asymptomatic or cause a variety of symptoms, ranging from those of a typical acute meningitis to cranial nerve impairment to seizures.

- *Meningovascular involvement* of the spinal cord and sometimes the brain with resulting infarction (in essence these are small strokes, and symptoms will depend entirely on their location) is a less common manifestation of early neurosyphilis. Behavioral and personality changes, headache, and dizziness, likely due to mild meningitis, often precede and herald actual infarction by days to weeks. In at-risk populations, syphilis should be considered as a cause of large-vessel stroke.

- *Ocular symptoms* (loss of vision or blurry vision due most often to posterior uveitis or panuveitis) and *otic symptoms* (hearing loss) can also occur at this stage.

Late Neurosyphilis. The manifestations of late neurosyphilis appear at least 10 years and often several decades after infection. The major manifestations are *general paresis, tabes dorsalis, gummatous disease,* and *chronic meningitis.* These are rarely seen since the advent of modern diagnostic techniques and antibiotic therapy.

- *General paresis,* aka *syphilis dementia,* is a gradual-onset dementia characterized by a constellation of symptoms that typically evolve 10 to 20 years after the initial infection. The mnemonic PARESIS is useful for remembering the domains that are affected:

Personality (labile, paranoid, disinhibited)
Affect (flat, depressed, euphoric, manic)
Reflexes (hyperactive deep tendon reflexes)
Eye (large, unequal pupils that react slowly to light and accommodation; eventually patients may develop **Argyll Robertson pupils** [although these are more commonly seen with tabes dorsalis], which are small and irregular, unreactive to light but able to constrict with accommodation)
Sensorium (delusions, illusions, hallucination)
Intellect (impaired memory, judgment, and insight)
Speech (slurred)

- *Tabes dorsalis* will not usually develop until at least 20 years after infection. Involvement of the posterior (aka dorsal) columns of the spinal cord and the dorsal root ganglia (*tabes dorsalis* roughly translates from Latin as "dorsal decay") results in gradual sensory loss in the lower extremities, hyporeflexia, and lightning-like lancinating pains of the face, trunk, and/or extremities. The loss of pain and proprioception can lead to joint destruction (Charcot joints) and traumatic ulcers. Other manifestations of tabes dorsalis include sensory ataxia, bladder dysfunction, gastrointestinal upset, and pupillary abnormalities, including Argyll Robertson pupils.

- *Gummas* are a type of granulomatous lesion that develop in the brain or spinal cord late in the course of tertiary syphilis. They present like mass lesions (see page 390).

- *Chronic meningitis* can also occur and is thought to be the cause of the dementia seen with general paresis.

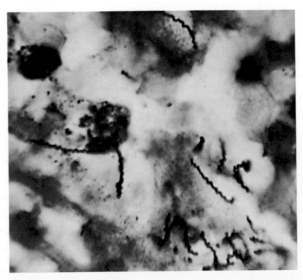

Immunostaining demonstrates numerous spirochetes. (Reprinted from Rubin R, Strayer DS. *Rubin's Pathology: Clinicopathologic Foundations of Medicine.* 5th ed. Lippincott Williams & Wilkins; 2008.)

Diagnosis. A combination of the following three items establishes the diagnosis of neurosyphilis:

1. clinical symptoms,

2. a positive CSF serology—the test used most often is the VDRL,[5] and

3. an elevated CSF cell count or protein.

However, not all patients with neurosyphilis will meet all three criteria; that's where clinical judgment comes in. Patients with a positive blood serology, whether a nonspecific test (*e.g.*, VDRL or RPR) or specific treponemal test (*e.g.*, FTA-ABS), plus any of the above criteria, warrant serious consideration for the diagnosis of neurosyphilis.

Patients with neurologic, ocular, or otalgic symptoms consistent with syphilis should undergo lumbar puncture even if their syphilis history is uncertain and the results of serologic testing are not confirmatory.

In addition, some patients have *asymptomatic* neurosyphilis. These patients have evidence of primary or secondary syphilis but without any neurologic signs or symptoms. Guidelines vary, but a lumbar puncture may still be recommended if these patients are at high risk for neurosyphilis, that is, if they are HIV positive, have a high RPR titer and a low (<350/μL) CD4+ T cell count, and have not been treated with antiretroviral therapy. A positive CSF VDRL confirms the diagnosis. Even without a positive CSF VDRL, an elevated CSF white cell count and/or protein is consistent with neurosyphilis, although it can also be caused by HIV itself. Most guidelines recommend treating these patients as though they have neurosyphilis.

Treatment. Syphilis in any phase is responsive to penicillin; resistance to penicillin has not been a problem. Unlike patients with primary syphilis, which can be treated with a single intramuscular (IM) injection, patients with neurosyphilis should receive a 10- to 14-day course of either IV or IM penicillin. Penicillin-allergic patients should be desensitized to penicillin if possible; if not, ceftriaxone is an alternative option.

The success of therapy is judged both by clinical improvement and by normalization of CSF abnormalities. Following the course of treatment, patients should have a repeat CSF analysis performed every 3 to 6 months. Failure of the cell count to decrease by 6 months or of the CSF VDRL to decline at least 4-fold by 1 year are indications for repeat treatment.

---

[5]Keep in mind that the CSF VDRL test lacks sensitivity: whereas a reactive test is confirmatory (most of the time), a negative test does not exclude the diagnosis. The FTA-ABS test is the opposite: sensitive but not specific. PCR testing of the CSF is also available, but it is not nearly sensitive enough to be widely used.

Lyme Disease: Neurologic Manifestations

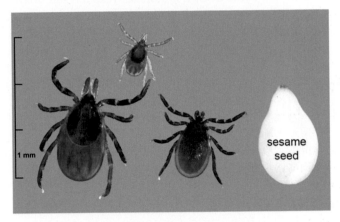

Lyme is spread through the bite of infected Ixodes ticks. The sesame seed shows relative size. (Reprinted from Engleberg NC, DiRita VJ, Dermody TS. *Schaechter's Mechanisms of Microbial Disease*. 5th ed. Wolters Kluwer Health/Lippincott Williams & Wilkins; 2012.)

Like *Treponema pallidum*, *Borrelia burgdorferi*, the cause of Lyme disease, is a spirochete. Similar to syphilis, when the primary infection goes untreated, the organism can disseminate to other organs. Other than the skin and joints, the nervous system is the most commonly affected organ system. Reminiscent of neurosyphilis, nervous system involvement in Lyme disease can present in several ways.

- ***Central nervous system involvement.*** *Meningeal seeding* presents like a typical aseptic meningitis. Symptoms include fever, headache, neck stiffness, and photophobia. If CSF analysis is performed, it will show mild pleocytosis, moderate elevation in protein, and normal glucose. Far less commonly, patients can develop signs and symptoms of *encephalopathy* or *encephalomyelitis*, with brain and spinal cord involvement. However, most patients with Lyme disease who complain of headache, mild cognitive impairment, or memory deficits probably do not have actual infection of the CNS; rather, just as with other nonspecific symptoms such as fever and fatigue, these patients are probably experiencing symptoms that frequently accompany any inflammatory process.

- ***Peripheral nervous system involvement*** is common. Any cranial nerve can be affected, but most often it is the seventh cranial nerve that is involved, producing a facial palsy. In endemic areas, patients with facial palsy should be tested for Lyme disease. Most cases are unilateral, but bilateral involvement does occur. Other peripheral nerves can be affected as well. *Radiculoneuritis* typically presents with pain, often accompanied by sensory or motor findings and hyporeflexia; the clinical picture can mimic typical mechanical radiculopathies (see Chapter 11) such as sciatica.

The diagnosis of nervous system Lyme disease requires clinical evidence of neurologic involvement along with a potential tick exposure and a positive blood serology. CSF analysis is typically not performed in patients with peripheral nerve involvement or mild nonspecific symptoms, but it is recommended in patients with meningitis if only to rule out other more threatening pathogens. The CSF will usually, but not always, test positive for Lyme antibodies. As with neurosyphilis, the sensitivity of PCR testing is too low to be useful.

All patients with confirmed Lyme disease should be treated. Oral doxycycline remains the drug of choice even for patients with neurologic involvement, with the exception of those rare patients with encephalitis; they require treatment with IV ceftriaxone.

Box 8.6 Post-Lyme Syndrome

Some patients who have been treated appropriately for Lyme disease continue to experience nonspecific symptoms that may have a neurologic flavor—headache, generalized weakness, and impaired cognitive function. These patients are suffering and their symptoms should be taken seriously, but there is no evidence that they have ongoing infection. The cause of their symptoms is not currently understood. Additional antibiotic therapy will not be helpful.

 COVID-19: Neurologic Manifestations

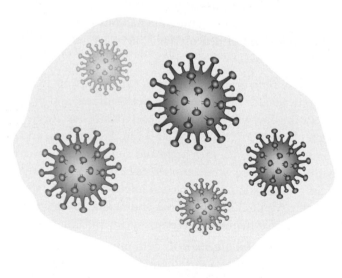

The by now all-too-familiar picture of the SARS-CoV-2 virus.

The neurologic manifestations of COVID-19, the disease associated with the SARS-CoV-2 virus, are, like everything associated with this pathogen, protean to say the least. It is easiest to group them into several categories:

• Secondary manifestations of the underlying disease, such as headache and dizziness (just as one might see with any febrile illness)

- Encephalopathy/encephalitis. Many patients present with altered mental status, but it remains unclear if this is the result of true CNS infection (encephalitis) or is simply secondary to the effects of systemic infection and consequent metabolic derangements (encephalopathy). Nonspecific but very real and debilitating cognitive symptoms may persist for many months in some patients.

- An increased risk of both ischemic and hemorrhagic stroke, even in young patients. This appears to reflect the hypercoagulable state associated with the excess inflammatory response that is responsible for so many of the severe complications of the disease.

- Peripheral and cranial nerve involvement, including, in many patients with COVID-19, a loss of taste and smell

- Skeletal muscle damage, which can lead to rhabdomyolysis

A Few Other CNS Infections to Know About

Neurocysticercosis

Neurocysticercosis (NCC) is caused by the larval stage of the pork tapeworm, *Taenia solium*. NCC is the most common parasitic disease of the central nervous system and the most common cause of acquired epilepsy in the world. It is endemic in Latin America, Asia, Africa, and India.

The cysticercosis life cycle results in 3 phases of disease: (1) the initial (or viable) phase is usually asymptomatic; (2) the degenerating phase is symptomatic owing to an induced inflammatory response; and (3) the nonviable phase, in which the cysticerci resolve and calcify. Intraparenchymal NCC is the most common form, characterized by one or more cysts within the brain parenchyma. Symptoms vary based on cyst location, but seizures are the most common presentation. Fever is often absent. Extraparenchymal forms include intraventricular, subarachnoid, ocular, and spinal disease. The diagnosis is based on clinical symptoms, epidemiologic exposure, and consistent neuroimaging findings.

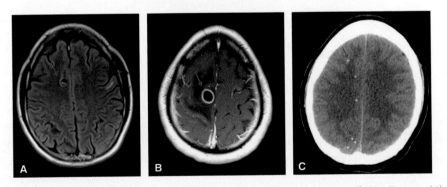

Scans from different patients with NCC, showing the different stages of the disease: (*A*) the viable stage on FLAIR MRI, with a single nonenhancing cyst; (*B*) the degenerating (*i.e.*, enhancing) stage on postcontrast MRI, with a single enhancing cyst surrounded by significant edema; and (*C*) the nonviable (*i.e.*, calcified) stage on CT, with several scattered calcified cysts. (Courtesy of Jonathan Howard.)

Initial treatment should be focused on the management of elevated intracranial pressure, the result of diffuse edema caused by a high cyst burden (steroids are first-line therapy), and seizure control. Antiparasitic therapy with albendazole and praziquantel is indicated for patients with viable or degenerating cysts on imaging, but should be avoided in those with a high cyst burden because of the danger of worsening the inflammation.

Leprosy

Leprosy was for thousands of years believed to be, in various forms, a hereditary disease, a curse, or a punishment from God. We've learned a few things over the years and now know that the disease is caused by *Mycobacterium leprae*, an acid-fast bacillus that was identified in the 1870s by Dr. Gerhard Henrik Armauer Hansen (leprosy is also known as Hansen disease). Despite everything we now understand about leprosy, and in part because of the dramatically reduced prevalence of the disease over the past several decades (most clinicians in the United States will never see a single case), it remains a feared and largely misunderstood illness. Leprosy is rarely life-threatening. It is not highly contagious, and treatment is effective.

Today, the majority of cases occur in developing countries. Risk factors include older age, prolonged close contact with affected patients, and exposure to wild armadillos (the mechanism of transmission from armadillo to human is unclear, but armadillos in the southern United States comprise a large reservoir of *M. leprae*). Putting aside armadillos, transmission in most cases is thought to occur via respiratory secretions. Cutaneous lesions and peripheral nerve damage are the major clinical manifestations; *Mycobacterium leprae* grows best in cooler temperatures, hence its predilection for the skin and superficial nerves.

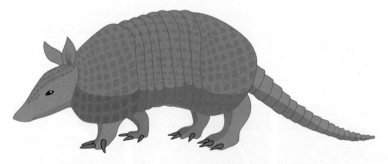

An armadillo. It is unclear if this one carries leprosy.

There are numerous types of leprosy, but two in particular are important to know. The **tuberculoid form** of the disease is limited to hypopigmented skin lesions that are associated with tender enlarged nerves and predominantly sensory nerve damage, which causes areas of decreased sensation typically in and around the skin lesions. The **lepromatous form** of the disease, a more diffuse form that's seen most often in immunocompromised patients, characteristically causes more widespread cutaneous lesions with more extensive sensory loss that can result in severe body and digital deformities. Motor neuropathies, body hair loss (predominantly affecting the eyebrows and eyelashes), and collapse of the nasal septum can also occur.

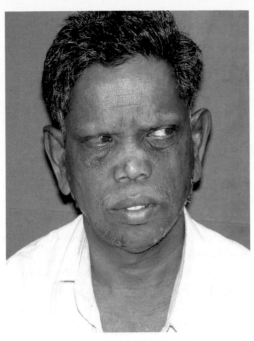

Lepromatous leprosy can cause the loss of eyebrows and eyelashes as well as nasal septal perforation and collapse. (Reprinted from Garg SJ. *Uveitis*. 2nd ed. Wolters Kluwer; 2018.)

The diagnosis is based predominantly on clinical findings; skin biopsy and tissue PCR testing can help confirm the diagnosis. There are no reliable blood tests. Multidrug therapy with dapsone and rifampin is first line; clofazimine is added for lepromatous disease. Treatment is effective, but it may take several years for the cutaneous lesions to fully resolve.

Poliomyelitis

As of this writing, there are only two remaining polio-endemic countries: Afghanistan and Pakistan. Vaccination has eliminated the disease from the United States and other developed countries, and the number of cases in less developed regions is vanishing as well.

Poliovirus (an enterovirus species) is most often asymptomatic. It can also cause a mild febrile illness and aseptic meningitis. Far less often, it can attack the motor neurons of the brainstem and spinal cord, resulting in poliomyelitis. *Acute, asymmetric flaccid paralysis* is the hallmark of the disease, often preceded by meningeal signs including neck stiffness, headache, and fever. CSF examination is critical for diagnosis and will show an aseptic meningitis profile with a moderate pleocytosis, as well as a positive poliovirus culture or PCR. Treatment is supportive.

Approximately two-thirds of patients with poliomyelitis are left with residual deficits. Although you are likely to never see a patient with the acute illness, patients who contracted polio prior to widespread vaccination may present to you with progressive fatigue and muscle weakness, a condition known as *post-polio syndrome*. Typically, symptoms develop at least 15 years after the acute infection. The pathogenesis is not fully understood. An electromyography (EMG) will confirm lower motor neuron involvement, and treatment is supportive.

Non-polio enteroviruses (such as echoviruses and coxsackievirus) and *arboviruses* (including West Nile, as mentioned above) can also cause acute flaccid paralysis, mimicking poliomyelitis.

Botulism

Botulism is caused by the bacterium *Clostridium botulinum*. Descending paralysis and cranial neuropathies, often preceded by gastrointestinal symptoms, are the result of blockade of the presynaptic acetylcholine receptors. This disease is discussed further in Chapter 12 (see page 316).

 Brain Abscess

Brain abscesses are infectious in nature, but they present most often like mass lesions, with headache, seizures, and focal neurologic deficits. The location, size, and rate of growth of the abscess will determine the precise symptomatology. Fever is present in only about 50% of cases. The differential diagnosis therefore includes both CNS infections and other mass lesions, including hematomas and tumors.

A brain abscess can develop either via hematogenous spread from a distant site of infection or as a result of extension from a contiguous source of infection (*e.g.*, sinusitis, mastoiditis, or a dental infection). Operative procedures and head trauma can also be responsible. Bacteria are by far the most common etiologic agents—staphylococcal species, streptococcal species, and enterobacteriaceae top the list—but other pathogens, such as fungi, mycobacteria, and parasites can be responsible as well, particularly in immunocompromised patients. For example, HIV infection is a major risk factor for brain abscess caused by *Toxoplasma gondii* and *Mycobacterium tuberculosis.*

All patients with suspected brain abscess should undergo imaging. MRI with gadolinium is the preferred test and is particularly good at distinguishing brain abscess from malignancy. Blood cultures should always be sent, and lumbar puncture for CSF cultures should be performed if not contraindicated owing to the risk of elevated intracranial pressure and subsequent herniation.

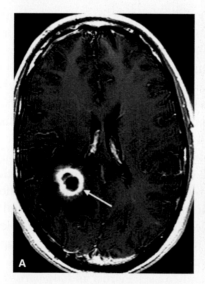 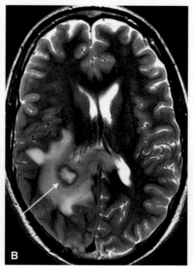

MRI postcontrast T1 (*A*) and T2 (*B*) sequences showing a cerebral ring-enhancing abscess with significant surrounding vasogenic edema. White arrows point to the abscess. Reprinted from Farrell TA. Radiology 101, 5th Edition. Philadelphia: Wolters Kluwer, 2019.

Treatment includes antimicrobial therapy, and the sooner it is instituted the better the outcome. Typical courses range from 4 to 8 weeks of IV antibiotics. Stereotactic aspiration is also often indicated for diagnosis and drainage.

Potential complications of brain abscesses include seizures, hydrocephalus (particularly with lesions in the posterior fossa), and rupture into the ventricular system. Mortality has improved greatly in the past few years—it is now about 15%—and the majority of patients make a good recovery.

Box 8.7 Spinal Epidural Abscess

Spinal epidural abscess is rare and the result of hematogenous spread, neurosurgical procedures, or spinal injection. Most patients have underlying risk factors, notably diabetes and IV drug use. *Staphylococcus aureus* is the pathogen identified most often. Fever, focal back pain, and neurologic dysfunction, including sensorimotor deficits and bowel and bladder dysfunction, can occur. Treatment includes IV antibiotics and, in a majority of cases, neurosurgical drainage. Most patients do well, but a small number of patients end up with some degree of paralysis. Mortality is less than 10%.

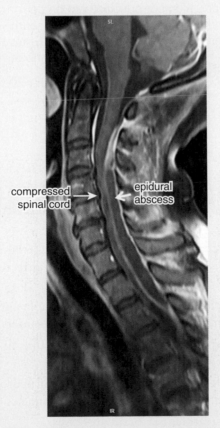

Postcontrast T1-weighted MRI showing a large epidural abscess with enhancement of the surrounding wall causing severe displacement and compression of the spinal cord. (Modified from Peterson JJ. *Berquist's Musculoskeletal Imaging Companion*. 3rd ed. Wolters Kluwer; 2017.)

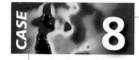

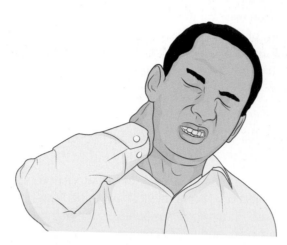

Follow-up on Your Patient: Amir presented with several hours of headache, fever, chills, and photophobia, and your examination confirmed nuchal rigidity. You suspect he might have meningitis and, given delays in getting him to the hospital, start him immediately on IV antibiotics (ceftriaxone and vancomycin) and dexamethasone even before a lumbar puncture can be performed. The CSF ultimately shows an increased opening pressure, a high leukocyte count with a neutrophilic predominance, an elevated protein, and a low glucose. Gram stain is positive for Streptococcus pneumoniae. He improves rapidly with antibiotics and recovers without any neurologic complications.

You now know:

- | How to recognize and diagnose bacterial meningitis, a true medical emergency.
- | The specific features of bacterial meningitis associated with the most common pathogens.
- | How CSF analysis can help you distinguish bacterial meningitis from meningitis due to viruses as well as from other infectious and noninfectious causes.
- | When to suspect chronic meningitis, which can result from infection, malignancy, and autoimmune/inflammatory disorders.
- | When to suspect encephalitis, and specific features of herpes encephalitis and arthropod-borne encephalitis.
- | The clinical manifestations and management of neurosyphilis, Lyme disease, COVID-19, and other infections with important neurologic manifestations.
- | The features and treatment of brain abscesses.

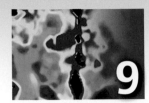

9 Multiple Sclerosis (and Other Immunologic Diseases of the Central Nervous System)

In this chapter, you will learn:

1 | How to diagnose multiple sclerosis

2 | How to sort through the complicated differential diagnosis of multiple sclerosis

3 | How to treat exacerbations of multiple sclerosis and reduce the risk and severity of recurrent attacks

4 | The differential diagnosis of optic neuritis

5 | How to diagnose and manage several less common but nevertheless important immunologic CNS disorders

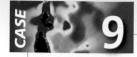

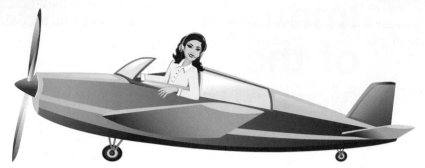

Your Patient: Emma, a previously healthy 33-year-old airline pilot, comes to see you because of double vision that has lasted about 36 hours and that occurs whenever she looks to her left. She went on the internet, looked up the diagnostic possibilities, and is concerned that she might have multiple sclerosis. She recalls that a year ago she experienced numbness in her left leg that lasted several days and then gradually resolved just as mysteriously as it appeared. What is the next step in your management?

Internuclear Ophthalmoplegia (INO)
on left gaze (right MLF lesion)

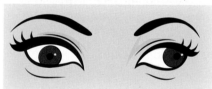

Internuclear ophthalmoplegia (INO). Your examination of Emma reveals the eye findings shown here. This is an example of internuclear ophthalmoplegia (INO), caused by a lesion in the medial longitudinal fasciculus (MLF). The MLF is a tract of fibers in the brainstem that yokes together the nuclei of the third and sixth cranial nerves to allow for conjugate horizontal gaze. For instance, to look to the left, the left nucleus of the sixth cranial nerve fires, resulting in abduction of the left eye and, via the MLF, simultaneous adduction of the right eye.

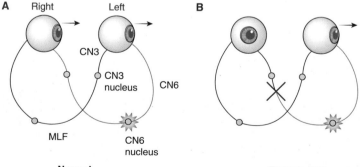

If the MLF is damaged, as in the case of Emma (and as illustrated in the diagram above), the right eye cannot adduct beyond the midline when she tries to look to the left. The left eye, which can abduct, would show marked nystagmus. A quick note on naming: Emma's INO would be called a RIGHT INO. It's confusing because the MLF itself crosses the midline, but convention dictates that the lesion is named after the eye that fails to move completely (in this case, the right eye).

The immune system is an impressive but imperfect construct that sometimes attacks healthy host cells and tissues when it really should be busy taking care of foreign invaders such as viruses and bacteria or eliminating cancerous cells before they get out of control. The nervous system is not exempt from this sort of misguided autoimmune attack. One of these autoimmune diseases, multiple sclerosis (MS), is quite common, with a prevalence in some regions of greater than 100 per 100,000 people.

 ## *Multiple Sclerosis*

Not that long ago, the diagnosis of MS was justly feared. Although some patients did well and experienced little or no disability, many others got worse—usually in fits and starts, sometimes relentlessly—and went on to develop diffuse and often devastating neurologic deficits and disability. Little could be done to alter its natural course. This is no longer the case. Many medications, all immune modulators of one kind or another, are now available, and these, combined with lifestyle interventions and symptomatic treatments, have significantly altered the prognosis for the better.

The greatest challenge often lies in making the diagnosis. The disease can strike anywhere in the CNS and can therefore manifest itself in myriad ways. Many patients come to see their healthcare provider with minor neurologic complaints, far less dramatic than Emma above, and it can be difficult to figure out who needs an evaluation for MS and who does not. It is important not to dismiss these seemingly inconsequential complaints without a careful history and physical examination, because early diagnosis and treatment of MS can slow the progression of the disease and limit disability.

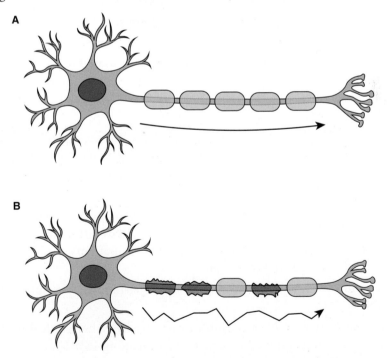

The pathophysiology of MS is complex and not completely understood but in most cases appears to involve inflammation directed against the myelin sheath within the CNS, leading to demyelination and, ultimately, axonal degeneration. The axon at the top (A) shows healthy myelination, whereas the one below (B) has been damaged by MS.

Some Basic Background Facts

- MS is three times as common in females as in males
- It presents most often between the ages of 20 and 50 years
  - A word to the wise—these first two facts should not be misconstrued to mean that MS *only* occurs in young females; it can and does occur in men and can and does occur in children and older patients as well, just less often.
- Risk factors for MS include both genetic and environmental factors
  - Hundreds of genetic variants have been identified that are associated with an increased risk of MS. However, no one gene or constellation of several genes is sufficient to account for the disease; the interaction between genetic predisposition and various environmental factors appears to be essential.
  - Environmental risk factors include obesity, smoking, prior infection with Epstein Barr virus, and geographical location. MS has a unique geographic distribution, becoming more common as one moves farther from the equator (*i.e.*, at high latitudes). No one knows for certain why this is. Hypotheses include lower levels of UV radiation exposure or lower serum levels of vitamin D among populations at higher latitudes.
  - *Important*: Neither a history of trauma nor any vaccine (none!) has been definitively associated with an increased risk of MS.

Defining MS

There is no one specific test that establishes the diagnosis of MS. Classically, the diagnosis of MS requires:

- At least two episodes of neurologic dysfunction **disseminated in space and time** within the CNS. In other words, at least two neurologic deficits must appear over two distinct periods of time and must be localizable to two different anatomic regions (i.e., 'space') within the CNS.

This definition still applies, but has been, and continues to be, expanded as our understanding of the disease has grown and our imaging techniques have improved. The most recent 2017 iteration of **the McDonald criteria** (the gold-standard criteria used for MS diagnosis) requires five things for the diagnosis of MS:

- A "typical" clinical syndrome (see page 236 for details; it is important to remember that the McDonald criteria are only validated in patients who present with symptoms consistent with MS), as opposed to patients with nonspecific symptoms such as headache or fatigue
- Objective clinical evidence on neurologic examination (for example, Emma's INO)
- Dissemination in space (this criterion can be met by either clinical findings OR the presence of lesions on magnetic resonance imaging [MRI])

- Dissemination in time (this criterion, too, can be met by either clinical or MRI findings or, entirely unrelated to time but an appropriate surrogate according to the most recent criteria, by the presence of cerebrospinal fluid (CSF)-unique oligoclonal bands in the CSF; more on these later)

- Lack of a better explanation for the patient's presentation (*i.e.*, the overall clinical picture is not better explained by a different inflammatory or infectious etiology). This is an important caveat in that we still need to ensure that other etiologies are not missed.

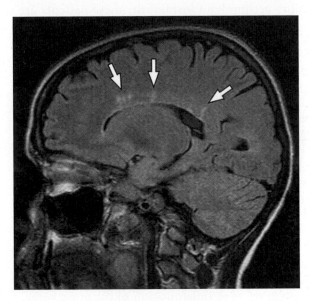

A sagittal MRI of the brain in a patient with MS. Note the periventricular demyelinating plaques that radiate away from the lateral ventricle at approximately 90-degree angles. These are colloquially referred to as Dawson fingers and are characteristic of MS. (Reprinted from Lee E. *Pediatric Radiology: Practical Imaging Evaluation of Infants and Children*. Wolters Kluwer; 2017.)

MS comes in two basic clinical phenotypes:

- **_Relapsing remitting MS_**—85% of patients have this form of MS, which is characterized by intermittent attacks of neurologic dysfunction involving different sites in the CNS. These flares are variably referred to as relapses, attacks, or exacerbations; don't be confused, these terms all refer to the same thing. Patients may recover completely from each attack or experience some degree of residual neurologic compromise and disability.

  - Patients presenting with a first clinical attack are said to have **clinically isolated syndrome (CIS).** Although these patients do not fulfill the classic definition of MS (remember, you need dissemination in space and time), many do meet current MS criteria (based on radiographic or CSF evidence; see the above discussion). Those who do not meet the criteria for MS are at high risk for conversion to clinically definite MS.

- There is also an entity termed **radiologically isolated syndrome (RIS)**, in which 2 lesions consistent with MS are seen incidentally on an MRI in a patient without any clinical symptoms of MS whatsoever. As many as 40% of these individuals will experience their first clinical attack within 5 years.

- *Primary progressive MS*—this type of MS is less common; it evolves gradually, without discrete episodes of acute dysfunction and recovery. Some patients with the relapsing, remitting type of MS will evolve into this type of clinical picture, and when disability accumulates insidiously, these patients are then said to have **secondary progressive MS.**

Box 9.1

The distinction between relapsing remitting MS and progressive MS is an important one, since the treatment and prognosis are very different.

Clinical Signs and Symptoms

Now that we've defined MS, let's look at its clinical manifestations. What are the "typical" symptoms? They are many and varied, as you would expect from a disease that can cause damage anywhere in the CNS, so let's focus on the most common ones.

Optic Neuritis. This term refers to inflammation of the optic nerve. Symptoms include unilateral vision loss that typically progresses over several days to weeks. The loss of vision may be total or just some mild blurring. Color vision is often lost preferentially over acuity. Ocular pain is common and is often exacerbated by eye movements. The most common finding on physical examination is an afferent pupillary defect, or APD (see Box 9.2).

Funduscopic examination may reveal papillitis (a swollen optic nerve head), but in the majority of cases the inflammation of the optic nerve involves only the retrobulbar (meaning behind the eyeball) part of the nerve and therefore cannot be visualized. As part of your bedside examination you will likely be able to demonstrate decreased visual acuity and compromised visual fields (the classic finding is a central scotoma, or dark spot, in the center of vision). In any patient with optic neuritis, obtain an MRI with gadolinium of the orbits and the brain, which may reveal enhancement and swelling of the affected optic nerve as well as other lesions consistent with prior, clinically silent demyelinating attacks. Approximately 20% of patients with a first attack of optic neuritis and an otherwise normal MRI will go on to develop MS; if, however, the MRI shows evidence of prior demyelination consistent with MS, that number jumps to 80%.

Most patients will recover adequate visual function within several weeks to months after an acute attack.

Box 9.2 Afferent Pupillary Defect

One of the characteristic findings of optic neuritis is an *afferent pupillary defect* (APD). Swing a flashlight back and forth between the good eye and the bad one. When the light swings back to the bad eye, the pupil, which you would ordinarily expect to constrict, will instead dilate. This occurs because the pupillary reflex is consensual: in other words, light in one eye causes both pupils to constrict. Thus, when light illuminates the good eye, both eyes constrict consensually in the normal way, but when the light illuminates the bad eye, overall light perception is compromised and the pupils appear to dilate.

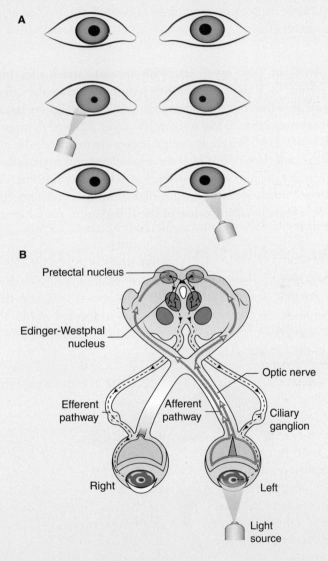

(*A*) Demonstration of an afferent pupillary defect. (*B*) Anatomy of the pupillary reflex pathway. (*1*) The afferent limb of the reflex: light hits the retina, activating the ipsilateral optic nerve, which projects to the two bilateral Edinger-Westphal (EW) nuclei of the oculomotor nerves (thus the consensual nature of the reflex). (*2*) The efferent limb of the reflex: parasympathetic fibers running within the oculomotor nerve (CN3) project from the EW nuclei to the ciliary ganglion, where they activate the short ciliary nerves that innervate the sphincter pupillae, causing bilateral pupillary constriction.

Box 9.3 The Differential Diagnosis of Optic Neuritis

Although it is most commonly associated with MS, optic neuritis has many other possible causes. In general, *bilateral optic neuritis* or *optic neuritis associated with new neurologic or systemic symptoms* should prompt a more thorough investigation into other etiologies. A few important ones to be aware of include:

- Neuromyelitis optica spectrum disorder (NMOSD) (see page 243)
- Chronic relapsing inflammatory optic neuritis (CRION)
- Connective tissue diseases (*e.g.*, systemic lupus erythematosus and sarcoidosis)
- Paraneoplastic optic neuropathy (most often associated with the CRMP5 autoantibody)
- Infectious syndromes (*e.g.*, Lyme disease, syphilis, cytomegalovirus)

Spinal Cord Involvement, (i.e., myelitis). With an acute attack affecting the spinal cord, patients may experience focal motor or sensory symptoms below the affected spinal level. Although symptoms are often not perfectly symmetric, both legs are usually involved to some extent. Patients may initially feel a tightness at the affected dermatome level; this has been called the "*MS hug.*" When motor pathways are involved, the affected muscles may initially be weak and flaccid, but over time spasticity and hyperreflexia will develop. Spinal cord involvement can also lead to urinary and bowel symptoms. An MRI of the spine typically shows "short-segment" lesions, that is, lesions involving fewer than 3 vertebral levels. For a more detailed review of the spinal cord, see Chapter 10.

Box 9.4 The Lhermitte Sign

The Lhermitte sign is a characteristic feature of MS that is often highlighted in lectures and on rounds. The patient describes an electrical sensation that shoots down the spine when the neck is flexed. Although suggestive of MS, the Lhermitte sign is not pathognomonic and can be seen in other diseases that affect the dorsal column fibers in the cervical spinal cord.

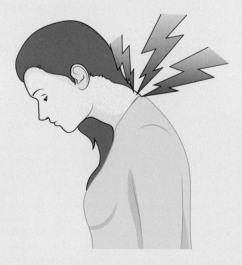

The Lhermitte sign.

Brainstem and Cerebellar Syndromes. Oculomotor abnormalities are far less common than optic neuritis. However, double vision can occur, often from internuclear ophthalmoplegia (INO), as in the case of Emma, which began this chapter, or from palsy of a single nerve (usually the sixth cranial nerve). MS can also cause trigeminal neuralgia (see page 108). Cerebellar involvement can cause vertigo or ataxia.

Cerebral, Cognitive Deficits. These deficits usually develop with advanced disease affecting multiple areas in the cerebrum. Short-term memory, executive function, visuospatial function, and the speed at which one thinks and communicates can be compromised; the last is colloquially known as *"MS brain fog."*

Over time, in addition to cognitive deficits and mood dysfunction, patients may develop disabling symptoms from irreversible axonal injury. Among these are:

- Neurogenic bladder (incontinence, frequency, urgency)
- Neurogenic bowel (incontinence, constipation)
- Sexual dysfunction
- Neuropathic pain
- Chronic fatigue
- Spasticity (increased muscle tone, often with superimposed spasms)
- Altered gait

How to Make the Diagnosis

Let's restate the major diagnostic criterion for MS: *evidence of neurologic deficits disseminated in space and time.* The first attack, as we've already mentioned, is referred to as *clinically isolated syndrome*, although evaluation at that time may reveal other lesions that qualify for the full diagnosis of MS. A thorough history and physical examination are therefore essential.

Perform a Complete History and Neurologic Examination. In particular, ask about the most common manifestations of MS. Prompt the patient to try to recall any other event that may have been ignored or forgotten but that may have been a sentinel MS event that completely resolved. Next, carry out a careful neurologic examination. You may uncover a subtle finding that even the patient is unaware of (*e.g.,* eye movement abnormalities, subtle sensory loss or abnormal reflexes).

Get an MRI. If you suspect the diagnosis, get an MRI of the brain. Contrast is necessary if the patient is presenting with new, active symptoms; otherwise, there's no need for gadolinium. Virtually all MRI centers use a standardized MS protocol. If a brain MRI is inconclusive, or if there are signs or symptoms of spinal cord involvement, then the cord should be imaged as well.

Box 9.5 Spinal Cord Imaging

Key point: if you are interested in the spinal cord itself—which, in the case of MS you are (remember, it is a disease of, and only of, the central nervous system)—order cervical and thoracic spine MRIs. There is no need for a lumbar scan. Remember: the cord itself ends at approximately L1; thus, a lumbar spine MRI does not visualize the spinal cord, only the bundle of spinal nerves and nerve roots we refer to as the cauda equina.

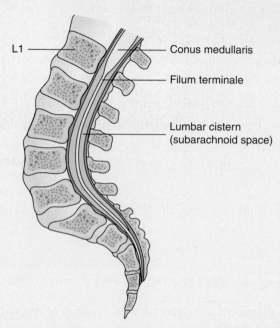

The lumbar spine. Note how the cord ends at the level of L1.

White matter lesions on MRI can be seen in many diseases, not just MS. Long-standing cerebrovascular disease and, perhaps surprisingly, migraine, are the two most common potential mimics (see page 98, Box 3.3). However, there are specific MRI criteria that, if met, make MS the most likely diagnosis. The classic MS lesions are ovoid as opposed to round and tend to occur in four specific locations:

- Periventricular
- Juxtacortical (and cortical, a recent addition to the 2017 McDonald criteria)
- Infratentorial (brainstem and cerebellum)
- Spinal cord

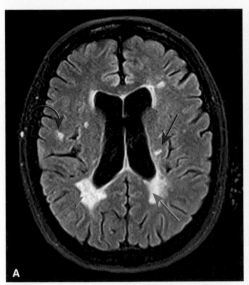
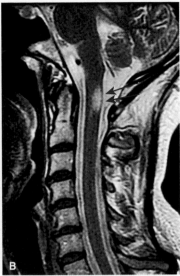

(*A*) Juxtacortical (*blue arrow*) and periventricular (*purple arrow*) MS lesions. The more confluent white matter disease (pink arrows) is characteristic of long-standing microvascular disease (*i.e.*, due to uncontrolled hypertension, hyperlipidemia, *etc.*); these areas do not represent MS plaques. (*B*) High cervical spine MS lesion (*red arrows*). (*A*, modified in part from Sanelli PC, Schaefer PW, Loevner LA. *Neuroimaging: The Essentials*. Wolters Kluwer; 2016; and *B*, reprinted from Barkovich AJ, Raybaud C. *Pediatric Neuroimaging*. 6th ed. Wolters Kluwer; 2018.)

All MS lesions (old or new) are hyperintense on T2 imaging. Active lesions are gadolinium enhancing (and continue to enhance for approximately 1 month); old lesions are not enhancing and can, over time, form so-called black holes on T1 imaging indicative of axonal loss. Therefore, if you see both enhancing and nonenhancing lesions, you have evidence for dissemination in time as well as space. The MRI can also assess the severity of the disease and to some degree help predict the patient's prognosis.

Look at the CSF. If the diagnosis is still uncertain, CSF analysis is the next step. What you are looking for are (1) *CSF-specific oligoclonal bands*, which are present in the majority of patients with MS, plus (2) an *increased IgG synthesis rate*. The former refers to bands on electrophoresis that are not present in the serum. The latter refers to the rate at which IgG is manufactured within the CSF. These findings are not specific to MS, so they must be assessed within the overall clinical context. However, the absence of CSF-specific oligoclonal bands suggests that the patient may not have MS (in suspected MS, only 2% to 3% of patients will prove to actually have the disease in the absence of oligoclonal bands). The number of white blood cells in the CSF is usually normal (less than 5) but can be elevated, although it rarely exceeds 50.

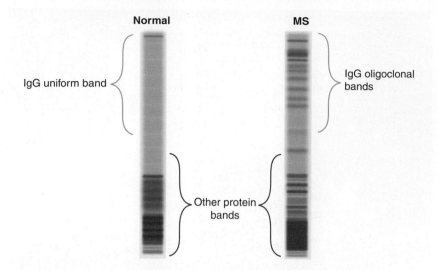

Oligoclonal bands on electrophoresis. The first shows a normal electrophoresis. The second is from a patient with MS.

If You Are Still Not Sure What Is Going on. Although rarely used anymore, *visual and somatosensory evoked potentials* measure the speed of nerve conduction, and they will prove to be abnormal in some patients with MS. Their accuracy isn't great, but in the right clinical context an abnormal evoked potential may, in difficult cases, reveal local dysfunction in a CNS region such as the optic nerve and thus be the final piece of evidence that makes you reasonably confident that your patient has MS.

Differential Diagnosis

The differential diagnosis of MS is extensive given the manifold ways in which it can present. Among the most important confounders are:

- Other inflammatory diseases that affect the CNS (including NMOSD, ADEM, Neurosarcoidosis and Susac Syndrome; see discussion below, pages 243-244)
- Vascular diseases—CNS vasculitis can cause a scattering of neurologic deficits often due to small bleeds or strokes that may mimic some of the features of MS (see page 88)
- Infections—Lyme disease should be considered (although fulminant neuroborreliosis is rare), HIV and syphilis
- Metabolic diseases—Think vitamin B12, copper, and zinc deficiencies
- CNS malignancies—Among these, you need to consider lymphoma, primary neoplasms, and paraneoplastic syndromes (see Chapter 16)
- Psychiatric disorders—Consider depression or anxiety with somatic features (*e.g.*, tingling, fatigue, and brain fog); these can mimic symptoms of MS but will not be associated with objective findings on neurologic examination, and imaging will be normal

Several primary inflammatory conditions can affect the CNS and closely mimic the way MS presents and evolves. Although less common than MS, these are important for you to know.

- ***Neuromyelitis optica spectrum disorder** (NMOSD)* comprises several related but distinct entities that present most commonly with optic neuritis or transverse myelitis (see page 267) and less often with hiccups or intractable emesis (the result of involvement of the area postrema in the medulla). Nearly all cases are associated with the **aquaporin-4 (AQP4)-IgG autoantibody** (aquaporin is a water channel protein present throughout the body, including the CNS); a smaller percentage are seropositive for myelin oligodendrocyte glycoprotein (MOG).[1]

- NMOSD can cause severe attacks and profound disability. NMO-related optic neuritis, for instance, is typically much more severe than MS-related optic neuritis, with a more rapid course and a more devastating outcome if left untreated.

- To diagnose NMOSD:

  - Suspect the disease because of the clinical picture as well as the appearance of the lesions on MRI. A brain MRI is often unremarkable, but the spinal cord may reveal thick, long lesions spanning multiple vertebral levels (unlike the "short-segment" lesions characteristic of MS).

  - Test the blood for AQP4 autoantibodies (more sensitive than testing the CSF) and, if negative, for MOG antibodies. Unlike in MS, the CSF often shows an elevated white cell count and oligoclonal bands are usually absent. Accurate diagnosis is important, because, compared with MS, NMOSD often requires significantly longer courses of corticosteroid therapy (often with additional plasmapheresis, commonly referred to as PLEX) to prevent relapses and does not respond to the disease-modifying medications that are used for MS. Rituximab and eculizumab, among others, are used instead, although evidence of their efficacy in this setting is still relatively sparse.

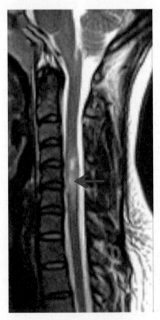

NMO lesion in the cervical spinal cord (*arrow*). Contrast this with the smaller MS spinal cord lesion pictured in figure B on page 241. (Reprinted from Sanelli P, Schaefer P, Laurie Loevner L. *Neuroimaging: The Essentials*. Wolters Kluwer; 2015.)

[1]MOG antibody disease represents an overlapping but likely clinically distinct syndrome that can be associated with both monophasic and relapsing attacks of demyelination. It can closely resemble AQP4 disease, but it tends to affect younger patients and often has a more favorable outcome, with a generally good response to steroid therapy.

- *Acute disseminated encephalomyelitis (ADEM)* is an acute, rapidly progressive, and typically monophasic disease caused by autoimmune demyelination. It is most often seen in children following a bacterial or viral infection. The presentation is variable but typically includes both new, focal neurologic deficits and systemic symptoms such as fever, headache, and nausea. Unlike the relatively well-circumscribed ovoid lesions on MRI characteristic of MS, the lesions associated with ADEM are bigger and more diffuse (often described as "fluffy") and, importantly, tend to enhance with contrast all at once. The CSF will show a lymphocytic pleocytosis (although typically less than 100 cells) and, like NMOSD, will not demonstrate oligoclonal bands. Treatment is with high-dose corticosteroids, followed by plasma exchange if needed.

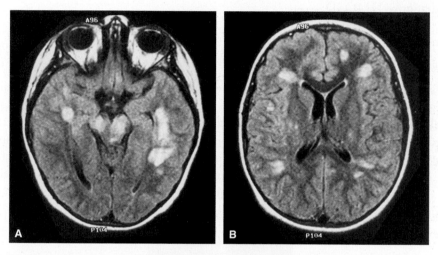

The "fluffy" lesions characteristic of ADEM. (Reprinted from Brant WE, Helms CA. *Brant and Helms Solution*. Wolters Kluwer; 2006.)

- These are a host of still other immunologic/inflammatory disorders that can mimic MS but that are even rarer than NMOSD and ADEM. Two you should be aware of are:

  - *Neurosarcoidosis*, the neurologic manifestation of sarcoidosis. Like MS, it can affect the brain, optic nerve, and spinal cord. Unlike MS, neurosarcoidosis can affect just about everything else in the nervous system, including the peripheral nerves and meninges.

  - *Susac syndrome* is an even less common disorder. It is an inflammatory vascular disease that most often presents with sensorineural hearing loss, encephalopathy, and retinal artery occlusions. Susac can look very similar to MS on MRI but has a particular predilection for the corpus callosum.

Clinical Course

The most common course for MS is one of relapse and remission. With treatment, most patients will do very well for many years. A significant minority of patients, even without therapy, will only have one or several attacks and will suffer very little disability. However, without treatment, about half of patients will evolve into secondary progressive MS.

A **relapse** or **exacerbation** is defined as an episode of new neurologic deficit or disability that develops over several hours, persists for more than 24 hours, and occurs in the absence of fever or infection. Recovery occurs slowly over weeks to months but may not be total, and many patients will have some degree of residual neurologic deficit. The frequency and severity of relapses is unpredictable and varies greatly. Fortunately, treatment can greatly improve the overall prognosis.

Box 9.6 Pseudorelapse

A relapse must be distinguished from a *"pseudorelapse,"* a worsening of neurologic symptoms from already existing deficits. Many patients will experience a pseudorelapse with an increase in body temperature caused by exercise, hot weather, infection, or fever. This type of pseudorelapse is called the *Uhthoff phenomenon*. It does not signify a new attack or lesion, just a further decrease in electrical conductivity caused by the increased temperature. These events are typically transient, and patients will return to their baseline once they cool down. Stress and infection are other common triggers that can cause pseudorelapses.

Patients with primary progressive MS have a steadier decline. This diagnosis is made by documenting progressive neurologic disability without relapses over a period of at least 1 year.

Treatment

The treatment of MS is 3-fold: treat the acute attacks, reduce the risk of future attacks and disability, and manage symptoms. Key point: Patients with clinically isolated syndrome (CIS) who are at high risk of progression to full-blown MS should also be offered disease-modifying therapy (see prognostic factors below).

Treating Acute Exacerbations. High-dose corticosteroids remain the mainstay of treatment for an acute relapse. Steroids accelerate recovery but do not have any definitive impact on a patient's long-term prognosis or risk of future attacks. Oral and parenteral formulations are equally effective and safe, but patients with severe exacerbations causing acute disability are generally hospitalized for intravenous (IV) steroids and close monitoring. As always, when dealing with high-dose steroids, blood glucose levels must be carefully tracked and a proton-pump inhibitor prophylactically prescribed for gastric protection. Insomnia, agitation, and psychosis are other important side effects of high-dose steroids. For an exacerbation that does not respond to steroids, plasmapheresis is the second-line option.

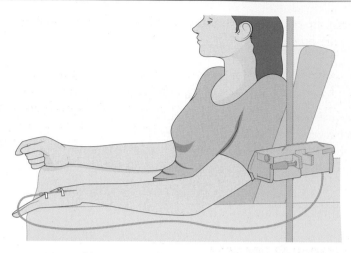

IV steroids are generally given in a hospital setting.

Modifying the Disease Course. Your mantra: *treat early*. Disease modifying therapy reduces the risk of recurrent attacks, the appearance of new lesions on MRI, and disability. Disease modifying drugs also reduce the risk that patients with CIS will progress to MS. Disease modifying drugs should not be used to treat acute exacerbations and do not reduce existing symptomatology.

Several classes of drugs are now available to treat relapsing remitting disease:

- *Injectable agents*: *Interferon beta* was the first effective disease modifying drug. The interferons are still sometimes used because of their proven safety record, but they are less effective than the newer oral drugs. *Glatiramer acetate* is another injectable drug that's also been around for many years and can work well with few serious side effects.

- *Oral agents:* Many patients prefer oral agents to injectable ones, and there are now several on the market. Depending on the particular agent, patients need to have their complete blood count and liver function tests monitored periodically. *Fingolimod, dimethyl fumarate*, and *teriflunomide* are three of the more commonly prescribed.

- *Monoclonal antibodies*: These agents are given via IV infusion. They are highly effective but carry more risk. *Natalizumab* (directed against alpha4-integrin, Natalizumab binds and prevents lymphocyte adherence to vessel walls, thereby reducing lymphocyte entry into the CNS) and *ocrelizumab* (directed against the B cell surface antigen CD20) are the two most commonly prescribed. Natalizumab in particular requires regular monitoring of JC virus antibody status, because patients who have been exposed to JC virus (approximately half of the general population) are at significantly higher risk of developing progressive multifocal leukoencephalopathy (PML, see page 218) and must be switched to another medication.

In general, the more effective the drug, the greater the risk of potentially serious side effects. However, these medications are well tolerated by the vast majority of patients.

Until recently we had no disease-modifying agents for primary progressive MS. However, *ocrelizumab* has been found to reduce the percentage of patients who experience disability and disease progression. The most common side effect is infection, particularly upper respiratory infections. PML can also occur. Another drug, *siponimod,* appears to be effective in limiting disability in secondary progressive MS.

Symptomatic Treatment. Patients who develop long-term complications of MS often require additional help to manage their symptomatic burden. There is a long list of lifestyle interventions and medications that can be helpful. Anticholinergic drugs (for example, oxybutynin) are often prescribed for urinary incontinence; baclofen is one of the most common medications prescribed for spasticity; gabapentin is used to treat neuropathic pain.

What about *cannabinoids?* The data here are far from ideal, but evidence is slowly mounting that cannabinoids can be at least modestly effective for reducing spasticity and neuropathic pain in MS (as of this writing, cannabinoids are not US Food and Drug Administration approved for this indication in the United States).

Box 9.7 Vitamin D For MS?

Various vitamins and dietary interventions have been studied, and no consistent benefit has been found, with one possible exception. The association of low levels of vitamin D with an increased risk of MS in Caucasian populations would suggest that supplementation might be useful. Although the benefits haven't been as profound as investigators had hoped, in at least some patients vitamin D supplementation does appear to reduce the appearance of new lesions on MRI as well as the rate of relapse and progression to disability. Most patients are therefore placed on vitamin D therapy, aiming for levels within the normal range.

Prognosis

MS is a treatable disease. The goal for all patients is what neurologists term *"no evidence of disease activity"* (NEDA) in the first year after diagnosis. NEDA means no clinical relapses, no new lesions on MRI, and no accumulation of disability. As the years go by, however, this goal becomes more and more difficult to maintain.

It is virtually impossible to predict the course of the disease in any given patient; however, favorable prognostic features include:

- female sex,
- younger age at diagnosis, and
- little disability at 5 years after diagnosis

Optic neuritis as the first symptom portends a more favorable prognosis in the short term, but long-term disability is no better or worse than in patients with other presentations.

Poorer prognostic features include:

- male sex,
- older age at diagnosis,
- frequent attacks early in the course,
- progressive disease from the start, and
- cerebellar symptoms as the first clinical evidence of the disease.

Initiating therapy with the more aggressive medications is often recommended for patients with poor prognostic features or multiple MRI lesions because they are at greatest risk of accumulating disability.

MS and Pregnancy

Women with MS can have normal pregnancies and breastfeed safely.

Pregnancy appears to decrease the frequency of MS exacerbations, but an increase in the number of exacerbations in the postpartum period essentially balances out the equation. Pregnancy does not change the long-term prognosis of the disease. Women with MS have a slightly increased rate of caesarian deliveries and low birth weight babies, but there does not appear to be an increase in stillbirths, ectopic pregnancies, birth defects, or spontaneous abortions. When possible, women should not be on disease modifying drugs during pregnancy, but this recommendation has not been adequately studied. Exacerbations are treated with corticosteroids.

The take-away is that pregnancy is not contraindicated by MS, but risks and benefits should be weighed in patients with severe disease in whom temporarily stopping or significantly altering treatment poses high risk.

Breastfeeding is safe with some disease modifying drugs, but the data are limited for the newer drugs, so consult with an MS specialist and obstetrician to guide management. MS itself is not a contraindication to breastfeeding.

Autoimmune Encephalitis: One Other Immunologic CNS Disease You Should Know

For a long time, we thought of encephalitis as principally an infectious disease, most commonly caused by herpes simplex virus or mosquito- or tick-borne pathogens (see page 215). But encephalitis can also be caused by the body's own immune system attacking the brain. As it turns out, autoimmune encephalitis is nearly as common as its infectious counterpart. Consideration of this diagnosis is crucial, as rapid treatment results in significantly better outcomes.

There are two main types of encephalitis that are considered to be immune mediated:

- *Paraneoplastic encephalitis*, which is invariably malignancy related (although it often presents prior to the patient having any awareness of an underlying malignancy), caused not by the cancer itself but by the immunologic reaction (*i.e.*, antibodies) that the cancer provokes.

- *Autoimmune encephalitis*, which is most often due to autoantibodies directed against neuronal surface antigens.

The nomenclature is a little misleading, as paraneoplastic encephalitis is by definition autoimmune, and autoimmune encephalitis can be paraneoplastic. Don't worry too much about the classification. Here's what you should know:

Presentation

In general, immune-mediated encephalitis presents subacutely, over weeks to months, although it can sometimes evolve much more rapidly. There are three main anatomical targets.

• *Limbic encephalitis*, as the name implies, involves the structures of the limbic system, including the amygdala, hippocampus, hypothalamus, and limbic cortex[2]. It is considered a classic paraneoplastic syndrome but can occur without an underlying malignancy. Common symptoms include memory loss, cognitive and behavioral changes (these patients are often initially admitted to psychiatric wards owing to agitation, disinhibition, and various bizarre behaviors), focal seizures, and symptoms related to hypothalamic dysfunction such as hyperthermia and endocrine abnormalities. MRI can be normal, but often shows increased fluid-attenuated inversion recovery (FLAIR) signal in the mesial temporal lobes.

One form of limbic encephalitis, called **anti-NMDA receptor encephalitis**, is most often seen in young women and is caused by autoantibodies directed against the glutamatergic NMDA (N-methyl-D-aspartate) receptor. Orofacial dyskinesias (which look like choreoathetoid chewing movements, see page 346), as well as severe autonomic instability, are common. Anti-NMDA antibodies are most frequently associated with ovarian teratomas. A second form of limbic encephalitis, **anti-LGII encephalitis**, is more likely to be seen in older patients and in men. It presents more often with faciobrachial dystonic seizures, peripheral neuropathy, and hyponatremia. LGII antibodies are typically not associated with an underlying neoplasm.

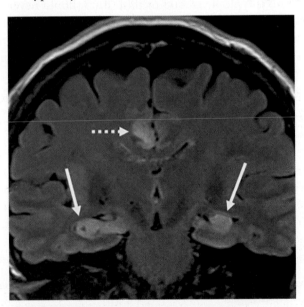

Coronal MRI demonstrates prominent FLAIR hyperintensities in the bilateral mesial temporal lobes (solid arrow) and cingulate gyrus (dashed arrow), characteristic of limbic encephalitis. (Reprinted from Scheld WM, Whitley RJ, Marra CM. *Infections of the Central Nervous System*. 4th ed. Wolters Kluwer; 2014.)

• *Brainstem encephalitis* can present with a wide range of symptoms localized to the pons and medulla, including extraocular movement abnormalities, dysphagia, dysarthria, and vertigo. This disorder often occurs in conjunction with paraneoplastic cerebellar degeneration.

---

[2]The structures of the limbic system are involved in regulating behavior, emotions and establishing long-term memory.

- ***Encephalomyelitis*** presents with diffuse involvement of the nervous system including the regions listed above, the spinal cord, and the dorsal root ganglia. Most cases are associated with anti-Hu antibodies (which are also frequently associated with limbic encephalitis, sensory neuronopathy, and cerebellar degeneration). Small cell lung cancer is the most commonly associated malignancy.

- Other, less common targets include the optic nerves, retina, and the dorsal root ganglia.

Diagnosis

Workup should include an MRI, EEG, and both serum and CSF serologic testing (most of the autoantibodies are best tested for in the serum, but some, most notably anti-NMDA, are more sensitive in the CSF). When appropriate, a comprehensive malignancy screen should be performed as well.

Treatment

Treatment with immunotherapy (most often corticosteroids, IV immunoglobulin, and plasmapheresis; rituximab is typically second or third line) should never be delayed by antibody characterization or malignancy diagnosis in patients presenting with a classic autoimmune encephalitis syndrome. Once the specific syndrome is identified, treatment can be narrowed and refined. Recovery is variable but can be complete or near complete if treatment is started early.

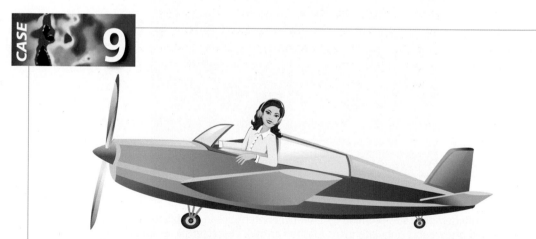

Your Patient's Follow-up: Emma presented with internuclear ophthalmoplegia, a finding that is highly suggestive of MS in a patient her age. Her history of an episode of leg numbness a year earlier would constitute a second lesion disseminated in time and space, but historical evidence has to be carefully scrutinized in all patients. Emma needed an MRI, and it confirmed the presence of several lesions, some clinically silent, consistent with MS. She was treated with high-dose glucocorticoids, and her double vision resolved. She was started on disease-modifying therapy soon after. Several years out she continues to do extremely well with only one mild attack of optic neuritis and no progressive disability.

You now know:

- | MS is the result of immune-mediated demyelination and axonal destruction of neurons in the CNS.

- | It is classically defined by the dissemination of clinical attacks in space and time; the use of MRI and testing for CSF-specific oligoclonal bands has broadened the definition. This is important, because early diagnosis allows for early treatment, which can modify the course of the disease.

- | Most patients with MS have relapsing remitting disease, for which there are many disease modifying medications; some patients will have primary progressive disease, and we now have medication for that as well.

- | One more time—early diagnosis and treatment matters, and even patients with clinically isolated syndrome (CIS) should be considered for disease modifying therapy.

- | Acute exacerbations are treated with several days of oral or IV corticosteroids, but steroids do not modify long-term outcome.

- | When chronic, disabling complications develop, symptomatic therapy is available that can, in many patients, significantly improve quality of life.

- | Women with MS can have normal pregnancies and safely breastfeed.

- | The differential diagnosis of MS is broad and includes neuromyelitis optica spectrum disorder (NMOSD) and acute disseminated encephalomyelitis (ADEM).

- | Autoimmune encephalitis comes in many varieties, and the list of relevant autoantibodies is growing by the day. The good news? The clinical presentation is often easily recognizable, and you do not need to wait for antibody confirmation to begin treatment.

The Spinal Cord

10

In this chapter, you will learn:

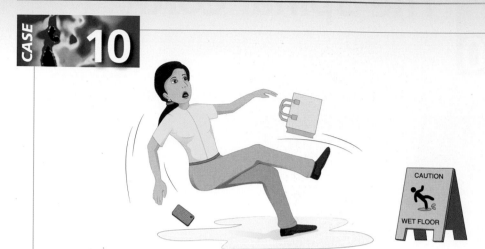

CASE 10

Your Patient: Priya, a 22-year-old marketing executive, presents to the emergency department after slipping and falling in the street this morning. She says she's been feeling weak for the past few days, with tingling in both her feet and progressive difficulty walking. When she woke up this morning her symptoms were worse, and she was on her way to see her doctor when she fell. When she got to his office, he sent her to the emergency department for an expedited workup. On examination, her vitals are stable. She is weak in both of her legs, left slightly worse than right, flexor muscles slightly worse than extensors. Her ankle jerk and patellar reflexes are brisk, and she has several beats of clonus at each ankle. Her sensation to light touch is decreased in both legs, and when you test pin prick sensation with a safety pin, you find that she feels the prick much less sharply everywhere from her toes up to a band that circles her waist just a few inches below her navel. She has no pain. What's the next step in your management?

In this chapter, we will focus on how to recognize spinal cord pathology, which is often serious and sometimes a medical emergency. Chapter 1 has already provided you with a detailed look at the motor and sensory tracts as they ascend and descend the cord, but as Chapter 1 is by now many pages in your past, let's start with a quick review of basic cord anatomy.

Basic Anatomy

The spinal cord begins where the brainstem ends, and extends (in adults) to approximately the L1 vertebra. The cord itself is part of the CNS, serving as a conduit between the brain and the rest of the body.

- There are 33 vertebrae. Twenty-four are articulating—7 cervical, 12 thoracic, and 5 lumbar vertebrae—and 9 are fused—5 sacral vertebrae (fused into the sacrum) and 4 coccygeal vertebrae (fused into the coccyx, or "tailbone").

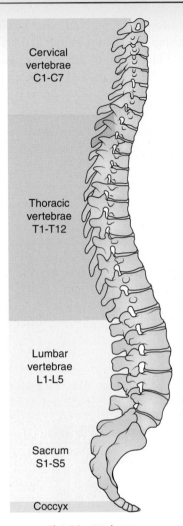

Cervical
vertebrae
C1-C7

Thoracic
vertebrae
T1-T12

Lumbar
vertebrae
L1-L5

Sacrum
S1-S5

Coccyx

The 33 vertebrae.

- There are 31 paired spinal nerves that exit the cord: 8 cervical, 12 thoracic, 5 lumbar, 5 sacral, and 1 coccygeal. The C1 to C7 spinal nerves exit the cord *above* their corresponding vertebrae (*e.g.*, the third cervical nerve, C3, exits between the second and third cervical vertebrae), whereas C8 on down exit *below* (*e.g.*, T2 exits between the second and third thoracic vertebrae). Each nerve contains a dorsal root (carrying sensory afferents) and a ventral root (carrying motor efferents).

- The lower extent of the cord contains 2 important structures. The first is the ***conus medullaris***, the very caudal tip of the cord, which terminates at approximately the L1 vertebra (in neonates, it is closer to L3). The second is the ***cauda equina***, a bundle of nerve roots derived from the second lumbar cord segment to the first coccygeal cord segment that extends below the cord (cauda equina is Latin for "horse's tail" reflecting its bundled and splayed appearance).

- Like the brain, the spinal cord is covered in 3 layers of meninges. The dura (the toughest, outermost layer) extends approximately to the S2 vertebral level (caudal to where the cord ends) and inserts into the coccyx. The arachnoid also extends to S2 but closes on itself, forming a sealed sac of cerebrospinal fluid (CSF) that bathes the cord. The pia (the most delicate, innermost layer) clings to the cord until it gathers together at L1 (where the cord ends) into a tight, string-like bundle called the ***filum terminale*** that helps to anchor the cord in place and, along with the dura, inserts into the coccyx at S2.

It is critical to distinguish *cord* levels from *vertebral* levels. The termination of the *cord* is at roughly the L1 *vertebral* level, whereas the arachnoid space extends to the S2 *vertebral* level, resulting in a large, safely accessible space from which to obtain CSF via lumbar puncture (see Chapter 1 for details).

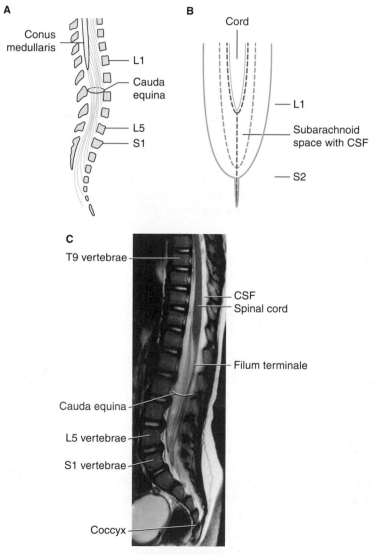

(*A*) The lower spinal cord. (*B*) The three layers of meninges surrounding the cord. The dura (pink) ends at S2 and inserts into the coccyx. The arachnoid (orange) forms a closed sac of CSF that bathes the cord. The pia (purple) gathers into the filum terminale and then, like the dura, inserts into the coccyx at S2. (*C*) What this all actually looks like on an MRI showing the lower thoracic and lumbar spine. You can see the splayed appearance of the bundle of nerve roots extending below the cord. (*C*, modified from Haines DE. *Neuroanatomy Atlas in Clinical Context*. 10th ed. Wolters Kluwer; 2018.)

- The major *motor tract* that descends through the cord is the corticospinal tract. These neurons start out in the motor cortex of the brain, run down the cord mostly in the lateral white matter, and synapse on lower motor neurons (LMNs; the anterior horn cells), which then exit the cord and travel to their target muscles. The two major *sensory tracts* are the dorsal column/medial lemniscus tract and spinothalamic tract, which carry pressure/vibration/proprioception and pain/temperature, respectively. See Chapter 1 for a detailed review.

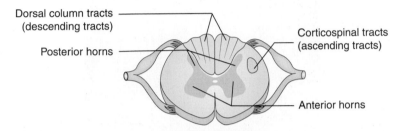

Dorsal column tracts (descending tracts)

Posterior horns

Corticospinal tracts (ascending tracts)

Anterior horns

The gray matter of the cord (shaped like a butterfly) is organized into two ventral (anterior) horns and two dorsal (posterior) horns. The surrounding white matter, which carries the ascending and descending tracts, includes the ventral, dorsal, and lateral funiculi. Note that this organization is opposite that which we see in the brain, where the gray matter of the cortex lies on the outside and the white matter tracts lie deeper within.

Acute Spinal Cord Compression

Acute cord compression is a true neurologic emergency. Despite improvements in early diagnosis and treatment, it remains an often devastating and debilitating event. Although treatment of cord compression is more often *neurosurgical* than neurological, it is important to understand the pathogenesis of cord compression and, especially, to be able to recognize it when you see it. You must know how to distinguish the acute-onset weakness or numbness caused by cord compression from that caused by confounding diagnoses such as stroke, Guillain-Barre syndrome, or seizure (among others) so you can quickly help to guide management. Treatment depends entirely on the underlying etiology.

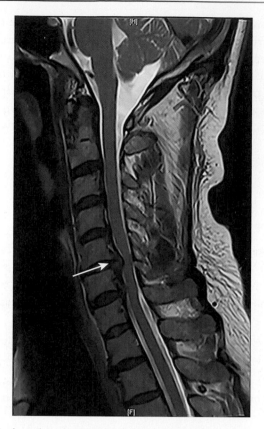

An example of cervical cord compression by a herniated disc (white arrow), on an MRI. (Modified from Grauer JN. OKU12 Orthopaedic Knowledge Update. Wolters Kluwer.)

Causes

Important causes of acute spinal cord compression include:

- *Trauma.* Motor vehicle accidents, sports injuries, falls, and gunshot wounds are the most common causes of traumatic spinal cord injury. Over 12,000 new cases of traumatic spinal cord injury occur every year in the United States.

- *Malignancy.* Almost any cancer can metastasize to the spine, but prostate, lung, and breast cancer as well as multiple myeloma are the most likely to involve the vertebrae. Once seeded within the vertebrae, these tumors can invade the epidural space, resulting in cord compression from both mass effect and pathologic compression fractures as well as from the obstruction of venous blood outflow and subsequent cord edema.

- *Epidural abscess.* Risk factors include intravenous (IV) drug abuse, immunocompromised state, spinal trauma, and spinal surgery. Epidural abscesses classically present with a triad of symptoms: fever, focal back pain, and neurologic deficits. *Staphylococcus aureus* is the most common causative organism.

- *Epidural hematoma.* Spinal epidural hematomas are usually the consequence of spinal trauma or surgery, often in patients with a baseline propensity to bleed, such as those on anticoagulation or who have thrombocytopenia. Spontaneous spinal epidural hematomas are rare. Because they are most often caused by venous (as opposed to arterial) bleeding, symptoms tend to evolve over hours to days, although they can sometimes present more acutely.

Clinical Presentation

Spinal cord anatomy is complicated, but recognizing acute cord compression is usually pretty clear-cut. The most common presenting symptoms are listed below. No matter what medical or surgical field you choose, *learn these red flags*: you will likely encounter hundreds if not thousands of patients with back pain over the course of your careers, the vast majority of whom are not experiencing acute cord compression, so knowing when to be worried for cord compression and when to initiate immediate evaluation and treatment is crucial.

- *Bilateral extremity weakness.* Patients who present with acute-onset weakness of both arms and/or both legs, without any facial weakness[1] have cord pathology until proven otherwise. The weakness is often asymmetric (*i.e.*, one leg is affected more than the other) and is often associated with at least 1 or 2 of the other features listed below. This is not to say that all patients with bilateral leg weakness have acute cord compression (Guillain-Barre syndrome, for instance, can cause this, although it typically progresses over the course of days, not hours; see page 284). But patients with bilateral weakness of the arms and/or legs almost always need an expedited workup to exclude cord compression before you consider other causes.

- *A sensory level.* A sensory level is defined as the most caudal (that is, the lowest, or furthest from the head) dermatomal level (see Box 10.2 on page 261) at which both light touch and pinprick are intact, and it indicates a possible cord lesion either AT or slightly ABOVE that level. Patients with decreased sensation to light touch and pinprick below their nipples, for instance, have a T4 sensory level, suggesting that their lesion is around T4 or above (more precisely, the lesion is likely closer to T6 or above, thanks to Lissauer tract: if you remember from Chapter 1, the first-order neurons of the spinothalamic tract run up alongside the cord in what's known as Lissauer tract for about 2 vertebral levels before they enter the cord. Don't worry too much about this; it is rarely clinically relevant).

---

[1]We need to make an important distinction here between facial weakness, which cannot be caused by a spinal cord lesion, and numbness, which can be. Because the nuclei of CN5 (which provide sensation to the face) are huge, spanning most of the brainstem into the cervical cord, cervical spine lesions can cause facial *numbness*. Thus, although face *weakness* cannot be attributed to a spinal cord lesion, face *numbness* can, albeit rarely.

Box 10.1 Bilateral ACA Pathology

Acute pathology affecting the bilateral anterior cerebral artery (ACA) territory in the brain is one other cause of sudden-onset bilateral lower extremity weakness (see homunculus below; the ACAs supply the cortex predominantly responsible for lower extremity movement). Rapidly expanding or bleeding parasagittal tumors are one possible cause. Strokes due to azygous ACA occlusion (a circle of Willis variant in which the anterior communicating artery is absent and the proximal segments of both ACAs form a single trunk) are another.

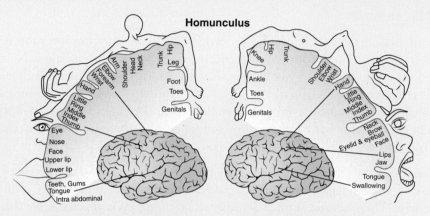

A reminder of the homunculus in the cerebral cortex, demonstrating the proximity of the two sides to each other where motor input to the lower extremities originates.

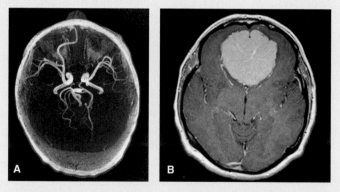

(*A*) An azygous ACA. If the single ACA trunk is occluded, both ACA territories are at risk of ischemia. (*B*) A big parasagittal meningioma. *A*, Courtesy of Dr. Roberto Schubert, Radiopaedia.org, rID: 17059. *B*, Reprinted from Haines DE. *Neuroanatomy Atlas in Clinical Context*. 10th ed. Wolters Kluwer; 2018.

• *Bowel or bladder dysfunction.* Depending on the etiology, patients with acute cord compression may present with underactivity, overactivity, or normal activity of bowel and bladder pathways. Trauma may cause a period of neurogenic spinal shock (see the Examination section on page 262) resulting in flaccid bowel and

Box 10.2 Dermatomal Landmarks

Here are some useful dermatome landmarks to know. A dermatome is an area of skin supplied by sensory nerves from a single spinal nerve root.

C3	High turtleneck
T4	Nipple
T10	Navel
L1	Inguinal ligament
L4	Patella

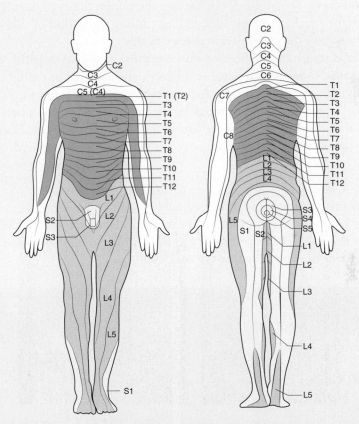

The dermatome person. You do not need to memorize this individual, but it will serve as a great reference.

bladder tone, which result in fecal impaction and overflow urinary incontinence. Other types of compression above the conus may disrupt coordination between the sphincters and the musculature of the bowel or bladder wall, leading to a combination of urgency and incomplete evacuation. Conus medullaris syndrome, discussed later, leads to flaccid tone resembling posttraumatic neurogenic shock.

Box 10.3 The ASIA Impairment Scale

The ASIA (American Spinal Injury Association) Impairment Scale is a standardized neurologic examination that assesses the distribution and degree of both motor and sensory dysfunction and is used to help classify injury severity and set goals for rehabilitation.

Examination

Immediately following acute spinal cord trauma, patients can present with **spinal shock**, the loss of all spinal cord function below the level of the lesion. Flaccid paralysis and areflexia are characteristic. Other symptoms include an atonic bladder with overflow incontinence, bowel distension with severe constipation, diminished rectal tone, and sometimes significant autonomic dysfunction. Spinal shock can last anywhere from hours to days before receding to reveal the patient's true neurologic function. So, during the period of shock, you cannot accurately prognosticate the patient's outcome or recovery.

With time, the examination will become what is referred to as a **myelopathic examination** (*i.e.,* an examination consistent with spinal cord injury), characterized by typical upper motor neuron (UMN) findings such as spasticity, hyperreflexia, and clonus below the level of the lesion. Spinal cord injury is primarily an upper motor neuron injury (with the exception of the few lower motor neurons that are affected at the level of the lesion), and thus the examination is characterized by upper motor neuron-type symptoms (see page 20 for a review).

Triage and Evaluation

Patients with traumatic spinal cord injuries should be immobilized and taken directly to a hospital setting. In any patient in whom you suspect cord compression, an MRI of the spine is almost always necessary. A CT will show you bone (and can therefore show narrowing of the spinal canal), but does not visualize the cord itself.

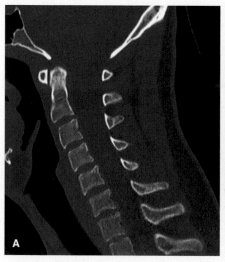 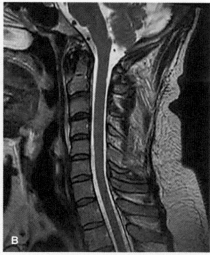

You can see the difference between the CT (*A*) of the cervical spine (which nicely visualizes the vertebrae, but can't tell you much of anything about the cord) and the MRI (*B*), which clearly delineates the cord and surrounding thecal space. (*A*, reprinted from Benzel EC. *Cervical Spine.* 5th ed. Wolters Kluwer; 2012. *B*, modified from Berquist TH. *MRI of the Musculoskeletal System.* 6th ed. Wolters Kluwer; 2012.)

We said this in Chapter 9, but it is worth repeating: if you are concerned about damage to the spinal *cord*, order cervical and thoracic spine MRIs. There is no need for a lumbar scan. The cord ends at approximately L1; thus, a lumbar spine MRI predominantly visualizes the cauda equina, not the cord. If you aren't sure where the lesion localizes, you can order an MRI of the entire spine (often called a "spinal survey"), but the quality tends to be worse than a dedicated cervical or thoracic scan. This should serve as an important reminder of why it's important to know your anatomy!

Once you diagnose cord compression, treatment depends entirely on the underlying cause. Trauma may require surgery; malignancy may require radiation; epidural abscess may require antibiotics and drainage.

Spinal Cord Syndromes

There are several specific syndromes resulting from spinal cord compression that deserve special mention because, if you recognize them, they can quickly help you localize the problem and institute rapid treatment where appropriate.

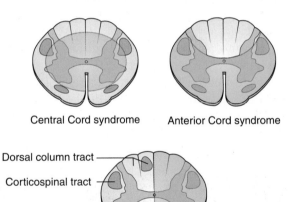

Central Cord syndrome   Anterior Cord syndrome

Dorsal column tract

Corticospinal tract

Spinothalamic tract

Brown-Séquard syndrome

Three important, incomplete spinal cord syndromes (the green areas show the site of the lesions).

Brown-Sequard Syndrome

Brown-Sequard syndrome results from hemisection of the spinal cord. It's worth looking back at Chapter 1 to review the anatomy of the sensory and motor tracts before trying to understand this syndrome. In most cases of spinal cord injury, the symptoms are often incomplete and mixed—the cord is rarely perfectly hemisected, and the damage is rarely perfectly symmetric—but the symptoms of a "textbook" case are listed in full below.

Below the level of the spinal cord lesion, you'd expect to see:

- Ipsilateral upper motor neuron (UMN) symptoms (due to corticospinal tract damage)
- Ipsilateral loss of vibration, pressure, and proprioception (dorsal column damage)
- Contralateral loss of pain and temperature (spinothalamic tract damage; remember, the spinothalamic tract crosses immediately when it enters the cord. Further, because of Lissauer tract, pain and temperature sensation should be lost a few levels *below* the lesion)

At the level of the lesion, you'd expect to see:

- Ipsilateral lower motor neuron (LMN) symptoms (anterior horn cell damage)
- Ipsilateral loss of all sensation (damage to the spinothalamic tract fibers as they cross)

Causes include trauma, extrinsic compressive lesions, tumors, and multiple sclerosis plaques. Treatment depends entirely on the underlying etiology.

Anterior and Central Cord Syndromes

Anterior cord syndrome is most commonly the result of trauma or infarction of the anterior spinal artery (which supplies blood flow to the anterior two-thirds of the cord). Symptoms include bilateral weakness and loss of pain and temperature sensation below the level of the lesion, with preservation of vibration, pressure, and proprioception due to sparing of the dorsal column tracts.

Central cord syndrome is most often seen in older patients with degenerative cervical spine disease and in younger patients with hyperextension injuries (*e.g.*, from a rear-end car collision); it can also be due to an expanding syrinx, a fluid-filled cavity within the cord (often seen in association with Chiari 1 malformations or as a consequence of previous cord trauma). A suspended sensory level (*i.e.*, a loss of sensation in a band- or cape-like distribution across the arms and upper back with retained sensory function in the trunk and legs) due to damage of the spinothalamic tract fibers as they cross is characteristic, although, if the lesion extends sufficiently outward to hit the ascending sensory tracts, central cord lesions can also cause bilateral loss of sensation below the level of the lesion. If weakness is present, it affects both upper extremities more than the lower extremities, because the fibers supplying the arms run more medially within the corticospinal tract than the fibers supplying the legs.

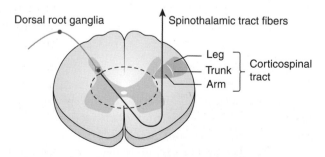

Central cord syndrome often only affects the crossing fibers of the spinothalamic tract, resulting in a suspended sensory level or cape-like loss of sensation at approximately the level(s) of the lesion, with intact sensation both above and below. Also note how the motor fibers of the lateral corticospinal tract supplying the arms run medially to those supplying the legs and are therefore more likely to be compromised.

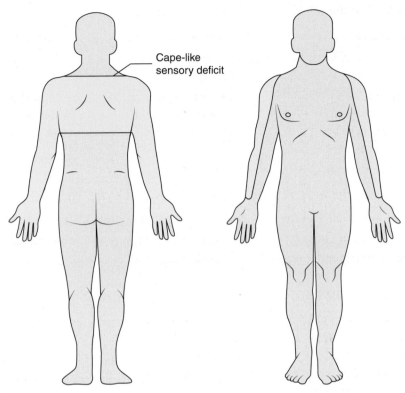

Cape-like
sensory deficit

The cape-like sensory loss that can be caused by central cord lesions.

Conus Medullaris and Cauda Equina Syndromes

Conus medullaris syndrome is a constellation of signs and symptoms attributed to injury of the conus; likewise, cauda equina syndrome is the result of injury to the cauda (and therefore technically not a true "cord" syndrome). As with Brown-Sequard, these syndromes are rarely complete and can have significant overlap, but understanding the differences is useful.

	Conus Medullaris Syndrome	Cauda Equina Syndrome
Due to	Compression at vertebral level L1/L2	Compression of 2/more spinal roots below L2
Characteristic presentation	Early bowel and bladder symptoms	Prominent lower back/leg pain
Motor symptoms	Mixed UMN/LMN (usually mild)	LMN (often asymmetric)
Sensory symptoms	Saddle anesthesia (S3-5 dermatomes)	Involves the dermatomes of whichever roots are affected
Autonomic symptoms	Urinary retention and overflow incontinence, impotence	Less common than with conus medullaris syndrome

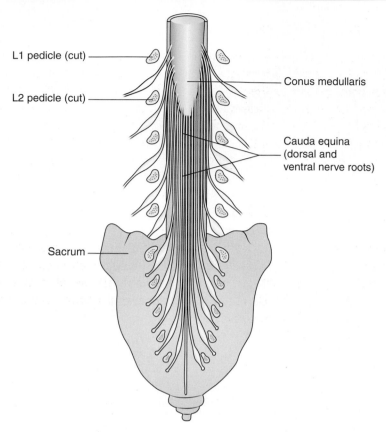

L1 pedicle (cut)

L2 pedicle (cut)

Conus medullaris

Cauda equina
(dorsal and
ventral nerve roots)

Sacrum

A quick reminder of what we're talking about.

The conus contains sacral cord segments and nerve roots. Compression, most commonly the result of vertebral fracture, trauma, or disc herniation (see Box 10.4), tends to present acutely, with early and prominent bowel and bladder dysfunction, typically mild and bilateral leg weakness (the lesion can and often does affect both the descending UMNs in the cord and the LMNs exiting the spinal column, since everything is crammed in together very tightly here), and saddle anesthesia.

Lesions at or below the L2 vertebrae can damage the cauda, which contains lumbar and sacral nerve roots. Causes include disc herniation (most commonly), lumbar spinal stenosis, epidural abscess and tumors, as well as a myriad of inflammatory causes including sarcoid and chronic inflammatory demyelinating polyneuropathy. Lower back pain and pain radiating down into the legs are common. Lower extremity weakness is more often asymmetric (the nerves are more spread out here), and sensory loss is in the dermatomal distribution of whichever nerve roots are affected (*e.g.*, if nerve roots S3–5 are affected, it will, as with conus, present with saddle anesthesia).

In either case, empiric steroids can be considered in an effort to limit edema, although the evidence regarding their efficacy is mixed and the risk of potential complications (particularly infectious complications) must be weighted against potential benefit. An MRI is almost always helpful for diagnosis. If an infectious or inflammatory condition is suspected, a lumbar puncture is also necessary. Treatment depends on the underlying etiology: surgery for disc herniation; radiation for cancer; steroids, plasmapheresis (PLEX), or IV immunoglobulin (IVIG) for an inflammatory demyelinating polyradiculopathy (see page 284); *etc.*

Box 10.4 Disc Herniation

Discs are located between the vertebrae and act like cushions to help support and protect the spinal column. They are composed of an outer fibrous ring (called the annulus fibrosus) and an inner, hydrated layer (the nucleus pulposus). Disc herniation occurs when the nucleus pulposus is squeezed out through a crack in the annulus fibrosus. Herniation can happen anywhere, but the lumbar spine is the most common location (hence disc herniation is high on the differential diagnosis for conus and cauda syndromes). Many disc herniations are asymptomatic. Symptomatic herniation usually starts with weeks to months of vague, aching back pain (due to gradual degeneration of the disc and the ligaments holding the disc in place), followed by the sudden onset of severe pain, tingling, and/or numbness that spreads into the ipsilateral leg due to spinal nerve compression, usually in the setting of exercise or a Valsalva maneuver (coughing and sneezing are common precipitants). Older patients are at higher risk, but disc herniation can occur in younger individuals, often athletes, as well. Treatment includes physical therapy, anti-inflammatories, and muscle relaxants. Many patients do well and improve on their own, but surgery is an option if these treatments fail.

 Transverse Myelitis

The term *transverse myelitis* refers to inflammation of the spinal cord. It tends to present subacutely, over hours to days, with progressive weakness of both arms and/or legs, paresthesias, a sensory level, autonomic symptoms including bowel and bladder incontinence, sexual dysfunction, and lower back and leg pain.

Transverse myelitis is merely a descriptive term, referring to segmental cord inflammation. Patients with transverse myelitis require an extensive evaluation to determine the actual etiologic diagnosis, which guides subsequent treatment. There are many potential underlying etiologies, so let's break them down into just a few categories:

- *Infectious* (West Nile virus, Zika virus, herpes simplex virus, HIV, human T cell leukemia virus type 1, Lyme disease, and syphilis are a few examples)
- *Systemic autoimmune diseases* (transverse myelitis can be associated with lupus, sarcoidosis, and Sjogren syndrome)
- *CNS autoimmune diseases* (multiple sclerosis, neuromyelitis optica, acute disseminated encephalomyelitis)
- *Paraneoplastic* (most often associated with anti-Hu and anti-CRMP5 antibodies; more on these in Chapter 16)
- *Spontaneous* (idiopathic; the cause of as many as 30% of cases remains unknown despite a comprehensive evaluation)

Diagnosis requires an MRI, which will show a discrete contrast-enhancing lesion in the cord spanning 1 or more vertebral segments (if the lesion spans 3 or more segments, it is termed *longitudinally extensive transverse myelitis,* or LETM[2]). The CSF should, in most cases, be inflammatory, with pleocytosis and elevated protein. A series of assays for viral nucleic acid, specific antibodies, oligoclonal bands, and immunoglobulin synthesis rates are performed on both the CSF and serum to further identify the etiology.

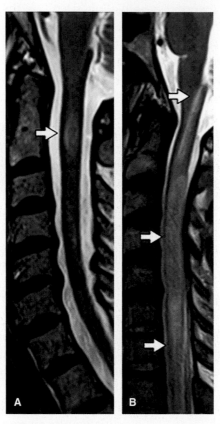

(*A*) Transverse myelitis in a patient with multiple sclerosis and (*B*) with neuromyelitis optica. Arrows are pointing at the hyperintense cord lesions consistent with transverse myelitis. (Reprinted from Louis ED, Mayer SA, Noble JM. *Merritt's Neurology*. 14th ed. Wolters Kluwer; 2021.)

Treatment depends on the underlying etiology, but as you can imagine, this is not always immediately apparent and the workup can take several days. When the cause is not known upfront, first-line treatment consists of high-dose IV corticosteroids, which should be given empirically and rapidly to prevent progressive symptoms. Plasmapheresis (PLEX) as well as immunosuppressive agents such as cyclosporine, mycophenolate, and rituximab are also used for refractory cases.

---

[2]If you remember from Chapter 9, cord lesions from multiple sclerosis tend to be small, or "short segment," whereas cord lesions associated with neuromyelitis optica typically fit into the "LETM" classification.

Toxic/Metabolic Spinal Cord Disorders

Vitamin B12 deficiency can result in degeneration of the dorsolateral white matter spinal columns, a disorder known as ***subacute combined degeneration***. This condition presents with a gradually progressive, upper motor neuron-type weakness (due to degeneration of the corticospinal tracts that run in the lateral white matter), paresthesias, and potentially disabling sensory ataxia (due to involvement of the sensory fibers that run in the dorsal column/medial lemniscus tract). An elevated serum methylmalonic acid is a more reliable diagnostic test than a decreased serum B12. MRI can show high T2 signal in the dorsolateral columns of the spinal cord. Aggressive treatment with B12 can stop progression of the disease. See page 281 for a review on the other sequelae of B12 deficiency.

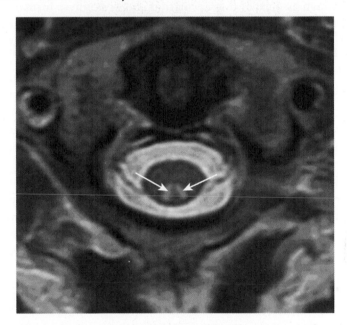

T2 hyperintensities (white arrows) involving the dorsolateral spinal columns on axial MRI, consistent with subacute combined degeneration. (Modified from Kumar A, Singh AK. Teaching neuroimage: inverted V sign in subacute combined degeneration of spinal cord. *Neurology*. 2009;72(1):e4.)

Copper deficiency, which results most commonly from malabsorption in the setting of gastrointestinal surgery (such as gastric bypass) or zinc toxicity (zinc inhibits copper absorption), can mimic subacute combined degeneration. Associated anemia (which can be micro, macro, or normocytic, as opposed to the megaloblastic macrocytic anemia caused by B12 deficiency) and leukopenia are common. Treatment is with copper supplementation.

Nitrous oxide is a common drug of abuse, in large part because it can be obtained so easily. It is, for example, used to fill balloons and as a propellant in cannisters of whipped cream. When inhaled, it creates a sense of euphoria (its use for entertainment gave rise to so-called laughing parties). However, it can also cause irreversible inactivation of vitamin B12.

This most often occurs after chronic exposure to nitrous oxide, but it can also occur quickly, even after a single exposure, in patients with baseline low levels of B12. The resulting dorsolateral spinal cord dysfunction is identical to that caused by B12 deficiency from other causes. Treatment requires immediate cessation of nitrous oxide exposure and high-dose B12 supplementation.

 ## Lumbar Spinal Stenosis

Lumbar spinal stenosis, or narrowing of the bony lumbar spinal canal, is not primarily a spinal *cord* problem, but it is an incredibly common cause of disability in the elderly population and one that you will likely encounter regardless of what field of medicine you choose. It is most often caused by degenerative disease (also called *spondylosis*) affecting the vertebrae. Although associated disc herniation and osteophyte formation can compress the cord (if the T12/L1 vertebrae are affected; remember, the cord ends at approximately L1) or the cauda equina, most often it impinges on the neural foramina where the spinal roots exit.

Radicular back and leg pain[3] that worsens with standing and walking and improves with sitting and leaning forward, known as *neurogenic claudication*, is characteristic. It is thought that walking and standing increase the metabolic demand of nerves and narrow the space within the lumbar canal, resulting in worsening ischemia and compression of already-injured nerves. Bilateral but often asymmetric sensory loss and weakness of the lower extremities are also common.

Diagnosis requires imaging demonstrating narrowing of the lumbar spinal canal (MRI is the gold standard) *as well as* characteristic clinical symptoms. Physical therapy and nonsteroidal anti-inflammatory drugs are first-line therapies; current evidence does not support the utility of epidural steroid injections. Surgery is typically reserved for those who do not respond to medical management and must be carefully considered on a case-by-case basis, as there is limited evidence demonstrating clear benefit.

Box 10.5 Cervical Stenosis

Cervical stenosis, like lumbar stenosis, is most often the result of degenerative vertebral disease. It tends to present gradually, with gait dysfunction and/or hand clumsiness; frank weakness is less common. Diagnosis and management are much the same as with lumbar stenosis. *Degenerative thoracic disease* is significantly less common than either cervical or lumbar disease.

---

[3]*Radiculopathy* refers to symptoms attributed to nerve *root* compression. Unlike lesions confined to the spinal cord, which don't tend to be painful, nerve root compression *hurts*. The pain is typically described as sharp with an almost electric quality, shooting down whichever nerve is affected (for more information, take a look at Box 11.8 in the upcoming chapter on Peripheral Neuropathies).

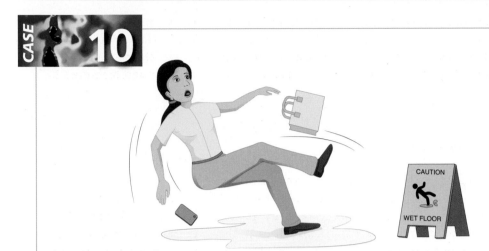

Your patient's follow-up: You are concerned about spinal cord injury and immediately order an MRI of the cervical and thoracic spine. You don't know what exactly is going on, but given Priya's bilateral lower extremity symptoms, sensory level, and hyperreflexia, you have been able to quickly localize whatever it is to the spinal cord. Luckily, the imaging is done quickly and shows a chunky T2 hyperintense lesion within the cord spanning several thoracic vertebral levels. She is started on empiric high-dose steroids and admitted. A few days later, her aquaporin-4 antibody comes back positive, confirming the diagnosis of neuromyelitis optica. She undergoes one course of PLEX following her steroid treatment, with significant improvement in her symptoms, and is discharged soon after with close follow-up.

You now know:

- | When to suspect acute cord compression, and what to do about it.
- | How to differentiate and diagnose conus medullaris syndrome and cauda equina syndrome.
- | How to recognize, diagnose, and treat lumbar spinal stenosis.
- | The many potential etiologies of transverse myelitis, including infectious, systemic autoimmune, CNS autoimmune, and paraneoplastic causes.
- | The presentation and treatment of vitamin B12 deficiency and other toxic/metabolic causes of subacute combined degeneration.

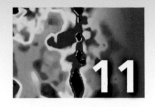

11 The Peripheral Neuropathies and Amyotrophic Lateral Sclerosis

In this chapter, you will learn:

1 | That amyotrophic lateral sclerosis (ALS) presents with weakness characterized by both upper and lower motor neuron findings

2 | That length-dependent sensorimotor neuropathy is extremely common and has multiple causes, but it can often be easily diagnosed with a basic neurologic examination and some simple laboratory tests

3 | When to suspect Guillain-Barre syndrome, and the importance of expediting evaluation and treatment

4 | How centering your diagnosis of peripheral neuropathy around a few key points—acute versus chronic, motor versus sensory, symmetric versus asymmetric—will allow you to figure out who does and does not need to be evaluated and treated quickly

5 | That mononeuropathies, such as carpal tunnel syndrome, often result from compression or injury, and how they should be managed

6 | All the different ways that diabetes can wreak havoc on the peripheral nervous system

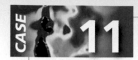

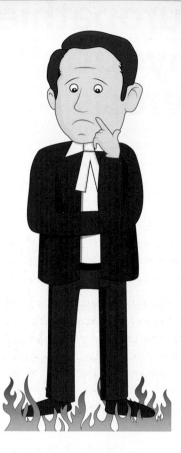

Your Patient: Allen, a 50-year-old lawyer, presents with numbness and tingling in his feet for the past year. He has no other symptoms, and his past medical history is benign. He is on no medications. He is mildly overweight. Your neurologic examination confirms decreased sensation to vibration in the lower extremities as well as diminished ankle reflexes. He is concerned that he might have diabetes—both his parents have type 2 diabetes—but his fasting glucose is 96 mg/dL and his hemoglobin A1c is 5.6%, both normal values. What are your next steps in his evaluation?

It seems as if the central nervous system gets all the attention. It is, after all, the essence of who we are. But don't be too quick to write off the peripheral nervous system (PNS). Without it, the CNS would be pretty helpless. We wouldn't be able to sense the world around us, feed and dress ourselves, or pound away at a computer keyboard to write these sentences.

This chapter is devoted to the peripheral neuropathies, and there are a lot of them. However, you will discover that their evaluation is straightforward. When confronted with a patient in whom you suspect a peripheral neuropathy, always ask yourself if the symptoms are:

- Acute or chronic?
- Symmetric or asymmetric?
- Predominantly sensory or motor? And finally,
- Localizable to one or multiple nerves?

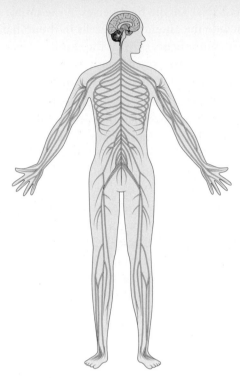

Remove the brain and spinal cord, and you are looking at the peripheral nervous system. Well, not exactly. This statement is a bit of an oversimplification. There are a few important exceptions: the cranial nerves (except for CN1 and CN2), as well as the anterior horn cells within the spinal cord (the cell bodies of lower motor neurons), are part of the peripheral nervous system as well.

We will start this chapter with an illness that afflicts *both* the CNS and PNS, a smooth transition for us, but a devastating illness for those who are afflicted.

Amyotrophic Lateral Sclerosis (ALS)

Amyotrophic lateral sclerosis (ALS) is a disease of unknown cause that affects both upper and lower motor neurons. It is progressive and uniformly fatal. Although there are some familial cases with an identifiable underlying genetic mutation, most cases are sporadic and idiopathic. ALS is rare, with an incidence of less than 3 per 100,000 person-years. However, this number has been slowly increasing over the past few decades, likely a result, at least in part, of our longer life expectancy.

Symptoms. The key to diagnosing ALS is to recognize the involvement of *both* upper and lower motor neurons. As a reminder from Chapter 1 (this material should look familiar!):

- *Upper motor neurons* (UMNs) include all neurons that run in the motor pathways above the lower motor neurons. These include the neurons in the corticospinal and corticobulbar tracts. Weakness, increased tone and spasticity, hyperreflexia, clonus, and upgoing toes (aka the Babinski sign) are classic UMN findings.

- *Lower motor neurons* (LMNs) are the final nerves in the motor pathways that innervate the muscles. These include the anterior horn cells in the spinal cord and the cranial nerves that have motor components (*i.e.*, all the cranial nerves except 1, 2, and 8). Like UMN disease, LMN disease presents with weakness, but it can also cause muscle atrophy, decreased muscle tone, hyporeflexia, and fasciculations (or muscle twitching).

Patients with ALS will all eventually have findings consistent with both UMN and LMN disease. Initially, however, there may be evidence of only upper or lower motor neuron disease, complicating the diagnosis. The most common presentation is asymmetric limb weakness, typically involving the hands and/or feet, although a significant minority (~20%) of patients will first present with weakness of the bulbar muscles.

Bulbar symptoms (*i.e.*, symptoms localizable to the medulla), such as dysarthria and dysphagia, are also common in ALS and can be caused by either UMN disease (specifically the corticobulbar tracts, which begin in the motor cortex and synapse on the motor nuclei of the cranial nerves in the brainstem) or LMN disease (the brainstem cranial nerves themselves: 9, 10, 11, and 12). *Pseudobulbar affect* is a common UMN bulbar symptom that's characterized by inappropriate laughing or crying, often triggered by stimuli that under normal conditions would not have elicited such responses. Spastic speech, increased masseter tone, and laryngospasm (often described as a brief squeezing sensation in the throat) are other common UMN bulbar symptoms. Tongue fasciculations are the most common LMN bulbar symptom.

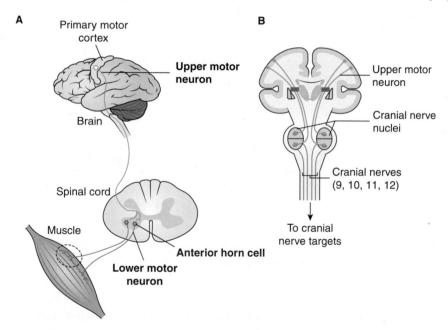

(*A*) The upper motor neurons of the corticospinal tract begin in the motor cortex and project downward, through the corona radiata, internal capsule, and brainstem (where they cross to the contralateral side) into the spinal cord where they synapse on lower motor neurons. (*B*) The upper motor neurons of the corticobulbar tract also begin in the motor cortex but synapse in the brainstem (again, after crossing) on the nuclei of CN9, CN10, CN11 and CN12.

About half of patients with ALS will ultimately exhibit some degree of cognitive impairment. Some patients may have sensory complaints, such as paresthesias, but the sensory examination is almost always normal. If not, you need to consider other diagnoses.

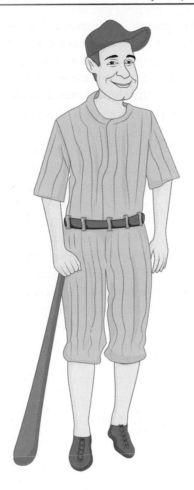

Lou Gehrig, the celebrated Hall of Fame baseball player who played 17 seasons for the New York Yankees, was diagnosed with ALS in his 30s. The disease is now commonly and colloquially referred to as Lou Gehrig disease.

Diagnosis. The diagnosis of ALS is made by history and neurologic examination, and it is confirmed by electromyography (EMG) and nerve conduction studies (NCS). Magnetic resonance imaging MRI of the brain and spinal cord are done in order to rule out other possible causes; MRI is usually normal in ALS, although you may (rarely) see T2 signal changes beginning in the motor cortex and extending down into the corticospinal tracts. Cerebrospinal fluid (CSF) analysis can also be useful to rule out other causes of polyneuropathy, such as inflammatory disorders, HIV infection, lymphoma, and Lyme disease.

Prognosis. The prognosis is poor. Median survival is 2 to 5 years, although there are some patients who live much longer, albeit with relentlessly progressive disability. Unlike multiple sclerosis (see Chapter 9), progression is not one of exacerbations and remissions but rather of linear decline. The most common cause of death is respiratory failure due to respiratory muscle involvement.

Treatment. Treatment is largely symptom based and requires multidisciplinary care. As the disease progresses, patients often require a feeding tube and tracheostomy with mechanical ventilation. There are medications approved specifically for patients with ALS; riluzole, a glutamate inhibitor, and edaravone, a free radical scavenger, can slow progression to a modest degree and may extend survival by several months.

Box 11.1 ALS Mimics and Variants

Several disorders, all even less common than ALS, need to be considered in the differential diagnosis of patients who present with a motor neuropathy.

ALS mimics include:

- *Multifocal motor neuropathy* (MMN), an autoimmune demyelinating disease that can present just like ALS but with exclusively lower motor neuron involvement. Patchy, often asymmetric weakness typically spares the cranial nerves and bulbar muscles. In many but not all patients MMN is associated with antibodies to ganglioside GM1. It is important to distinguish MMN from ALS because, unlike ALS, it responds to intravenous immunoglobulin (IVIG). EMG (along with the clinical picture) is critical to help differentiate these two conditions.
- *Stenosis of the cervical spine*, the result of progressive degeneration of the vertebrae and intervertebral discs of the cervical spine, usually from osteoarthritis. Patients may present with:
  - neck, shoulder, or arm pain
  - lower motor neuron findings in the upper extremities (which can occur at the level of cord compression, a result of damage to the anterior horn cells and/or nerve roots)
  - upper motor neuron findings in the upper and/or lower extremities (a result of damage to the corticospinal tract within the spinal cord)
  - sensory loss in the arms and decreased sensation below the level of the lesion (following a dermatomal pattern)
  - gait impairment, which is very common and is due to a combination of the sensory and motor deficits described above

The diagnosis of cervical stenosis is made by imaging and electrodiagnostic testing.

ALS variants include:

- *Primary lateral sclerosis:* This disorder presents with solely upper motor neuron signs and symptoms. Only late in the course do some patients exhibit lower motor neuron involvement. It progresses more slowly than ALS—patients need to be followed for several years before this diagnosis can be made—and their life expectancy is considerably better.
- *Progressive muscular atrophy:* This condition presents with solely lower motor neuron signs and symptoms, although late in the course some patients will also exhibit upper motor involvement. Survival may be a few months longer than with classic ALS.

For each of these disorders, history, neurologic examination, and EMG are critical to help distinguish them from ALS.

Peripheral Neuropathies: An Overview

Let's begin with a quick review of anatomy (just this paragraph, we promise!). The PNS is divided into two components: the *somatic division,* which includes the spinal nerves (the sensory afferents and motor efferents) and the *autonomic division,* which is further divided into the *parasympathetic* and *sympathetic* divisions. Keep in mind that the cranial nerves, with the exception of CN1 and CN2 are part of the PNS. Depending on the specific cranial nerve, they can be made up of sensory, motor, and/or autonomic components.

When we talk about peripheral neuropathies, we are talking about pathology affecting any of the above: the somatic sensory and motor nerves, yes, and also the autonomic and cranial nerves. Thus gastroparesis, orthostatic hypotension, and diplopia can all be due to peripheral neuropathy.

Peripheral neuropathies are very common. You will see patients with peripheral neuropathies no matter what branch of medicine you choose.

The term "peripheral neuropathy" actually encompasses a number of different disorders:

- *Polyneuropathy*—This is what most people think of when they use the term peripheral neuropathy. Polyneuropathy refers to damage of multiple nerves by a single disease process. Involvement is usually symmetrically bilateral and synchronous; that is, when symptoms progress, they do so on the right side and left side at more or less the same time. We will spend most of this chapter looking at these disorders, as they are by far the most common.

- *Mononeuritis multiplex*—This term refers to damage of at least two separate peripheral nerves; unlike polyneuropathy, it need not be symmetric and the damage to the various nerves does not need to occur at the same time.

- *Mononeuropathy*—This term means damage to a single nerve. These disorders are usually caused by trauma, entrapment, or compression. A common example is carpal tunnel syndrome (median neuropathy at the wrist). However, not all mononeuropathies are mechanical in origin; the big exception is cranial mononeuropathy, which is more often the result of an infectious/inflammatory process (*e.g.*, a CN7, or Bell palsy) or ischemic event (CN3 palsy).

- *Plexopathy*—Plexopathies affect either of two discrete networks of nerves, the brachial plexus, which innervates the muscles and skin of the shoulder and arm, or the lumbosacral plexus, which innervates the muscles and skin of the lower extremities.

Box 11.2 Peripheral Neuropathy Versus Radiculopathy

You will recall from Chapter 10 that the term *radiculopathy* refers to compression of a nerve root, often by a herniated disc or osteophyte. In general, *radiculopathies are painful,* whereas peripheral neuropathies by and large are not, or at least not predominantly so (one important exception to this rule is small fiber neuropathy; see page 288). Radiculopathies tend to cause *incomplete symptoms* (*i.e.*, mild weakness as opposed to total paralysis, because the involved muscles are also getting neurologic input from other nerve roots), whereas peripheral neuropathies are more likely to cause *complete symptoms*. Knowing your peripheral neuroanatomy here is crucial. Luckily, however, when your best neurologic examination leaves you uncertain, electrodiagnostic testing can help localize the lesion.

Polyneuropathies

One way to think of the polyneuropathies is to classify them into primary axonal and primary demyelinating disorders. Although this classification can be helpful from a pathophysiologic viewpoint, and we won't ignore this approach entirely, from a practical standpoint it is preferable to think in terms of what you are likely to see in the clinic. And this is surprisingly straightforward, easily broken down into only three categories:

- Length-dependent sensorimotor polyneuropathies
- Inflammatory demyelinating polyneuropathies
- Small fiber neuropathies

Length-Dependent Sensorimotor Polyneuropathies

These polyneuropathies are very, very common. They present with *bilateral, symmetric deficits*. Because the longest nerves in the body are preferentially affected, symptoms tend to start in the feet (and, to a lesser degree, the hands; when both hands and feet are affected, the patient's neuropathy is said to have a "stocking-glove" distribution) and then progress upward. Sensory deficits are the most common presentation, resulting in numbness and paresthesias, but motor abnormalities can be present and can even be the predominant feature. Absent or decreased deep tendon reflexes often accompany the sensory findings (remember, the peripheral motor nerves are LMNs!). Autonomic dysfunction may also develop. In most cases the neurologic deficits evolve slowly, over years.

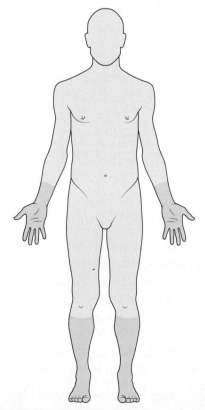

The classic stocking-glove distribution of a polyneuropathy.

Diabetes is by far and away the most commonly identified underlying etiology, but there are several others you should be familiar with. The most frequent alternative diagnoses are:

- *Infectious diseases* (such as HIV, hepatitis C, and Lyme disease)
- *Vitamin deficiencies* (including B1, B6, B12, D, and E)
- *Dysproteinemias* (such as multiple myeloma, Waldenstrom macroglobulinemia, and monoclonal gammopathy of undetermined significance)
- *Hereditary disorders* (most commonly Charcot-Marie Tooth disease)
- *Drug or toxin related* (chronic alcohol use, various chemotherapeutic agents and heavy metal exposures)
- *Less common causes*—but important ones not to miss!—include vasculitis, amyloidosis, paraneoplastic syndromes, and other systemic diseases such as hypothyroidism and end-stage renal disease.
- *Idiopathic*—by definition, no underlying cause can be found

Most of these polyneuropathies are considered predominantly axonal; however, some degree of demyelination is often present on electrophysiologic testing as well.

A typical neuropathy screen (i.e., blood work sent from the office for patients who present with classic length-dependent sensorimotor polyneuropathy) includes vitamin levels, serum protein electrophoresis and immunoelectrophoresis (to rule out dysproteinemias), and thyroid function tests. Screening for diseases like Lyme and HIV should be considered on a case-by-case basis, based on risk.

Let's take a quick look at a few of the more common etiologies of length-dependent sensorimotor polyneuropathies.

Diabetes. It is conventionally taught that it takes diabetes many years to cause neurologic damage, and it is true that the prevalence and severity of neuropathy correlate with the duration and severity of the patient's diabetes. However, more than 10% of patients will have evidence of neuropathy at the time their diabetes is first diagnosed, and as many as 25% of patients *without* diabetes but with impaired glucose tolerance will show electrodiagnostic changes consistent with diabetic neuropathy. The message here is simple: you should not dismiss the possibility of hyperglycemia as the cause of peripheral neuropathy in patients not previously diagnosed with diabetes or without laboratory criteria for frank diabetes. A glucose tolerance test may be worth doing, because it will be abnormal in some of these patients. Neurologists not uncommonly are the first to diagnose diabetes in patients for whom peripheral neuropathy is the presenting symptom.

In a patient with frank diabetes or impaired glucose intolerance and a distal, symmetric polyneuropathy, your evaluation is done. Patients typically complain of pain and paresthesias in their feet and/or hands, and your examination will show diminished distal sensation to vibration and decreased ankle reflexes. Motor weakness, if it develops at all, is a much later finding.

Tight glucose control, exercise, and management of each of the components of metabolic syndrome (obesity, hypertension, hyperlipidemia, *etc.*) can delay the progression of diabetic polyneuropathy and may improve symptoms. If needed, anticonvulsants (often gabapentin and pregabalin), tricyclic antidepressants and selective serotonin-norepinephrine reuptake inhibitors may help mitigate neuropathic pain in diabetic patients.

Vitamin B12 (Cobalamin) Deficiency. It takes several years to deplete hepatic stores of vitamin B12. The most common causes include pancreatic insufficiency, ileal damage (as can occur in patients with Crohn disease or following bariatric surgery), pernicious anemia, and various medications that interfere with B12 absorption (including metformin and proton pump inhibitors such as omeprazole). Adherence to a strict vegan diet can also result in B12 deficiency.

The major consequences of B12 deficiency include megaloblastic anemia, neuropsychiatric disturbances (including depression and cognitive slowing) and myelopathy due to dorsolateral spinal column disease (known as *subacute combined degeneration*; see page 269 for details). Peripheral neuropathy is also common, usually accompanied by signs of myelopathy. It tends to be distal and symmetric and can come on acutely. An elevated serum methylmalonic acid is a more reliable diagnostic test than a decreased serum B12 level (B12 functions as a cofactor for methylmalonyl CoA mutase, which catalyzes the conversion of methylmalonic acid to succinyl CoA; therefore, B12 deficiency results in elevated levels of methylmalonic acid). Supplementation with vitamin B12 will delay progression and improve the patient's symptoms within weeks.

Vitamin B12.

Vitamin B1 (Thiamine) Deficiency. Thiamine deficiency is most often seen in the setting of poor nutrition (in populations whose diet consists mainly of rice or cereals or in patients with anorexia, previous gastric bypass surgery, hyperemesis gravidarum, or chronic alcohol abuse) and in patients on hemodialysis. It causes two distinct clinical phenotypes: *Wernicke Korsakoff syndrome* (see page 380) and *Beriberi*.

Beriberi can present in both infants (mainly those who are breastfed by women who are thiamine deficient) and in adults. It has two forms: *dry beriberi*, which is characterized by a symmetric length-dependent sensorimotor polyneuropathy, and *wet beriberi*, which includes signs and symptoms of cardiac involvement along with polyneuropathy. Measuring whole blood thiamine is the best test, but even this has limited diagnostic sensitivity and specificity. The erythrocyte thiamine transketolase activity test is another option. Depending on the severity of the presentation, treatment is with either intravenous (IV) or oral thiamine supplementation.

Vitamin B1.

Paraproteinemias. Paraproteinemias are characterized by an excessive amount of paraproteins (*i.e.,* monoclonal immunoglobulins produced by a clonal population of mature B cells) in the blood. *Multiple myeloma, monoclonal gammopathy of undetermined significance (MGUS)* and *Waldenstrom macroglobulinemia* can all cause a polyneuropathy (usually due to amyloidosis) that, except for the presence of a monoclonal immunoglobulin spike in the serum, presents clinically no differently from those described above.

Hereditary transthyretin amyloid (hATTR) is a type of heritable, autosomal dominant amyloidosis due to deposition of transthyretin-derived fibrils (transthyretin is a transport protein for, among other thing, thyroxine). Neuropathy is often the presenting symptom (bilateral carpal tunnel syndrome is common), but spinal stenosis, biceps tendon rupture, and involvement of other organs also occur. In patients with neuropathy in addition to unexplained cardiac, renal, or pulmonary disease, hATTR is an important diagnosis to consider, both because it is autosomal dominant and thus carries important genetic repercussions and because there is effective treatment. Tafamidis was approved in 2019; it is believed to stabilize the transthyretin protein and reduce formation of TTR amyloid.

POEMS syndrome stands for *polyneuropathy, organomegaly, endocrinopathy, monoclonal protein,* and *skin changes.* Not all patients with POEMS have all of these components. The presence of a monoclonal plasma cell disorder and a relatively severe peripheral neuropathy are required for the diagnosis. POEMS neuropathy begins as a typical distal sensory neuropathy, but this is followed by an often debilitating motor neuropathy that spreads proximally. Suspect POEMS in a patient with a known paraprotein (either benign or malignant), neuropathy, and any of the other features of this syndrome.

Charcot-Marie-Tooth Syndrome. Many genetic disorders present with distal polyneuropathy as a prominent feature. Charcot-Marie-Tooth (CMT) is the most common of them. CMT encompasses a group of progressive, hereditary sensory and motor neuropathies that are due to various genetic mutations associated with defective production of proteins required for fully functional peripheral nerves.

Patients tend to present in adolescence or early adulthood. Unlike in diabetic polyneuropathy, motor findings often predominate. Distal extremity weakness (often manifesting as clumsiness and frequently sprained ankles) with altered gait and muscle wasting is the most common initial presentation. Frank foot drop usually appears later in the course. Distal sensory loss is present but usually less prominent. Characteristic features on examination include high foot arches (known as *pes cavus*), hammer toes, and "stork legs," a result of distal muscular atrophy. If you suspect CMT, always ask about a family history of similar complaints. The diagnosis can be confirmed with electrophysiologic testing and genetic analysis. There is no specific therapy.

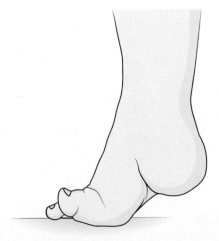

Pes cavus, or high arched foot, is a common feature of CMT.

Idiopathic Polyneuropathy. This disorder presents just like any other distal sensory polyneuropathy, but with no known cause. As many as 25% of patients with peripheral neuropathy will eventually be given this diagnosis. The good news is that the prognosis for these patients is generally excellent. The disease does not substantially progress in most patients, and motor weakness rarely develops.

Inflammatory Demyelinating Polyneuropathies (Guillain-Barre Syndrome)

The inflammatory demyelinating polyneuropathies are classified under the eponym *Guillain-Barre syndrome* (GBS), the names of two of the French neurologists who first described the disorder. Unlike the slowly progressive, predominantly sensory polyneuropathies described above, GBS most often presents as an acute to subacute monophasic, rapidly progressive and predominantly motor polyneuropathy or, more correctly, poly*radiculo*neuropathy, since the demyelination often begins at the nerve roots. There are several GBS variants—see the list below—but *acute inflammatory demyelinating polyradiculoneuropathy (AIDP)* is by far and away the most common, representing nearly 90% of all GBS cases.

Table 11.1 The Many Variants of GBS

Weakness Predominant	Weakness NOT Predominant
Acute inflammatory polyradiculo-neuropathy (AIDP)	Miller Fisher syndrome (MFS)
Acute motor axonal neuropathy (AMAN)	Bickerstaff Encephalitis
Acute motor and sensory axonal neuropathy (AMSAN)	Acute pandysautonomia
Pharyngeal-cervical-brachial variant	Pure sensory neuropathy

Acute Inflammatory Demyelinating Polyradiculoneuropathy. This is what most people mean when they talk about GBS. AIDP is an acute-onset, monophasic illness that progresses rapidly over the course of several days. *Molecular mimicry* is thought to be the pathophysiological mechanism in which, prompted by a prior infection, cross-reactive antibodies mistakenly attack the myelin of peripheral nerves.

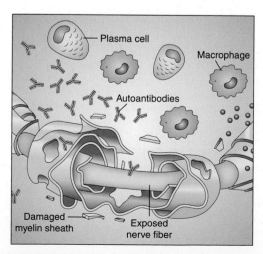

The immune system attacks the myelin lining of peripheral nerves in AIDP.

Symptoms. Symptoms are frequently preceded by a respiratory or gastrointestinal illness (*Campylobacter jejuni* is the most commonly identified precipitant, but a long list of viral infections, including Epstein-Barr virus, cytomegalovirus, influenza, and the Zika virus, and bacterial infections, including *Escherichia coli* and mycoplasma, have also been implicated).

Common symptoms include:

- Mild paresthesias in the hands and feet (often the initial symptom)
- Progressive, relatively symmetric weakness that begins in the lower extremities and ascends over hours to days; this ascending paralysis is the most characteristic feature of AIDP
- Depressed or absent reflexes
- Back and leg pain, due to nerve root inflammation
- Oculomotor, facial, and oropharyngeal weakness, due to cranial nerve involvement
- Respiratory muscle weakness (10% to 30% of patients ultimately require ventilatory support)
- Autonomic dysfunction, causing labile swings in heart rate, blood pressure, and potentially dangerous cardiac arrhythmias

Box 11.3 Can the Flu Vaccine Cause GBS?

If, and this is a very big if, the flu vaccine can cause GBS, the risk is extremely low, at most 1 to 2 cases per 1 million doses. This risk is far less than the risks associated with influenza itself (all you have to know is that 61,000 flu-related deaths occurred in the United States in 2017–2018, which was a typical flu season). Nevertheless, it is recommended that the flu vaccine not be given to persons who developed GBS within 6 weeks of a prior flu vaccination.

Diagnosis. Diagnosis is dependent on (1) physical examination, which should confirm profound, distal weakness with absent or depressed reflexes, and (2) CSF analysis, which will reveal an elevated protein and normal white count (known as "*albuminocytologic dissociation*"). Electrophysiologic testing can be valuable for confirming the diagnosis and distinguishing among the different GBS variants, which is important largely for establishing the patient's prognosis. It can take about 3 weeks to see changes on electromyography (EMG) and nerve conduction studies (NCS); if done too early, these tests will appear normal. Spinal MRI can be normal or show enhancement of the involved nerve roots. It is often necessary to rule out other spinal cord pathology that may be mimicking GBS. It is also a good idea to order the basic peripheral neuropathy blood work to definitively exclude other treatable causes.

Treatment. IV immunoglobulin (IVIG) and plasma exchange (PLEX) are equally effective first-line treatment options. Combining them does not improve outcomes, and there is no evidence that corticosteroids are helpful. Most patients begin to improve by 4 weeks, and 80% to 90% will make a full recovery, although it may take many months. Mortality is 5%, almost always from respiratory failure. Some patients may suffer relapses, and they are then said to have *chronic inflammatory demyelinating polyneuropathy* (see page 287).

Box 11.4 Tick Paralysis

One disease that can mimic GBS, although very rare, is tick paralysis. It is caused by neurotoxins produced by any of numerous tick vectors that block the release of acetylcholine from presynaptic nerve terminals. Ticks must have been feeding for at least 4 days to produce symptoms. Tick paralysis can present in many ways—asymmetric paralysis, facial and pharyngeal weakness, ataxia—but when the picture consists of paresthesias and ascending weakness it can mimic GBS. However, more often it is asymmetric, and CSF analysis will be normal. The key to diagnosis is to look for the tick, and the key to treatment is to remove it. Most patients will recover within hours to days upon removal. Treatment is otherwise supportive.

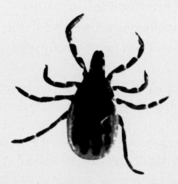

The lone star tick, one of many tick species that can cause tick paralysis. (Modified from Wolfson AB, Hendey GW, Ling LJ, et al. *Harwood-Nuss' Clinical Practice of Emergency Medicine*, 5th ed. Wolters Kluwer, 2009.)

Box 11.5 Other GBS Variants

Just a quick word on some important but far less common GBS variants:

- **Acute motor axonal neuropathy (AMAN)**: An acute, axonal form of GBS, AMAN occurs mostly in Asia and tends to affect younger adults. It progresses more rapidly than AIDP but has similar rates of recovery. It can be distinguished from AIDP by its lack of sensory involvement and its axonal pattern on electrophysiologic testing. It is often associated with the presence of ganglioside antibodies (including GM1, GD1a, and GalNac-GD1a).
- **Acute motor and sensory neuropathy (AMSAN):** A more severe form of AMAN, with both sensory and motor involvement. Prognosis is worse, with more protracted and often incomplete recovery.
- **Pharyngeal-cervical-brachial variant:** Characterized by weakness of the pharyngeal, neck, and shoulder muscles, with associated swallowing dysfunction. Leg strength and reflexes are usually preserved. Think of this as a localized, typically axonal GBS variant.
- **Miller Fisher syndrome (MFS):** Classically presents with the clinical triad of ataxia, areflexia, and ophthalmoplegia, although many patients will only actually

Box 11.5 Other GBS Variants   (Continued)

develop 2 of the 3 symptoms. Ganglioside antibodies against GQ1b are present in the majority of cases.

- **Bickerstaff encephalitis:** A brainstem encephalitis characterized by encephalopathy, hyperreflexia, and features of MFS including ataxia and ophthalmoplegia. Like MFS, it is also associated with GQ1b antibodies.
- **Pure sensory neuropathy:** This presents with significant sensory ataxia and areflexia, with either absent or very minor motor involvement.
- **Acute pandysautonomia:** Characterized by diffuse autonomic nerve involvement that can result in orthostatic hypotension, urinary retention, diarrhea, vomiting, decreased sweating, and pupillary abnormalities. Sensory abnormalities and diminished or absent reflexes may also be present.

Chronic Inflammatory Demyelinating Polyneuropathy. Chronic inflammatory demyelinating polyneuropathy (CIDP) can be thought of as the chronic form of AIDP. It is primarily distinguished both by its time course—by definition, symptoms must persist for at least 8 weeks—and its responsiveness to corticosteroid treatment (AIDP, you may recall, is not steroid responsive). It tends to be monophasic, with a relatively gradual onset and even more gradual recovery, but some patients can present with a relapsing and remitting course. Otherwise, CIDP closely resembles AIDP, with predominantly distal, symmetric, ascending motor weakness and decreased or absent reflexes. Albuminocytologic dissociation in the CSF is a hallmark finding, as with AIDP. IVIG, PLEX, or pulse high-dose corticosteroids are first-line treatment.

There are several CIDP variants, including sensory-predominant and pure motor forms, that can be harder to recognize and diagnose. CSF analysis and electrophysiologic testing are helpful.

Box 11.6 Electromyography and Nerve Conduction Studies

Electromyography (EMG) and nerve conduction studies (NCS) can help to distinguish peripheral nerve disorders from primarily muscular ones and axonal disorders from demyelinating ones. EMG measures the electrical activity of muscles. NCS (which assesses both sensory and motor nerves) measures how well and how fast nerves send signals. In general:

- Features of axonal disorders include reduced amplitude of evoked nerve action potentials (the "SNAP," or sensory nerve action potential, and "CMAP,' or compound muscle action potential), as well as abnormal spontaneous activity, including fibrillation potentials and sharp waves.
- Features of demyelinating disorders include slowed conduction velocities, prolonged distal latencies, and conduction block.

(Continued)

Box 11.6 Electromyography and Nerve Conduction Studies   (Continued)

Electrodiagnostic testing is often most useful when the diagnosis is uncertain.

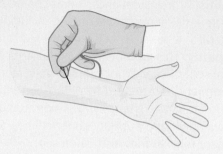

Performing an EMG involves the insertion of a tiny needle into different muscles.

Small Fiber Neuropathy

Small fiber neuropathy affects the small unmyelinated nerve fibers (known as "C" fibers) that transmit pain and temperature sensation. Patients typically present with distal burning pain and numbness involving the hands and feet. Neurologic examination is variable: you may find a length-dependent decrease in pinprick sensation, reduced ankle jerk reflexes or, not uncommonly, no objective abnormalities at all. Associated autonomic symptoms are common and can include dry mouth, urinary and bowel retention, and orthostatic hypotension. Diabetes is by far the most common underlying etiology, but the list of potential causes is long and includes:

- Vitamin B12 (cobalamin) deficiency
- Vitamin B6 (pyridoxine) toxicity
- Infectious etiologies (HIV, hepatitis C)
- Autoimmune conditions (Sjogren syndrome, sarcoidosis, systemic lupus erythematosus)
- Paraproteinemias (multiple myeloma)
- Paraneoplastic disorders

Electrophysiologic testing *will not detect* small fiber neuropathy; EMG and NCS will be normal. The lack of EMG/NCS abnormalities and a normal, or near-normal, neurologic examination in a patient with symptomatic neuropathy are what should lead you to suspect a small fiber neuropathy. Skin biopsy, which will show absent or diminished nerve endings, is the diagnostic test of choice. There is no specific treatment; various anticonvulsants and antidepressants can be used for pain control.

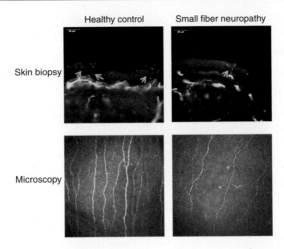

Examples of nerve fibers on skin punch biopsies and microscopy, from a healthy control and a patient with small fiber neuropathy. Note the lower density of nerve fibers in the patient with small fiber neuropathy. (Modified from Haüser W, Perrot S. *Fibromyalgia Syndrome and Widespread Pain*. Wolters Kluwer; 2018.)

 ## *Mononeuritis Multiplex*

Mononeuritis multiplex is unlike the polyneuropathies we have just discussed. The polyneuropathies evolve symmetrically, progressively, and continuously, whereas mononeuritis multiplex proceeds in a kind of scattershot accumulation of isolated, noncontiguous mononeuropathies. By definition, it must involve 2 or more noncontiguous nerves either simultaneously or sequentially. Mononeuritis multiplex is far less common than polyneuropathy.

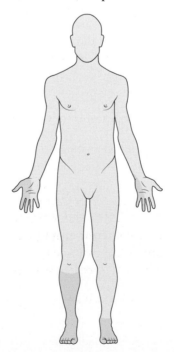

Multiplex. If you look quickly, the involved areas may resemble the stocking-glove distribution of a polyneuropathy. But a closer evaluation will reveal that the lesions are not symmetric and involve several distinct peripheral nerves. A careful examination will reveal the difference.

- *Vasculitis* is a common cause, most often the disorders associated with antineutrophil cytoplasmic autoantibodies (ANCA; such as granulomatosis with polyangiitis and microscopic polyangiitis), polyarteritis nodosa, cryoglobulinemia, and vasculitis associated with connective tissue diseases such as Sjogren syndrome.
- Other causes include:
  - *ischemic nerve damage* (*e.g.*, due to diabetes or sickle cell anemia)
  - *various infections* (mostly viral diseases such as hepatitis B, hepatitis C, HIV, and West Nile virus)
  - *neoplastic processes* (from tumor infiltration of nerves or as a result of a paraneoplastic syndrome).

Nerves of the lower extremities are typically affected first; foot drop due to peroneal nerve damage is the most common motor complaint. Over time, however, virtually any peripheral nerve can be affected, including those supplying strength and sensation to the upper extremities, the cranial nerves and autonomic nerves.

Nerve biopsy is often helpful to diagnose the underlying etiology; it can confirm a vasculitis and allow treatment to be initiated with corticosteroids, as well as rule out infiltrative disorders like lymphoma.

Management otherwise involves recognizing and treating the underlying condition, as well as pain control with the same medications used for the more common polyneuropathies.

 Plexopathies

The plexopathies involve multiple nerves but are caused by single lesions that involve a substantial part of or an entire plexus, either the brachial plexus or the lumbosacral plexus. These syndromes are rare and are most often caused by trauma, ischemia, inflammation, malignancy, diabetes, and radiation therapy.

Brachial Plexopathies

The brachial plexus is one of the most tested anatomical structures in the body. The mnemonic **R**eal **T**exans **D**rink **C**old **B**eer is often relied upon to help remember the anatomy:

- **R**oots (C5-T1)
- **T**runks (superior/upper: C5-6, middle: C7, inferior/lower: C8-T1)
- **D**ivisions (each trunk splits into anterior and posterior divisions)
- **C**ords (lateral, posterior, and medial)
- **B**ranches (the nerves given off by each cord)
  - Lateral cord → musculocutaneous nerve (C5-7), lateral root of the median nerve (C5-T1)
  - Posterior cord → axillary nerve (C5-6), radial nerve (C5-T1)
  - Medial cord → ulnar nerve (C8-T1), medial root of the median nerve (C5-T1)

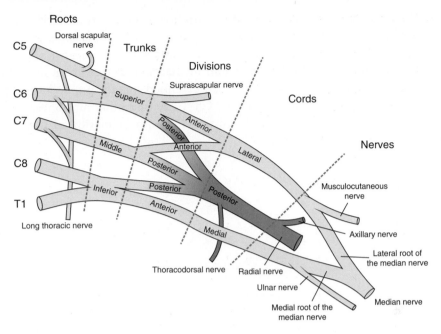

The brachial plexus.

Brachial plexopathies are typically classified into those that are traumatic (usually a result of sports injuries or motor vehicle accidents) and those that are not. A few specific syndromes involving the brachial plexus include:

- **Erb palsy** is caused by a tear of the superior or upper trunk of the brachial plexus (involving C5 and C6). This most often occurs in infants during delivery, a result of lateral traction on the neck of the baby due to shoulder dystocia. It presents with impaired shoulder abduction (due to deltoid and supraspinatus involvement; the arm hangs limply by the side), lateral rotation (infraspinatus involvement; the arm is medially rotated) and arm flexion and supination (biceps brachii involvement; the arm is extended and pronated). The majority of cases resolve with time and physical therapy. Surgical repair is second-line treatment if needed.

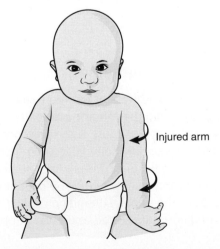

A summary of the common neurologic complications seen in infants with Erb palsy.

• **Klumpke palsy** is caused by a tear of the inferior or lower trunk of the brachial plexus (involving C8-T1). It is also typically caused by trauma during delivery but is less common than Erb palsy. This palsy presents with weakness in the intrinsic hand muscles innervated by the ulnar and median nerves (resulting in "claw hand," characterized by an extended wrist, extended metacarpophalangeal joints, and flexed distal interphalangeal joints), C8-T1 dermatomal numbness and, not uncommonly, Horner syndrome, due to the close approximation of the T1 nerve root to the sympathetic chain.

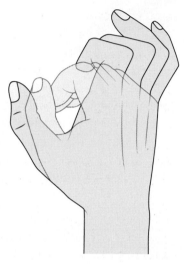

The "claw hand" of Klumpke palsy.

• **Parsonage-Turner syndrome** (also known as neuralgic amyotrophy) is an acute inflammatory brachial plexitis that can involve any portion of the brachial plexus. Most often it is idiopathic, but approximately 50% of patients report some sort of antecedent event, such as surgery or a viral illness. It classically presents with the acute onset of severe arm and shoulder pain followed within days to weeks by patchy upper extremity weakness. Most cases are unilateral, but bilateral involvement can occur. Recovery is gradual, often over months to years. There is no specific treatment.

Box 11.7 Thoracic Outlet Syndrome

Thoracic outlet syndrome refers to a group of disorders caused by compression of the nerves, arteries, and veins within the thoracic outlet (the space between the clavicle and first rib). The most common cause is the presence of anomalous ribs or an injury. The clinical picture is usually dominated by compression of the blood vessels, causing upper extremity edema. However, when the nerves of the brachial plexus are also involved (this is exceedingly rare!), the patient will complain of pain, numbness, and dysesthesias of the upper extremity provoked by elevating the arm or turning the neck. If the condition is untreated, muscular atrophy can develop.

Lumbosacral Plexopathies

These are uncommon, so we won't spend too much time here (and, happily, unlike with the brachial plexus, there is no need to learn the precise anatomy). There are a strikingly wide range of potential etiologies, including:

- *Diabetes. Diabetic amyotrophy* (also known as diabetic radiculoplexus neuropathy) typically presents acutely with asymmetric focal leg pain followed by proximal leg weakness. Associated autonomic symptoms are common. Partial recovery over weeks to months is standard.

- *Idiopathic.* Idiopathic lumbosacral plexopathy presents similarly to diabetic amyotrophy, but in patients without diabetes.

- *Neoplasm.* Neoplastic invasion of the lumbosacral plexus is most often due to direct extension of a tumor (nearly any form of carcinoma, melanoma, or lymphoma can be implicated), but it can also be caused by leptomeningeal involvement or hematogenous or lymphatic spread. Neoplastic lumbosacral plexopathy is nearly always painful, characterized by shock-like pains in the involved lower extremity.

- *Radiation.* Radiation lumbosacral plexopathy tends to occur months to years after pelvic radiation. It is often bilateral and rarely painful, presenting instead with weakness and, occasionally, sensory loss.

- *Retroperitoneal hematoma.* These typically develop within the psoas muscle and can occur spontaneously or following femoral arterial or venous catheterizations (most often in patients on anticoagulation). Severe back and leg pain and femoral neuropathy are common.

 Mononeuropathies

Mononeuropathy, the involvement of a single nerve, can result from almost any disease process. Any nerve can be affected, and we could list as many mononeuropathies as there are nerves in the body, but a few syndromes are common and deserve to be singled out:

- Median neuropathy at the wrist (carpal tunnel syndrome)
- Ulnar neuropathy at the elbow
- Peroneal and tibial neuropathies
- Bell palsy
- Meralgia paresthetica

Carpal Tunnel Syndrome

Carpal tunnel syndrome (CTS) is a form of median neuropathy due to entrapment of the median nerve (which is derived from spinal nerves C5-T1) within the narrow carpal tunnel in the wrist. This is usually caused by repetitive trauma from occupations that require frequent flexion and extension of the wrist (although, surprisingly, spending the day hammering away at a computer keyboard has not been convincingly found to cause CTS!). Other important risk factors to keep in mind include hypothyroidism (due to accumulation of mucinous material within the carpal tunnel), pregnancy (due to fluid accumulation and edema), and amyloidosis (due, no surprise, to amyloid deposition).

Patients will complain of numbness and paresthesias in the hand, often described as tingling and often worse at night. Examination will reveal that the sensory symptoms are limited to the first three digits of the hand and the medial side of the ring finger. Accompanying pain, however, need not be limited to the median nerve distribution and can radiate throughout the entire hand and even up the arm. Bilateral symptoms are surprisingly common, affecting more than half of patients with CTS.

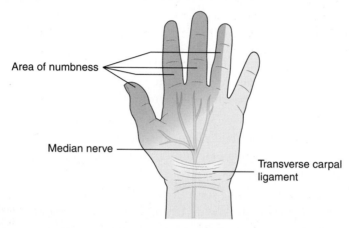

Compression of the median nerve within the carpal tunnel leads to sensory complaints in the first three digits and the medial side of the ring finger.

Various diagnostic maneuvers may help you make the diagnosis. The *Phalen test* involves having patients flex their wrist for 1 minute and seeing if that elicits or exacerbates their symptoms. The *Tinel test* involves tapping over the carpal tunnel and seeing if that produces symptoms in the fingers. If positive, both tests are suggestive of the diagnosis, but their sensitivity and specificity are limited (cited as around 50% to 80%). Wrist x-rays may be indicated to exclude other diagnoses, and electrophysiologic testing can be helpful when the diagnosis remains unclear.

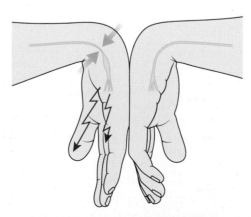

Phalen test for carpal tunnel syndrome.

Conservative treatment involves avoidance of the activity that is causing the problem (unfortunately not always possible) and the use of a wrist splint at night. Physical therapy and targeted exercises don't appear to add much. Some patients may benefit from local injection of a corticosteroid. For patients with persistent symptoms, surgical release of the carpal tunnel is a relatively simple procedure that can lead to complete resolution of symptoms.

Ulnar Neuropathy

Ulnar neuropathy is less common than median neuropathy. It can occur when the ulnar nerve (derived from spinal nerves C8-T1) is compressed at the elbow (in the cubital tunnel; this is the most common site) or the wrist (in Guyon canal). Sensory symptoms in the ulnar distribution tend to predominate in the former, whereas hand weakness, atrophy, and clumsiness predominate in the latter.

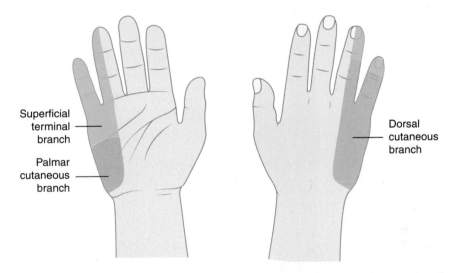

Sensory distribution of the ulnar nerve. Involvement of the palmar cutaneous or dorsal cutaneous branches indicates that the lesion is proximal to the wrist.

Peroneal and Tibial Neuropathies

The sciatic nerve is the largest nerve in the body, running from the hip all the way down into the toes. It is derived from spinal nerves L4 to S3. The sciatic nerve runs down the posterior thigh and then splits into two branches at the popliteal fossa: 1) the tibial nerve (L4-S3) and 2) the common peroneal, or fibular, nerve (L4-S2).

The common peroneal nerve runs laterally, wrapping itself around the lateral leg and fibula. It dorsiflexes and everts the foot and supplies sensation to the lateral leg and dorsum of the foot. Fibular neck fractures, lateral leg trauma, and significant weight loss can all cause peroneal neuropathy, which presents with foot drop, peroneal-distribution numbness, and a steppage (high-stepping) gait.

The tibial nerve runs medially. It inverts and plantar flexes the foot and supplies sensation to the sole of the foot. Tibial nerve injury is less common than peroneal nerve injury. Tibial nerve injury is most commonly caused by compression in the popliteal fossa (often due to a hematoma or a fluid-filled Baker cyst) or within the tarsal tunnel at the ankle.

The most helpful mnemonic to keep these two neuropathies straight that we were able to turn up is quite clever:

- Peroneal neuropathy: presents with **"foot dropPED"** (Peroneal, Everts, Dorsiflexes)
- Tibial neuropathy: presents with inability to stand on **TIP toes** (Tibial, Inverts, Plantarflexes)

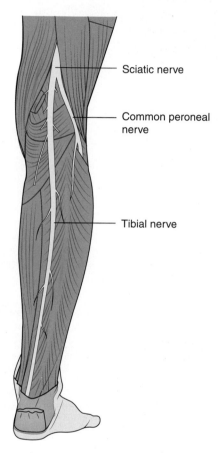

Sciatic nerve

Common peroneal nerve

Tibial nerve

Anatomy of the major nerves of the lower extremity.

Box 11.8 Sciatica

"Sciatica" is a colloquial term that refers to radicular back pain, *i.e.*, pain that radiates from the back into the leg along the dermatome (sensory distribution) of a nerve. It is a nonspecific term and is often used incorrectly to describe what is more accurately termed lumbosacral radiculopathy. Furthermore, the term sciatica is misleading, because radicular back pain can be the result of compression of any of the lumbosacral nerve roots, L1 through S4 (L5 and S1 are most commonly affected), whereas sciatic mononeuropathy (remember, the sciatic nerve is formed from the L4-S3 nerve roots) is relatively uncommon.

Box 11.8 Sciatica (Continued)

Lumbosacral radiculopathy is, on the other hand, extremely common. It is most often caused by either a herniated disc or spinal stenosis compressing part of the nerve root and causing inflammation. Pain that shoots from the lower back down into the leg, often with associated numbness and tingling, is the classic presentation. Most patients can be managed conservatively with physical therapy and a short course of acetaminophen or an anti-inflammatory medication such as ibuprofen. Epidural steroids are generally not recommended because of their limited efficacy and not inconsequential risks. Systemic glucocorticoids also appear to have little value. Surgical management is generally reserved for patients who develop frank weakness or who have persistent and debilitating pain despite conservative measures.

Bell Palsy

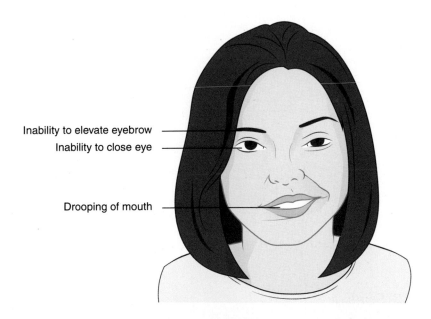

A patient with Bell palsy.

We are going to hold off on a full discussion of this common condition until Chapter 18, when we focus on disorders of the cranial nerves. For now, you should know that facial palsies come in two types: upper motor neuron (UMN) and lower motor neuron (LMN). LMN (or "peripheral") facial palsy, affecting the nucleus or axons of the seventh cranial nerve itself, is common, affecting up to 1 in 60 people during their lifetime. When the cause is unknown, peripheral facial nerve palsy is referred to as *Bell palsy.*

Peripheral facial nerve palsy presents with the acute onset of weakness on the ipsilateral side of the face (*i.e.*, a lesion of the left seventh nerve results in left-sided facial weakness), involving both the upper face (resulting in the patient's inability to close the eye or fully elevate the eyebrow) and the lower face (resulting in nasolabial fold flattening and drooping of the mouth). The forehead is spared in patients with UMN facial nerve palsies; again, all this will make more sense when we look at it in detail in Chapter 18.

Meralgia Paresthetica

This common mononeuropathy is the result of compression of the lateral femoral cutaneous nerve, a purely sensory branch of the lumbar plexus that supplies sensation to the anterolateral thigh. The majority of cases result from compression of the nerve as it passes beneath the inguinal ligament, often in the setting of pregnancy or obesity, or even just from wearing tight belts or waist bands. Patients complain of numbness, paresthesias, and pain in the anterolateral thigh. Because the lateral femoral cutaneous nerve is purely sensory, there should be no associated motor deficits.

Additional testing is almost never required. This is a diagnosis you can make by history and examination alone. Treatment involves avoiding precipitants (a new wardrobe may be in order), weight loss, and, for those patients with significant pain, the same medications that are useful for the polyneuropathies. Most patients recover within a few weeks to months.

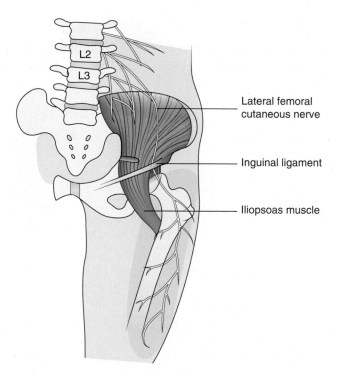

Damage to the lateral femoral cutaneous nerve can lead to numbness of the anterolateral thigh.

Box 11.9 The Peripheral Neurologic Manifestations of Diabetes Mellitus

As you have surely noticed by now, diabetes can wreak havoc on the peripheral nervous system in a number of ways. Here they all are, in one place, to help you keep them all straight:

- *Distal symmetric predominantly sensory peripheral neuropathy*, by far the most common
- *Autonomic neuropathy* can result in gastrointestinal symptoms, erectile dysfunction, and orthostatic hypotension. Also, and here's a small pearl, patients can lose the normal sinus arrhythmia of the heart, that is, the normal variation in heart rate with inspiration (faster) and expiration (slower); this can sometimes be the very first manifestation of diabetic neuropathy
- *Polyradiculopathy*—these include diabetic amyotrophy (just a fancy term for lumbosacral radiculopathy, with prominent pain, muscle weakness, and atrophy in the proximal lower extremity) and thoracic polyradiculopathy (which characteristically presents with abdominal pain in a band-like pattern around the trunk)
- *Mononeuropathy*—almost any nerve can be affected, but the most common are the cranial nerves (usually the oculomotor, trochlear, and abducens nerves, resulting in diplopia and ophthalmoplegia) and the median nerve (resulting in carpal tunnel syndrome)
- *Small fiber neuropathy*—characterized by distal burning pain and a normal neurologic examination; remember, skin biopsy is required for diagnosis because electrophysiologic testing will be normal

Box 11.10 Multiple Cranial Nerve Palsies

There are only a handful of things that can cause multiple cranial neuropathies simultaneously or within a short time frame of each other. It is worth going through the differential, because none of these are diagnoses you want to miss.

- *Infections*: Lyme, listeria, syphilis, and cryptococcus are most often implicated.
- *Autoimmune diseases*: Guillain-Barre syndrome and neurosarcoidosis are the two most commonly encountered.
- *Neoplastic disease*: Leptomeningeal carcinomatosis occurs when cancer cells spread into the leptomeninges (the pia and arachnoid) and cerebrospinal fluid and are thus disseminated throughout the neuraxis. This can present with severe headache (remember, the meninges are pain sensitive), polyradiculopathies (due to involvement of the spinal nerve roots as they exit the cord), and multiple cranial neuropathies (due to malignant invasion of the cranial nerves within the subarachnoid space). For more details, see Chapter 16.

(Continued)

Box 11.10 Multiple Cranial Nerve Palsies (Continued)

- *Cavernous sinus syndrome:* The two cavernous sinuses sit on either side of the pituitary gland and drain blood and CSF from the eye and superficial cortex into the internal jugular vein. Each sinus contains an internal carotid artery, third-order sympathetic neurons (that run on the surface of the carotid artery), and cranial nerves 3, 4, 5 (only the ophthalmic, V1, and maxillary, V2, branches), and 6. Thus, pathology within the cavernous sinus (often thrombosis, a mass, or fistula) presents with reduced facial sensation and ophthalmoplegia due to multiple cranial nerve involvement.

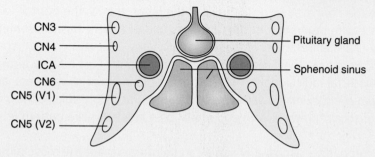

The cavernous sinus, which contains the internal carotid artery (ICA) and sympathetic nerves that run on its surface, as well as cranial nerves 3, 4, 5 (V1 and V2 branches only), and 6.

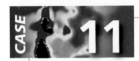

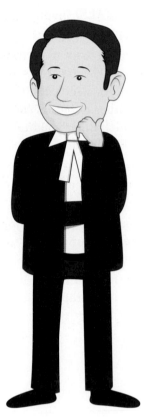

Your Patient's Follow-up: Allen, who presented with numbness and tingling in his feet, appears to have a typical distal sensory polyneuropathy. His fasting glucose and hemoglobin A1c were normal, so you order additional laboratory work including a vitamin B12/methylmalonic acid, SPEP and IEP (serum protein electrophoresis and immunoelectrophoresis, respectively; these will help rule out a paraproteinemia) and, because he lives in New England, Lyme antibody titers. All are normal. Despite his normal fasting glucose and hemoglobin A1c you still suspect impaired glucose tolerance because he is overweight, and a glucose tolerance test confirms your suspicion. No further workup is needed for the present moment. You encourage him to lose weight and together agree to consider starting metformin to improve his insulin sensitivity, delay the development of frank diabetes, and help him lose weight if lifestyle changes alone are insufficient. He returns to see you in 3 months having lost 8 pounds, and his neuropathic symptoms have improved.

You now know:

- | Amyotrophic lateral sclerosis (ALS) involves both upper and lower motor neurons and carries a grim prognosis.

- | There are various kinds of peripheral neuropathies, with varied etiologies and presentations (which you can now recognize).

- | Length-dependent sensorimotor neuropathies are most often caused by diabetes, but a long list of other potential causes must be considered in the absence of hyperglycemia, including hereditary conditions (such as Charcot-Marie-Tooth), and metabolic disorders (such as B12 deficiency).

- | The inflammatory neuropathies present with profound motor deficits; always think of Guillain-Barre syndrome and its many variants, as these are do-not-miss diagnoses.

- | Mononeuropathies can occur in multiples (mononeuritis multiplex) or as single nerve involvement (carpal tunnel syndrome, Bell palsy, and meralgia paresthetica prominent among them).

- | Diabetes can do almost anything to the peripheral nervous system; a stocking-glove distribution sensory polyneuropathy is the most common manifestation and can occur without overt hyperglycemia or other manifestations of diabetes.

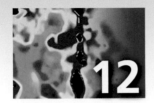

12 Diseases of the Muscles and the Neuromuscular Junction

In this chapter, you will learn:

1 | How to distinguish between disorders of the nerves, neuromuscular junction, and muscles

2 | How to recognize and treat diseases of the neuromuscular junction, such as myasthenia gravis

3 | How to recognize and treat inflammatory myopathies (*e.g.*, polymyositis) and noninflammatory myopathies (*e.g.*, muscular complaints caused by the use of lipid-lowering statins)

4 | How to diagnose and manage patients with rhabdomyolysis

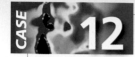

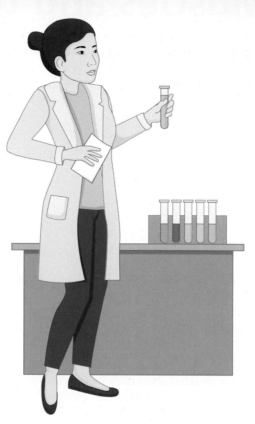

Your Patient: Carol, a 33-year-old laboratory technician, comes to see you for several episodes of double vision and droopy eyelids over the past few weeks. She has also started to experience occasional trouble swallowing and at the end of each day thinks her voice sounds funny—quieter than normal and more nasal-sounding. Despite these concerns, her examination in your office is normal. What is going on?

If you've been following along chapter by chapter, you may have noticed that we have been descending through the central nervous system and into the peripheral nervous system. We've now reached the outer provinces of neurology, the neuromuscular junction and the muscles themselves.

As you would expect, this is a chapter largely about weakness, and weakness has a pretty broad differential diagnosis. We've already seen that both central and peripheral nervous system disorders can lead to weakness, ranging from mild debility to full paralysis. How, then, are we to know when muscular disease itself, as opposed to disease of the central nervous system, peripheral nerves, or neuromuscular junction, is the culprit?

Figuring Out the Cause of Weakness

Weakness can be caused by disease processes extending anywhere from the cerebral cortex to the musculature. It can result from a host of genetic, infectious, inflammatory, toxic, metabolic, and malignant processes, in other words, diseases that are not primarily neurologic at all. Thus, patients with arthritis may describe their joint symptoms as weakness. Patients with the flu, chronic fatigue syndrome, chronic lung disease, or a sleep disorder may describe their primary symptom as weakness, although careful questioning may reveal that what they really mean is fatigue or lack of energy. And, of course, weakness can be a complaint of patients suffering from depression, anxiety, or just plain lack of motivation. How do we sort out all these possibilities? The good news is that if we rely on our neurologic toolbox, we will almost always be able to arrive at the correct diagnosis without too much delay.

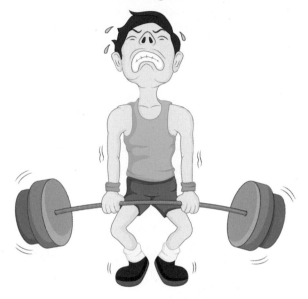

Weakness is in the eye (and body) of the beholder.

The *history* is always critical. One of the ways to separate out generalized weariness from true muscle weakness is to ask your patients if they feel weak all the time or just have difficulty with specific efforts (*e.g.*, climbing stairs or reaching overhead to get something down from a high shelf). The former often reflects an underlying systemic or psychosocial cause, whereas the latter is more suggestive of a neuromuscular issue. Certain complaints should be viewed as red flags for an urgent evaluation:

- Rapidly progressive weakness (over one or several days)
- Compromised ability to walk
- Shortness of breath
- Bulbar symptoms (meaning symptoms due to compromise of cranial nerves 9 to 12, such as dysphagia)
- Altered bowel or bladder function

The *physical examination* should always include strength testing and careful assessment for signs of both upper motor neuron and lower motor neuron compromise (see page 20). **As a general principle (and an important one to remember!), most primary muscle diseases (myopathies) affect the proximal musculature—the neck, back, deltoids, and hip flexors—whereas peripheral polyneuropathies predominantly affect the distal extremities, at least at first** (as you will see, however, this maxim is not written in stone). Most muscular diseases are symmetric, so finding focal lesions is more indicative of a neurologic process, for example, carpal tunnel syndrome or brachial or lumbar plexopathy.

Laboratory testing can rule in or out many of the potential causes of weakness. A primary muscular disease is suggested when serum muscle enzymes are elevated; these include aldolase, creatine kinase, the transaminases, and lactate dehydrogenase. Myoglobinuria is present with rhabdomyolysis. Screens for other causes of weakness include a thyroid stimulating hormone test (TSH, for thyroid disease), serum electrolytes (especially looking for hypokalemia, but also hypo- or hypernatremia and disturbances in calcium and phosphorus metabolism), urine toxicology screens, and testing for connective tissue disorders (such as poly/dermatomyositis and vasculitis). Genetic testing is indicated when you suspect one of the muscular dystrophies or other inherited disorders of the muscle. This is not a comprehensive list, and your clinical judgment should guide additional testing.

Finally, *nerve conduction studies (NCS) and electromyography (EMG)* can help pin down the type and site of the underlying disorder. *Imaging* is rarely useful. *Muscle biopsy* of an involved muscle can be helpful when an inflammatory myopathy, such as dermatomyositis, is suspected.

Causes of Weakness—An Anatomic Approach

Anatomic Site	Example
Upper motor neuron	Brain tumor
Lower motor neuron	Guillain-Barre, diabetic neuropathy
Upper and lower motor neuron	Amyotrophic lateral sclerosis
Neuromuscular junction	Myasthenia gravis
Muscle	See causes of myopathy below

Causes of Myopathy

(myopathy will be discussed starting on page 317)

General Classification	Examples
Inflammatory (see Box 12.1)	Polymyositis (PM)
	Dermatomyositis (DM)
	Inclusion body myositis (IBM)
	Immune-mediated necrotizing myopathy (IMNM)
Noninflammatory	Drug-Related: statins, steroids, alcohol
	Electrolyte disorders: hypokalemia, hypophosphatemia
	Infections: viral (HIV, influenza), bacterial (Lyme)
	Endocrine disorders: hypo- or hyperthyroidism
	Dystrophies: Duchenne, myotonic
	Metabolic: Glycogen and lipid storage diseases

Box 12.1 Updating the Way We Think About the Inflammatory Myopathies

There is a revised classification system for the inflammatory myopathies that is becoming increasingly preferred by experts in the field. Traditionally, the inflammatory myopathies have been classified as they are in the preceding table: polymyositis, dermatomyositis, inclusion body myositis, and immune-mediated necrotizing myopathy. However, these syndromes, once believed to represent unique and distinct entities, turn out to have significant overlap in terms of clinical phenotype and associated antibodies. A more recent classification system has proposed new divisions based on clinical manifestations and myositis-specific antibodies. This is not just an academic exercise, but may prove to have real clinical utility. The diagnostic categories that have emerged are:

- Dermatomyositis (most often associated with anti-Mi 2, anti-MDA5, or anti-TIF1y antibodies)
- Inclusion body myositis (associated with vacuolated fibers and mitochondrial abnormalities on histology)
- Immune-mediated necrotizing myopathy (associated with anti-SRP or anti-HMGCR)
- Antisynthetase syndrome (most often associated with anti-Jo1 or anti-PL7 antibodies; clinically this is very similar to dermatomyositis but is associated with significantly less severe muscle deficits)

Of interest, patients who have traditionally been classified as having polymyositis do not appear to represent a distinct subgroup of patients, and it has been suggested that this term ought to be discontinued. We have chosen to let the original categories stand, because much of the world still thinks this way, but it's important to be aware that this new classification exists, and that, in reality, polymyositis is a much less common syndrome, if it exists at all, than previously believed. We'll get to all the important details of the various myopathies in a bit.

Diseases of the Neuromuscular Junction

Myasthenia Gravis

Clinical Manifestations. Myasthenia gravis stands out from all the other causes of weakness because of one notable clinical feature: **fatigability**. What do we mean by this? Simply that muscle weakness worsens with repeated use. No other disorder, no neuropathy or myopathy, causes this phenomenon. You, the examiner, can miss this unless you look specifically for it, because the weakness typically varies throughout the day; in some patients it can appear and disappear over a matter of minutes. The weakness is usually worse after exercise and later in the day. The most commonly affected muscles include:

- *Ocular muscles.* Almost all patients with myasthenia will have ocular muscle weakness, which typically presents as either ptosis or diplopia. Unlike limb muscle weakness, ocular muscle weakness is often asymmetric. A small percentage of patients with myasthenia experience *only* ocular symptoms (this entity is termed "ocular myasthenia"; interestingly, around 50% of these patients are seronegative for antibodies against the acetylcholine receptor; see page 311).

Box 12.2 The Ocular Muscles

The ocular muscles include those that are responsible for eye movement (the superior, inferior, medial and lateral recti, and the superior and inferior obliques), involvement of which can cause diplopia, and the levator palpebrae, which is responsible for superior eyelid opening and which can cause ptosis when affected. Ocular myasthenia can also affect the orbicularis oculi muscle, which closes the eyes, resulting in weak eyelid closure.

- *Bulbar muscles.* Symptoms include dysarthria and dysphagia. Patients often report a change in the quality of their voice (often described as "nasal" sounding), difficulty drinking through a straw, inability to whistle, a sensation of food getting stuck in the throat, and jaw muscle weakness.
- *Neck muscles.* Neck flexion is usually affected more than extension, which can result in "dropped head" syndrome, an inability to keep the head upright, often most apparent at the end of the day.
- *Limb muscles.* As with other muscle diseases, the proximal muscles are predominantly affected.
- *Respiratory muscles.* As you can imagine, involvement of the respiratory muscles can be dangerous. Severe respiratory muscle weakness resulting in respiratory failure that requires intubation and mechanical ventilation is called "myasthenic crisis"; more on this in a bit.

Box 12.3 Vital Capacity, Negative Inspiratory Force, and Positive Expiratory Force

Don't worry, you haven't accidently picked up a pulmonology textbook. But permit us just a quick word on these parameters, since they are the best way to monitor for impending respiratory failure in patients with myasthenia. Inspiratory force is measured by both *vital capacity* (VC) and *negative inspiratory force* (NIF); expiratory force is measured by *positive expiratory force* (PEF). Myasthenia can affect both inspiratory muscles (primarily the diaphragm and external intercostals) and expiratory muscles (primarily passive, but abdominal and internal intercostals can be recruited). As a result, all patients who are admitted to the hospital with a myasthenic flare should have these parameters checked at least once if not two or even three times a day, depending on the severity of their presentation. The **20-30-40 rule** is a good one to remember: VC less than 20 mL/kg, an NIF less than 30 cm H_2O, or a PEF less than 40 cm H_2O can all indicate impending respiratory failure and should prompt immediate evaluation for intubation.

On examination, **neck flexor weakness** and something called the **single breath test** have both been shown to be good surrogate markers of respiratory function. The single breath test is performed by having patients take a deep breath in and then, on the exhale, count as high as possible until they run out of breath (the ability to reach 50 indicates normal respiratory function).

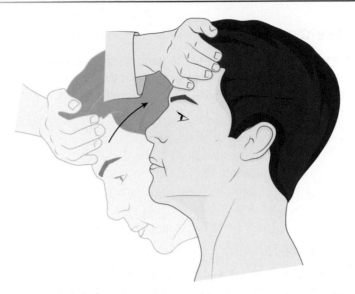

Testing neck flexor strength. The patient should push forward into your hand, while you actively push against them.

Box 12.4 Ptosis

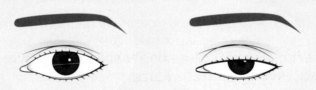

Ptosis of the eyelid.

The differential diagnosis for the underlying causes of ptosis is a good one to file away: it's short, for one, and includes relatively common diagnoses that are important to sort out.

- *Myasthenia gravis.*
- *Third cranial nerve palsy.* This classically presents with a "down and out" eye, mydriasis, and ptosis (often complete ptosis in which the eye appears fully closed) due to dysfunction of the levator palpebrae muscle. Patients most often report horizontal diplopia. We will discuss this in depth in Chapter 18.
- *Horner syndrome.* This is characterized by the classic triad of ipsilateral ptosis (usually incomplete), miosis, and facial anhidrosis. It can be caused by a lesion anywhere along the sympathetic pathway (see Box 12.5).
- *Aponeurotic, or senile, ptosis.* This entity is quite common and is caused most often by changes in the levator aponeurosis (part of the apparatus that elevates the eyelid) as we age. The absence of any other neurologic findings in an older patient should suggest this diagnosis.

Box 12.5 Horner Syndrome

Take a look at the anatomical drawing of the sympathetic nervous system that pertains to Horner Syndrome below. Gives you pause, no? But the anatomy underlying Horner syndrome isn't as complicated as it looks. It's a 3-step pathway.

- The *first-order neurons* travel from the hypothalamus down into the brainstem and cervical spinal cord and synapse on the:
- *Second-order neurons* in the lateral horn of the spinal cord (at the ciliospinal center of budge, usually around C8–T2). The second-order (or preganglionic) neurons then exit the cord and loop back up through the brachial plexus, over the apex of the lung and underneath the subclavian artery, to synapse on the third-order neurons in the superior cervical ganglion.
- The *third-order* (or postganglionic) neurons run on the surface of the common carotid artery and ultimately separate out toward their specific targets; these include the facial sweat glands, pupillary dilator muscle, and the superior tarsal muscle (Muller muscle), which helps to elevate the upper eyelid.

Common causes of Horner syndrome include:

1. Lesions of first-order neurons: brainstem strokes or tumors, spinal cord lesions above T1
2. Lesions of second-order neurons: pancoast tumors (tumors of the superior pulmonary sulcus), thyroid cancer
3. Lesions of third-order neurons: carotid dissection, cavernous sinus thrombosis

Finally, for those of you who love nothing more than a deep dive into neuroanatomy, you will want to note that the sympathetic sweat fibers split from the other sympathetic fibers near the level of the carotid bifurcation. The fibers traveling toward the pupillary dilator muscle and Muller muscle continue to run on the internal carotid artery, whereas those headed toward the sweat glands branch off to run on the external carotid artery. Therefore, lesions above this point will present with ptosis and miosis but not anhidrosis.

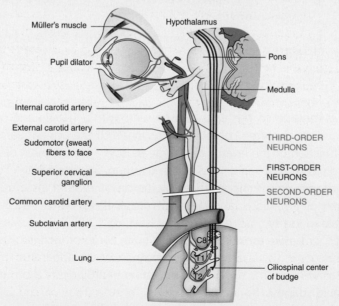

The anatomy underlying Horner syndrome; the first-order neuron is in red, the second-order in orange, and the third-order in blue.

Pathogenesis. Acetylcholine binds to two types of receptors: the nicotinic receptor (located - most importantly, for our purposes - at the neuromuscular junction), and the muscarinic receptor (located on the parasympathetic target end-organs). Myasthenia gravis is caused by autoantibodies that block the postsynaptic nicotininc acetylcholine receptors (AChRs) at the neuromuscular junction, thereby reducing neurochemical transmission across the synapse. Approximately 80% of cases are associated with AChR antibodies. In cases that are *not* associated with AChR antibodies, approximately one-third will be found to have muscle-specific tyrosine kinase (MuSK) antibodies, which are thought to mediate clustering of the acetylcholine receptors during development. Still other patients are considered "seronegative" (although other autoantibodies, including anti-LRP4, anti-titin, and anti-ryanodine receptor antibodies have been found in these patients). Not surprisingly, myasthenia gravis is sometimes seen along with other autoimmune conditions (such as thyroiditis, lupus, and rheumatoid arthritis).

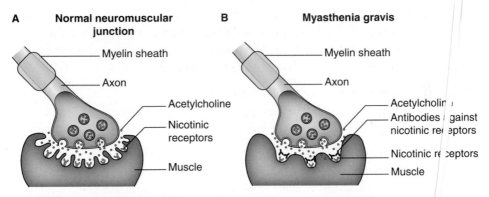

(*A*) Transmission across a normal neuromuscular junction. (*B*) Transmission is blocked by the presence of antibodies to the postsynaptic acetylcholine receptors.

Box 12.6 Drug-Induced Myasthenia

Myasthenia can be caused by various drugs, including penicillamine (used to treat Wilson disease or rheumatoid arthritis), alpha interferons, and immune checkpoint inhibitors (immunomodulatory drugs used to treat several different malignancies). The checkpoint inhibitors work by promoting an enhanced T cell–mediated immune response to cancer cells, but unfortunately, they can also cause a host of side effects due to immune system activation, including myasthenia, dermatomyositis, and polymyositis. Unsurprisingly, they can also significantly worsen pre-existing myasthenia. See Chapter 16 for more on the checkpoint inhibitors.

Myasthenia gravis is often associated with thymic pathology, including thymic hyperplasia or, in about 10% of patients, thymoma. The precise role of the thymus in myasthenia gravis is not understood; it may contain the antigens that initiate the autoimmune process or, via a T cell–mediated mechanism, elicit autoantibody production. It is important to appreciate that not all patients with myasthenia have thymic abnormalities, and not all patients with thymic abnormalities develop myasthenia. Of interest, thymectomy improves the disease in patients both with and without a thymoma and, when feasible, should be performed as soon as possible because (1) there is no compelling reason to wait if the patient is a good surgical candidate and (2) it can be curative.

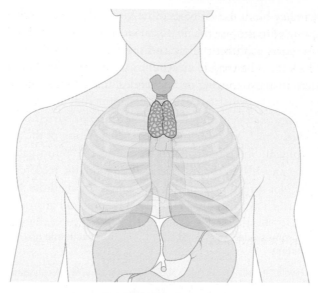

Location of a thymoma.

Diagnosis. Suspect myasthenia gravis in patients who complain of fatigable weakness, particularly when accompanied by ocular or bulbar findings. The diagnosis is confirmed by a combination of clinical, serologic, and, if needed, electrophysiologic evaluations.

1. *Neurologic examination and bedside tests.* Various bedside tests can be used to confirm fatigable weakness. Look for difficulty with sustained upgaze and increasing weakness with repeated strength testing. As mentioned earlier, checking neck flexor weakness and asking the patient to perform a single breath test are reliable surrogate measures of respiratory function. The sensory examination and deep tendon reflexes should be normal. There are two other old-school bedside tests for patients who present with ptosis:

   a. **The ice pack test.** Apply an ice pack to the ptotic eyelid for approximately 2 minutes. Improvement of 2 mm or more in the patient's ptosis is considered positive for myasthenia. This test has a high diagnostic sensitivity and specificity for distinguishing myasthenia-related ptosis from other causes. It is thought that the cooling inhibits the activity of acetylcholinesterase, the enzyme that breaks down acetylcholine.

   b. **The edrophonium test.** Edrophonium is a fast-acting acetylcholinesterase inhibitor. You give it in small, incremental doses and watch for improvement. For many years this was the test of choice, but this drug is no longer available for clinical use in the United States.

A
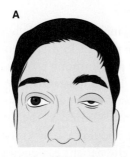

B
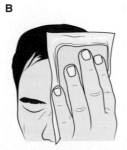

C
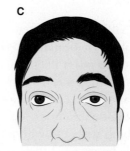

A positive ice pack test.

2. *Laboratory and serologic tests.* Levels of creatine kinase (CK) and inflammatory markers are typically normal. Detection of AChR antibodies or other antibodies associated with myasthenia gravis confirms the diagnosis. False positives are extremely rare. These serologic markers should be used for diagnostic purposes only; they are not useful to track disease activity, assess severity, or measure response to treatment over time.

3. *Electrophysiologic studies.* EMG and NCS are most helpful in *seronegative* patients to confirm the diagnosis; they are often otherwise unnecessary. Single-fiber EMG is the most sensitive electrophysiologic test, but repetitive nerve stimulation is less technically demanding and is therefore performed more often. The demonstration of decreased muscle action potential amplitude with slow rates of repetitive stimulation (*i.e.*, a "decremental response") is supportive of the diagnosis.

4. *Imaging.* All patients should have mediastinal imaging (typically with a CT of the chest) to assess their thymic status.

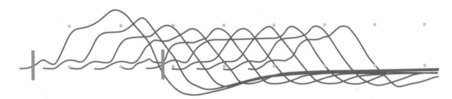

EMG in a patient with myasthenia gravis shows decreasing action potential amplitudes with repeated stimulation.

Treatment. *Acetylcholinesterase inhibitors (AChEIs)*, usually pyridostigmine, are first-line therapy. Acetylcholinesterase is an enzyme that rapidly breaks down acetylcholine. Blocking this enzyme therefore increases the concentration of acetylcholine in the synapse and effectively overpowers the immunologic blockade of the postsynaptic acetylcholine receptor. These are symptomatic medications; they do not modify the course of the disease or alter the long-term prognosis. Common side effects are those that you'd expect from excess parasympathetic activity (the mnemonic DUMBBELLS can help you remember these, see Box 12.7).

Box 12.7 Cholinergic Effects: DUMBBELLS

Diarrhea (and abdominal cramping)

Urination (frequency and incontinence)

Miosis

Bradycardia

Bronchospasm

Excitation of skeletal muscles (fasciculations, twitching, paralysis)

Lacrimation

Lethargy

Salivation

Note that all except the "E" are due to muscarinic (i.e., affecting the parasympathetic end-organs) effects. The nicotinic effects, due to excess acetylcholine at the neuromuscular junction, can be the most devastating.

Most patients will require *immunosuppressive therapy* as well. Corticosteroids are first line for patients who require more than AChEIs alone. Steroids have a relatively rapid onset, generally over 2 to 3 weeks, but can actually worsen symptoms initially. Common long-term "steroid-sparing" agents include azathioprine and mycophenolate. Rituximab, a monoclonal antibody which targets the CD20 antigen on most B cells, is usually reserved for patients with severe or refractory disease and is more effective in patients with MuSK myasthenia. Eculizumab, a more recently approved medication for refractory myasthenia that acts by inhibiting complement activation, is another option. Intravenous immunoglobulin (IVIG) or plasma exchange (PLEX) can also be used chronically in patients who do not respond to, or cannot tolerate, oral medications.

Patients with thymoma, whatever the severity of their disease, should undergo *thymectomy.* Thymectomy also appears to benefit most patients without a thymoma who have generalized disease, increasing the likelihood of remission and leading to clinical improvement while reducing the need for immunosuppressive therapy. Patients with MuSK myasthenia, however, typically do not respond to thymectomy.

The prognosis is favorable. Approximately 10% of patients do not respond to or are unable to tolerate pharmacologic therapy. The risk of refractory disease is highest in those with MuSK antibodies, an underlying thymoma, younger age at disease onset, and female sex.

Myasthenic Crisis. Myasthenic crisis occurs in about 15% of all patients with myasthenia. It is a true neurologic emergency that needs to be treated in an intensive care setting. Myasthenic crisis is due to severe weakness of the diaphragm and accessory breathing muscles, resulting in acute respiratory failure requiring ventilatory support. Common triggers include surgery, respiratory or other systemic infections, and various medications, most notably beta blockers, magnesium, and several antibiotics (aminoglycosides and fluoroquinolones are two of the most common culprits). Treatment consists of either IVIG or PLEX (these two modalities are thought to be equally effective, although plasmapheresis is believed to have a slightly quicker onset of action), as well as steroids.

Myasthenic crisis can sometimes be clinically confused with cholinergic crisis, which can happen (although rarely!) when patients take an excess of their AChEIs, resulting in oversaturation of the acetylcholine receptors to the point that the muscles stop responding. Although both can present with severe muscle weakness, cholinergic crisis will also be associated with the DUMBBELLS symptom constellation.

Box 12.8 IV Immunoglobulin and Plasmapheresis

A quick word on these two therapies. They come up frequently in neurology, and not just in the management of myasthenia gravis.

IV immunoglobulin (IVIG) consists of a pooled mixture of antibodies derived from donor plasma (a single dose can contain plasma from up to 100,000 donors!). It is used to treat people with immunoglobulin deficiencies (which makes sense) as well as those with autoimmune diseases, such as myasthenia and Guillain-Barre syndrome (which makes less sense; there are many theorized mechanisms but no one knows for sure how it works in these settings). Major adverse effects include volume overload (be careful in patients with congestive heart failure or chronic kidney disease), hypercoagulability, and transient aseptic meningitis. Patients who are IgA deficient are at risk for anaphylactic reactions to IVIG (as they may have pre-existing antibodies against IgA), and thus you must either check an IgA level prior to treatment or use an IgA-depleted formulation.

Box 12.8 IV Immunoglobulin and Plasmapheresis (Continued)

Plasmapheresis, also known as plasma exchange (PLEX), is an extracorporeal treatment, like hemodialysis, that selectively removes plasma and replaces it with another fluid, usually donor plasma, colloid, or crystalloid. The mechanism here is more straightforward: it works by removing the pathologic substance (in the case of myasthenia gravis, the AChR antibodies) from circulation. Side effects include hypotension, coagulopathy, and paresthesias. Unlike IVIG, which is typically given every day for 3 to 5 days via a peripheral IV, PLEX is given every other day, typically for about a week, and requires a central line.

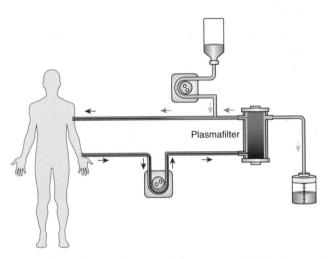

Plasmapheresis exchanges donor plasma, colloid, or crystalloid for the patient's plasma.

Other Diseases of the Neuromuscular Junction

There are several other diseases that can cause the rapid onset of pure motor weakness that also affect the neuromuscular junction. These are much less common than myasthenia gravis, but here are a few you should be aware of:

Lambert-Eaton Syndrome. Lambert-Eaton is caused by autoantibodies directed against the presynaptic calcium channels that are responsible for the release of acetylcholine into the synapse. About half of cases of Lambert-Eaton syndrome are paraneoplastic, most often associated with small cell carcinoma of the lung, and clinical manifestations typically precede the diagnosis of the cancer, often by years. Other cases appear to arise spontaneously.

Like myasthenia, patients present with fluctuating, predominantly proximal weakness. Unlike myasthenia, **muscle weakness improves with use**, cranial nerve involvement is uncommon, and hyporeflexia is present. Autonomic symptoms, including dry mouth and constipation, are common. An EMG will show facilitation with repeated stimulation at fast rates, thus distinguishing it from myasthenia; a single stimulus to a peripheral nerve after 10 seconds of isometric exercise can lead to an increment of more than 100% in the amplitude of the motor response. All patients diagnosed with Lambert-Eaton syndrome should be evaluated for malignancy for up to 5 years after the initial diagnosis.

The best therapy is to treat the underlying malignancy. Symptomatic relief can be obtained with IV immunoglobulin or 3,4 diaminopyridine, a potassium channel blocker.

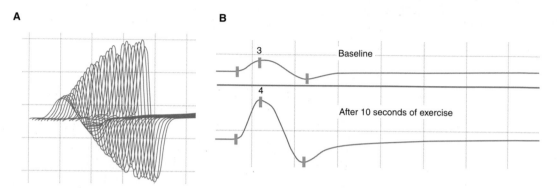

(*A*) An EMG tracing showing incremental increase in the size of action potentials with repeated stimulation and (*B*) increment after 10 seconds of exercise.

Botulism. The botulinum neurotoxin causes paralysis by completely blocking both the neuromuscular junction (the nicotinic acetylcholine receptors) and the parasympathetic nervous system (the muscarinic acetylcholine receptors).

Like Lambert-Eaton, the neurologic manifestations of botulism are the result of the blockade of *presynaptic* acetylcholine release. The neurotoxin is produced by the bacterium *Clostridium botulinum* and is most often acquired through contaminated food, particularly as a result of home canning, although wound infections and inhalation of aerosolized toxin (hence the putative interest of nefarious parties in using this as a weapon of bioterrorism) can be responsible. Cases are rare, averaging 100 or so per year in the United States. However, because infants are preferentially affected (about 70% of all cases, most often from contaminated honey), the disease can be particularly devastating.

When food poisoning is the source, gastrointestinal symptoms usually occur first, followed within 12 to 36 hours after ingestion by cranial nerve palsies and a descending flaccid paralysis, often with dry mouth, nausea, and vomiting. Because the neurologic process can progress so rapidly, leading to respiratory failure and death, treatment with antitoxin therapy should be given before the diagnosis is confirmed by EMG (which will show an incremental response of muscle action potentials to rapid, repetitive stimulation) and isolation of the toxin from the serum or stool.

If you suspect botulism, contact your local health department right away to help with testing and treatment. Any case of botulism is a public health emergency because of the risk of further cases originating from a single contaminated source.

Box 12.9 The Positive Side of Botulinum Toxin

Botulinum toxin, which can be so devastating, has also been harnessed for good. Formulations of the neurotoxin are now used in multiple clinical settings where relaxation of the musculature can be beneficial. Best known for its cosmetic uses (reducing "frown lines" and the like), it is also used to treat chronic migraine, blepharospasm, cervical dystonia, and more. The beneficial effect is only temporary, and thus treatments must be repeated every few months.

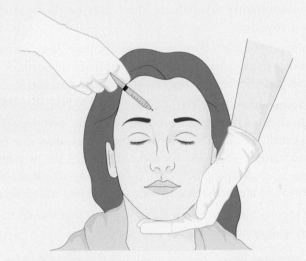

Injection of botulinum toxin to reduce chronic migraine.

Organophosphate Poisoning. The organophosphate insecticides are long-acting acetylcholinesterase inhibitors that cause excess acetylcholine to accumulate at muscarinic synapses and neuromuscular junctions.

The clinical picture is one of parasympathetic overdrive: the DUMBBELLS constellation of symptoms can, if severe, progress to confusion, seizures, and coma. Although the pathology here is essentially the opposite of that seen in myasthenia—too much versus too little stimulation of the acetylcholine receptors—they can look identical, since an excess of acetylcholine can effectively saturate the receptors, resulting in fasciculations, weakness, and, ultimately, paralysis.

Treatment is with atropine (an antimuscarinic agent that will reverse the muscarinic but not the nicotinic effects) and pralidoxime (which can regenerate acetylcholinesterase if given early after exposure).

 ## Myopathies

So here we are—we've traveled as far as we can down the motor pathways, across the neuromuscular junction, to arrive at the muscles themselves. Before we get into the specific primary muscle disorders that you should know, let's ask a fundamental question—*how do we know if a disease is primarily neurologic or muscular?*

Distinguishing Neurologic From Muscular Disease. The answer is not always simple, and you may need to resort to electrodiagnostic testing and muscle biopsy to pin down the diagnosis. But in many situations the history and examination will serve as reliable guides. Some key points:

- If there are sensory abnormalities or depressed (or increased) reflexes early in the disease process, you are almost certainly dealing with a neurologic disorder. The manifestations of myopathies are purely motor.

- Myopathies are usually symmetric and tend to be proximal; neuropathies can be asymmetric and are often distal.

- In the case of inflammatory myopathies, there may be (but not always) tenderness over the involved muscles.

- ALS (see page 275) and Guillain-Barre syndrome (see page 284), because they are predominantly motor in presentation, can mimic primary myopathies. But their distinctive histories and clinical presentations will usually lead you in the right direction.

- What about neuromuscular disease versus myopathy? The distinction between neuromuscular diseases, such as myasthenia gravis, and the myopathies that we are going to discuss next is usually not difficult if for no other reason than that myasthenia has a number of unique features, all spelled out above. But when the presentation is not classic, the distinction can be challenging. Rely on your neurologic toolbox—your examination, as well as laboratory and electrodiagnostic testing—and you will arrive at the answer.

We can group the myopathies into two major categories that should help you keep things straight: inflammatory and noninflammatory myopathies.

The Inflammatory Myopathies

These include *dermatomyositis, inclusion body myositis,* and *immune-mediated necrotizing myopathy.* We will include *polymyositis* here as well, but as per our earlier discussion (see Box 12.1 on page 307), please keep in mind that polymyositis is actually a much less common syndrome than previously believed. Patients with an inflammatory myopathy complain chiefly of weakness and mild myalgias.

Polymyositis and Dermatomyositis. Polymyositis is an autoimmune disease that affects the skeletal muscles. If the skin is also affected (see images below), we call the disease dermatomyositis.

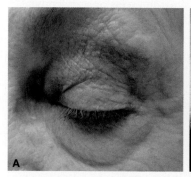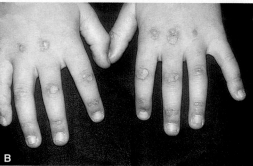

Examples of (*A*) the classic facial heliotrope rash of dermatomyositis, and (*B*) Gottron papules that can occur over the extensor surfaces of the hands. (*A,* reprinted from Council ML, Sheinbein D, Corneliu LA. *The Washington Manual of Dermatology Diagnostics.* Wolters Kluwer; 2016; and *B,* reprinted from Goodheart HP. *Goodheart's Same-Site Differential Diagnosis: A Rapid Method of Diagnosing and Treating Common Skin Disorders.* Wolters Kluwer; 2010.)

Clinical Manifestations. Patients present with progressive, symmetric, and predominantly proximal muscle weakness. They will often report difficulty climbing stairs or getting up from a chair. Patients may also experience flu-like symptoms (low-grade fevers, malaise, and fatigue). About half of patients have muscle tenderness. Interstitial lung disease and cardiac myositis can develop. Nearly half of patients with dermatomyositis (far fewer with polymyositis) have an underlying malignancy that is usually apparent within 2 years of the diagnosis of the myopathy. Women are affected nearly twice as often as men.

Laboratory Studies. Muscle enzymes (creatine kinase, transaminases, and aldolase) and nonspecific inflammatory markers (erythrocyte sedimentation rate [ESR] and C-reactive protein [CRP]) will be elevated. Testing should also be performed for antinuclear antibodies (ANA), which can be detected in about 60% of patients, as well as myositis-specific antibodies, such as anti-Mi2, anti-MDA5, and anti-TIF1y.

Biopsy and EMG. The diagnosis can be confirmed by muscle biopsy, which will also help distinguish polymyositis from dermatomyositis: the former will show endomysial inflammation, the latter perimysial inflammation (think dermatomyositis = inflammation that's closer to the skin; see the picture below).

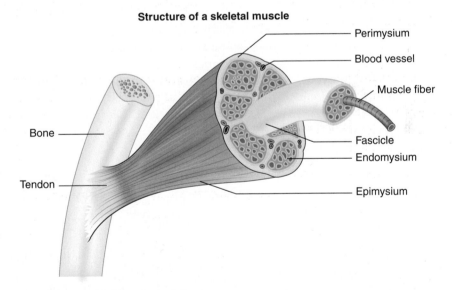

The perimysium surrounds a collection of muscle fibers, grouping them into bundles; the endomysium surrounds each fiber and lies deeper within the muscle.

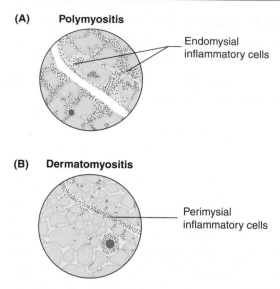

(A) **Polymyositis**

Endomysial
inflammatory cells

(B) **Dermatomyositis**

Perimysial
inflammatory cells

The differing pathologies of polymyositis and dermatomyositis on muscle biopsy.

Treatment. Initial therapy with corticosteroids is usually effective. Other immunosuppressive drugs are used when the disease is resistant to steroid therapy. The 10-year survival rate is now over 80% with current therapeutic regimens.

Inclusion Body Myositis. Inclusion body myositis presents with *both proximal and distal muscle weakness.* The distal weakness can be asymmetric and may be detected on examination by finding subtle weakness in the patient's grip or in the finger flexors. This is an insidious disease that progresses slowly. The diagnosis is generally made many years after the initial complaint of weakness.

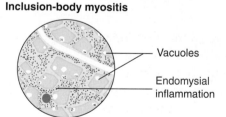

Inclusion-body myositis

Vacuoles

Endomysial
inflammation

Typical findings on muscle biopsy in patients with inclusion body myositis, including endomysial inflammation, vacuolated fibers, and mitochondrial abnormalities.

There are several ways in which inclusion body myositis differs from polymyositis and dermatomyositis:

- It is more common in men, and the average age of onset is older (60 years, as compared with 45 years).
- It affects both proximal *and distal* muscles (nearly 95% of patients will have some degree of distal finger flexor weakness on examination).
- The CK may or may not be elevated, but almost never as high as the levels that can be seen with polymyositis.

- Inflammatory markers, ESR and CRP, are not elevated.
- Muscle biopsy is distinct, revealing endomysial inflammation, rimmed bubble-like vacuoles, and, under electron microscopy, inclusion bodies.

Drug therapy has not been successful; the disease does not respond to steroids. Patients slowly become disabled over a course of many years.

Immune-Mediated Necrotizing Myopathy. This is the least common of the inflammatory myopathies. It can occur as either a paraneoplastic disorder or in association with certain drugs—most often, statins.

Immune-mediated necrotizing myopathy (IMNM) can be associated with anti-SRP antibodies or, when statin-associated, anti-HMGCR antibodies. Histology shows only scattered necrotic muscle fibers without the significant perimysial or endomysial inflammation seen with the other inflammatory myopathies. When statin associated, symptoms do not improve with discontinuation of the statin (see discussion below). Despite the lack of a significant inflammatory infiltrate on muscle biopsy, IMNM often responds to immunosuppressive therapies.

Noninflammatory Myopathies

Drug-Induced Myopathies. Numerous drugs can be directly toxic to the muscles. Among them are alcohol, glucocorticoids, interferons, amiodarone, antimalarial drugs, and anti-HIV agents. Others, such as diuretics, can cause weakness by causing hypokalemia.

One of the most common drug-induced myopathies is that produced by the *HMG-CoA reductase inhibitors (aka the statins)* that are used to treat hyperlipidemia.

Statin Myopathy. Statins are among the most commonly prescribed drugs, so it is important to understand their potential side effects. There are several ways in which these drugs can cause myopathy. We can organize these into four distinct clinical scenarios:

1. *Mild myalgias.* This mild form of statin-induced muscle toxicity occurs in 10% to 20% of patients on statin therapy. Patients will describe muscle aches and soreness, but there will be no objective weakness on examination. CK can be normal or mildly elevated. It's not always necessary to stop the statin, but temporary discontinuation, especially in the setting of moderate to severe pain, is often helpful. Many patients can then restart the same drug or a different statin without recurrence of their myalgias.

2. *Toxin-related myopathy.* This is the statin-induced *noninflammatory* myopathy that truly belongs in this section of the book. Patients complain of mild pain *that's associated with proximal muscle weakness*, distinguishing it from the more common clinical scenario above. The CK is elevated. Patients can almost always be successfully managed by stopping the drug and either switching to another statin or continuing the same one at a lower dose or given less frequently (*e.g.,* twice a week instead of daily). Improvement is usually seen within a few weeks of stopping the initial statin.

3. *Immune-mediated necrotizing myopathy.* Rarely, statins can cause a type of *inflammatory* myopathy, as mentioned in the section above, thought to be mediated by antibodies

against HMG-CoA reductase. Clinically, this can appear indistinguishable from toxin-related myopathy, but unlike toxin-related myopathy, symptoms do not improve when the statin is stopped. Immunosuppressive therapy is often necessary.

4. *Rhabdomyolysis.* Those very rare patients who develop signs of possible rhabdomyolysis (see Box 12.11 page 326) with severe muscle symptoms, dark urine, and a serum CK more than 10 times normal must stop their statin immediately; treatment to prevent renal damage must be undertaken at once.

Statins have many drug–drug interactions, and some of these may inhibit statin metabolism and increase statin levels in the blood, thereby increasing the risk of toxicity. The drugs most often implicated are the macrolide antibiotics, primarily because they are so widely prescribed, and gemfibrozil, which is used to lower triglycerides and therefore is frequently combined with statins in patients with hyperlipidemia. The risk of myopathy is greater with lipophilic statins (*e.g.*, simvastatin) than with hydrophilic statins (*e.g.*, rosuvastatin).

Routine monitoring of CK is not recommended for patients on a statin, but if you happen to discover an elevated CK in a patient who is asymptomatic, the drug does not have to be stopped as long as the CK is less than 10 times normal.

Steroid Myopathy. Corticosteroids are another common cause of drug-related myopathy. Steroid myopathy typically develops gradually, anywhere from several weeks to several months after steroid therapy is begun. The higher the dose of steroids, the greater the risk.

Patients report progressive proximal muscle weakness *without* myalgias or tenderness. The diagnosis is largely one of exclusion: muscle enzymes are normal, EMG is normal (or, less commonly, can show low-amplitude motor unit potentials), and muscle biopsy shows nonspecific type II fiber atrophy. Patients can improve within 3 to 4 weeks of discontinuing the steroid, but some, depending on the degree of weakness, may take significantly longer. Physical therapy is often helpful.

Endocrine Myopathies. Many endocrine disorders can cause myopathy, but most of the time you will already know that the patient has an endocrinopathy, so determining the cause of the patient's weakness should not be a challenge. Examples include:

- Hypo- and hyperthyroidism
- Hypo- and hypercortisolism (the latter often from exogenous steroids)
- Hyperparathyroidism
- Acromegaly (excess growth hormone in the adult)

Except for hypothyroidism, the CK is usually normal, and EMG may either be normal or show myopathic changes. The key to diagnosis, if you don't already know that the patient has an endocrine disorder, is to recognize other symptoms suggestive of an endocrinopathy and order the appropriate hormonal tests. Treatment involves treating the underlying endocrine disorder.

Myopathies Caused by Viral and Bacterial Illness. Many viral (including influenza, HIV, and SARS-CoV-2) and bacterial (Lyme disease) infections can cause myopathy, with symptoms ranging from benign myalgias to muscle tenderness, weakness, and, rarely, rhabdomyolysis. In most cases, the history of a preceding infection is enough to make the diagnosis. A CK and urinalysis should be checked to rule out rhabdomyolysis in severe cases. Muscle biopsy is rarely necessary but is sometimes done to exclude other causes of myopathy, including inflammatory and genetic diseases. Almost all cases are self-limited.

Inherited Myopathies. These diseases can be divided into the muscular dystrophies and metabolic myopathies. The muscular dystrophies are a group of hereditary disorders characterized by progressive weakness and wasting of muscles. The metabolic myopathies result from genetic defects in muscle energy metabolism.

Muscular Dystrophies

Duchenne Muscular Dystrophy (DMD). Duchenne muscular dystrophy is the most common muscular dystrophy that causes significant disability and early death. It is the result of an X-linked recessive gene mutation that codes for dystrophin, a protein that is critical for maintaining the integrity of the cytoskeleton of muscle fibers. Chorionic villus sampling can detect DMD by 12 weeks' gestation. The disease can be familial or the result of a sporadic mutation.

Presentation. Patients present in childhood (usually between 2 and 3 years old) with delayed motor milestones and mild hypotonia. Parents may note that their child is unable to keep up with his peers with running and jumping. By age 5 years, most patients will have clear-cut proximal weakness, and the muscles of the calves, shoulders, and buttocks may appear enlarged as muscle tissue is gradually replaced by connective and fatty tissue, a process termed *pseudohypertrophy*. By the onset of their teenage years, patients will have difficulty walking without assistance. The disease is accompanied by cognitive deficits and learning difficulties. Dilated cardiomyopathy often appears in the teenage years and can cause arrhythmias, congestive heart failure, and death.

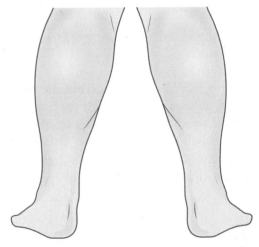

Pseudohypertrophy of the legs in a patient with Duchenne muscular dystrophy.

Diagnosis. By age 5 years, as the proximal weakness becomes unmistakable, a CK should be checked. If it is elevated, the patient should undergo DNA analysis or muscle biopsy (which will reveal absent or abnormal dystrophin). Because DMD is X-linked, it occurs mostly in males, although female carriers of the mutation may show some weakness and are at risk of developing cardiomyopathy.

Treatment. Muscle strength and function as well as mobility can be improved with daily glucocorticoid therapy. There is also evidence that creatine supplementation can improve muscle strength. Angiotensin converting enzyme inhibitors are cardioprotective and improve all-cause mortality. A newer agent, eteplirsen, is specifically designed to target the involved exon to allow production of a truncated form of dystrophin and can improve muscle strength.

Prognosis. DMD is relentlessly progressive. With current therapies, most patients today will survive their teenage years. Almost half of patients will survive to age 25 years, and some, with assistive ventilation, can live into their thirties.

Box 12.10 Becker Muscular Dystrophy

Becker muscular dystrophy is similar to Duchenne muscular dystrophy, but the skeletal muscular involvement tends to be milder (the dystrophin mutation is incomplete, resulting in some remaining functional protein), the onset of the disease is later, and cognitive difficulties are significantly less common. Most patients remain ambulatory well into adulthood. Cardiomyopathy, however, is evident in most patients usually by the teenage years, leading to high-grade conduction blocks and congestive heart failure.

There are many other muscular dystrophies, too many to cover in this text. Here, though, are two you should be familiar with.

Fascioscapulohumeral dystrophy (FSHD). Is an autosomal dominant disease. It progresses more slowly than DMD, with significant symptoms first appearing in adolescence. Characteristic signs include facial weakness, scapular winging, and abnormalities of the shoulder girdle. Weakness of the lower abdominal muscles can result in a positive Beevor sign (not unique to FSHD, but often associated with it), in which there is upward movement of the umbilicus upon neck flexion while in a supine position.

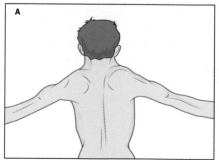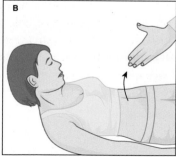

(A) Scapular winging and (B) Beevor sign in patients with FSHD.

Myotonic dystrophy. Comes in two major types, DM1 and the less severe DM2. Both are autosomal dominant. The former is the result of an expanded cytosine-thymine-guanine (CTG) repeat in the myotonic dystrophy protein kinase gene, the latter of an expanded CCTG repeat in a zinc finger protein.

Both types of myotonic dystrophy are characterized by progressive skeletal muscle weakness and *myotonia,* a term that refers to impaired relaxation of the muscles following contraction. One way to test this is to have patients grip your finger and then try to release their grip; the relaxation phase will be noticeably delayed. An EMG will show abnormal, spontaneous myotonic discharges (classically described as sounding like a "dive bomber") that occur at rest and after relaxation begins. Other associated features include cataracts, cardiomyopathy, frontal baldness and various endocrine disorders. EMG and DNA analysis will confirm the diagnosis.

To help you distinguish between DM1 and DM2:

- DM1 is the more severe form. Weakness is typically distal rather than proximal and characteristically affects the facial muscles, intrinsic hand muscles, and foot dorsiflexors, causing foot drop. Ptosis, impaired extraocular movements, dysphagia, and dysarthria are common.

- DM2 predominantly causes proximal weakness. Pain is more common, but cardiomyopathy and endocrine abnormalities are rare.

Life expectancy can be reduced for patients with severe forms of DM1, but both forms can be compatible with long life.

Metabolic Myopathies

These rare disorders result from defects in energy metabolism. If, for a moment, we can ask you to reach back to your halcyon days in biochemistry class, you will recall that ATP, the primary source of cellular energy, is generated by the breakdown of glycogen, glucose, and free fatty acids. When an inherited mutation compromises one of the enzymes that is critical for one of these pathways, the resulting energy deficit can lead to significant weakness. Some patients first present in infancy, some in adulthood.

Think of these disorders when you have a patient with unexplained exercise intolerance. There are three main categories of metabolic myopathy to be familiar with (many of these are discussed further in Chapter 17).

1. ***Disorders of glycogen metabolism.*** These are autosomal recessive disorders caused by impaired glycogen breakdown. The key feature is exercise intolerance; both isometric exercise and sustained aerobic activities bring on fatigue, cramps, and myalgias. The CK is elevated even at rest. Diagnosis relies upon clinical presentation, family history, laboratory abnormalities and, increasingly, genetic testing. Treatment varies, but often centers on diet modification and enzyme replacement therapy.

2. ***Disorders of lipid metabolism.*** The most common of these are the result of various defects in the carnitine cycle, resulting in abnormal fatty acid oxidation. The most common is *carnitine palmitoyltransferase II deficiency.* The infantile form is rapidly fatal, whereas the adult-onset form is less severe and presents with exercise intolerance and episodes of rhabdomyolysis. A high carbohydrate diet can prevent symptomatic attacks.

3. ***Mitochondrial myopathies.*** These disorders are due to mutations in mitochondrial DNA and can present with a wide range of symptoms. The myopathy can be isolated or can be just one component of an illness that impacts multiple organ systems. The myopathy itself can range from mild exercise intolerance presenting in adulthood to fatal infantile forms. Resting levels of lactate are almost always elevated and key to making the diagnosis.

Box 12.11 Rhabdomyolysis

The acute breakdown of muscle cells with the resultant release of their intracellular contents into the circulation is termed rhabdomyolysis. CK levels can go sky high, and myoglobinuria is present. The release of intracellular muscle contents can lead to severe electrolyte imbalances and acute renal failure. Potential triggers are numerous and include:

- Many of the disorders we've discussed in this chapter, including both inflammatory (rare) and noninflammatory (most common with the metabolic) myopathies; always consider statin-induced rhabdomyolysis in anyone taking one of these drugs.
- Acute trauma, such as crush injuries and lightning strikes
- Prolonged immobilization
- Compartment syndrome
- Extreme physical exertion (running a marathon in hot, humid weather)
  - Especially common in untrained or undertrained individuals, but anyone can get heat stroke with rhabdomyolysis if the stress is great enough
- Near drowning, probably from prolonged hypothermia
- Prolonged generalized tonic-clonic seizures
- Delirium tremens
- Overdosing on drugs, including amphetamines and cocaine
- Malignant hyperthermia
- Neuroleptic malignant syndrome
- Hypokalemia
- Hypophosphatemia

Box 12.11 Rhabdomyolysis (Continued)

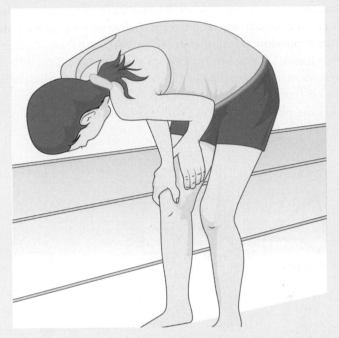

Rhabdomyolosis can occur from extreme exertion.

In patients with trauma, the nature of the trauma will dominate the clinical picture, but in most other settings the chief complaint will be myalgias, and patients may describe passing bright red urine. Muscles will be tender on examination.

Laboratory testing will reveal elevated muscle enzymes and myoglobinuria. The CK takes several hours before it will be seen to rise, peaking in 1 to 3 days and then declining over the next few days. Myoglobin has a half-life of only 2 to 3 hours, so it may not be present by the time you see the patient. Just a reminder—myoglobin will be read as blood on a urine dipstick, but microscopy will reveal an absence of red blood cells. Electrolytes should be checked—in particular, anticipate the possibility of hyperkalemia, which can cause serious cardiac arrhythmias. The most feared complication of rhabdomyolosis is acute renal failure. Renal injury in rhabdomyolysis can have many causes, including myoglobin itself, which is toxic to the kidneys.

Intensive fluid replacement is essential to successful management. Electrolyte disturbances should be monitored and treated if needed.

Critical Illness Myopathy. We can't leave the subject of myopathy without briefly discussing a common source of weakness seen in patients who are critically ill. The word "common" is actually an understatement: it has been estimated that as many as 11% of patients develop some degree of *critical illness myopathy* (CIM) within 1 day of being admitted to an intensive care unit, a number that rises to 67% for patients who are on mechanical ventilation for at least 10 days.

CIM typically presents as flaccid predominantly proximal muscle weakness of the limbs and respiratory muscles; the latter can make it difficult to wean patients off of mechanical ventilation. *Critical illness polyneuropathy* (CIP) can also develop, characterized by a distal, symmetric stocking-glove sensory-motor polyneuropathy with diminished deep tendon reflexes. Some patients develop a combination of the two.

The pathogenesis is not known, but hypotheses abound, including inflammation, immobilization, nutritional deficiencies, and the toxic effects of medications used in the intensive care unit (particularly corticosteroids and neuromuscular blocking agents). Generally, the sicker the patient (*e.g.*, those with sepsis or multiorgan failure), the greater the risk of developing CIM or CIP.

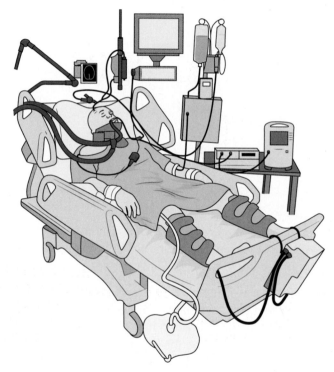

A significant number of patients admitted to the ICU will develop myopathy.

Definitive diagnosis can be made by EMG, but often the clinical setting, routine neurologic examination, and standard laboratory testing are sufficient to rule out other correctable causes and establish CIM/CIP as the likely culprit in these very ill patients.

There is no specific treatment. The best approach is to try to prevent the development of these symptoms with early mobilization, physical therapy, and adequate nutrition, but the evidence supporting these modalities is not as robust as we would like.

Patients usually recover within weeks to months of discharge, but about half will have some degree of persistent weakness.

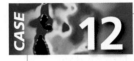

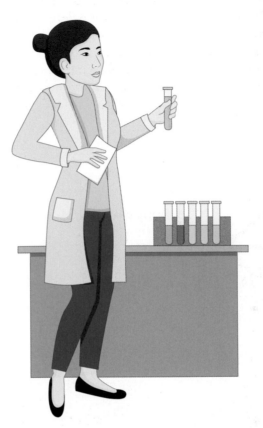

Follow-up on Your Patient: Carol's basic neurologic examination is normal, but because you suspect a neuromuscular junction disorder based on the symptoms she has reported to you, you do a thorough evaluation and note difficulty with sustained upgaze and fatigable shoulder weakness with repeated strength testing. She tests positive for AChR antibodies. Carol has myasthenia gravis. Treatment with an acetylcholinesterase inhibitor and immunosuppressive therapy relieves much of her symptomatology.

You now know:

- | How to sort out neurogenic, neuromuscular, and myopathic causes of weakness
- | The diagnosis and management of the most common disorder of the neuromuscular junction, myasthenia gravis
- | How to evaluate patients with primary myopathies, and discriminate between inflammatory and noninflammatory causes
- | The many causes of noninflammatory myopathy, among them drug-induced myopathies, endocrine myopathies, and inherited myopathies
- | How to recognize and evaluate patients with rhabdomyolysis

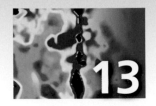

Parkinson Disease and Other Movement Disorders

13

In this chapter, you will learn:

1 | How to recognize and treat Parkinson disease

2 | How to diagnose the different types of tremor

3 | How to distinguish Parkinson disease from other *hypokinetic* movement disorders; in other words, from diseases associated with partial or complete loss of movement

4 | How to recognize and treat the common *hyperkinetic* movement disorders, that is, diseases associated with involuntary movements such as myoclonus and chorea

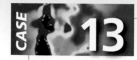

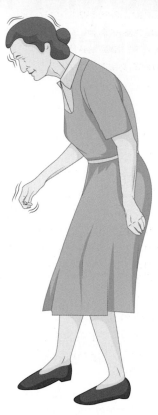

Your Patient: Suzanne, a 71-year-old family practice nurse, comes to your office and asks you to help her with a tremor in her right hand that has gradually become quite bothersome. One glance at her slow, shuffling gait tells you something is wrong. What are the next steps in her evaluation and management?

 Parkinson Disease

After Alzheimer disease, Parkinson disease (PD) is the most common neurodegenerative disorder, affecting more than 6 million people worldwide, and its prevalence is increasing rapidly. Whatever field of medicine you choose to pursue, you will have patients with PD. Although current treatment does not alter the natural history of PD, by recognizing the disease and instituting treatment early on you can help patients avoid unnecessary testing and greatly improve their quality of life.

Box 13.1

Why is the prevalence of Parkinson disease rising? Partly this is due to the aging population and improved diagnosis, particularly of patients in the early stages of the disease. However, there is also concern that environmental exposures, such as pesticides, herbicides, heavy metals, and various industrial solvents, may be playing a role as well.

One quick pearl: You probably think of PD as a disease of the elderly, and age certainly is a major risk factor. It affects only about 40/100,000 people between the ages of 40 and 50 years, whereas it affects over 1000/100,000 people between the ages of 70 and 79 years and over 2000/100,000 over the age of 80 years. However, because it can occur in young adults, don't be too quick to dismiss seemingly benign neurologic complaints, such as tremor (see below), in younger patients without first performing a careful evaluation.

Risk factors besides age include a family history of PD and the environmental factors mentioned in Box 13.1 above. Familial forms of PD are rare, and most cases appear to be sporadic. The jury is still out on whether repetitive head trauma is a risk factor for PD. Depression has been cited as a possible risk factor, but this association may only represent the overlap of two common disorders.

Etiology

The underlying cause of PD is not known. The pathology involves the loss of primarily *dopaminergic* neurons within the substantia nigra (a part of the basal ganglia located in the midbrain), as well as the destruction of neurons, both dopaminergic and otherwise, in other areas of the brain. *Lewy bodies*, which are eosinophilic cytoplasmic inclusion bodies containing the protein *alpha synuclein*, can be found in the affected regions of the brain. The role of alpha synuclein in the healthy brain is not well understood, but it is believed that it can be toxic to nerve cells when present in aberrant conformations.

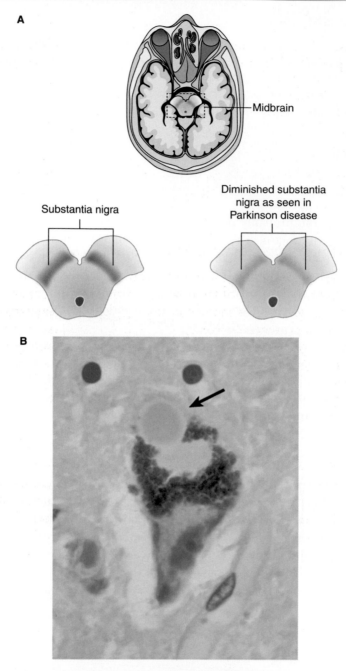

(A) The primary locus of pathology in PD is the substantia nigra, a part of the basal ganglia located in the midbrain. (B) Neuropathology from a patient with PD showing a Lewy body (black arrow) within the substantia nigra. Lewy bodies are often surrounded by a thin, clear halo. (B, reprinted from Rubin E, Reisner H. *Essentials of Rubin's Pathology*. 6th ed. Wolters Kluwer; 2013.)

Clinical Presentation

PD causes four classic physical signs that are the result of involvement of the extrapyramidal motor system, the part of the motor system involved in modulation and regulation of movement:

- Tremor
- Rigidity
- Bradykinesia
- Postural instability

If you like mnemonics, try TRAP (yes, we recognize that there is no A in the list above, but never doubt the ingenuity of neurologists who, in this case, substitute *akinesia* for the often more accurate bradykinesia).

Box 13.2 The Extrapyramidal Motor System

The term "extrapyramidal" distinguishes this part of the motor system from the pyramidal system. The tracts of the pyramidal system (the corticospinal and corticobulbar tracts) begin in the motor cortex and descend to their targets through the medullary pyramids (hence the name). The extrapyramidal system is everything else that impacts movement, and includes neurons within the basal ganglia and cerebellum. In general, the pyramidal system causes voluntary movement, whereas the extrapyramidal system causes involuntary movement, indirectly regulating and modulating the activity of the pyramidal system. See page 18 for a more comprehensive review of motor system anatomy.

The **tremor** of PD is classically described as a "pill rolling" tremor. It is primarily a resting tremor, most easily seen in the upper extremities, but it can also be postural (*i.e.*, most evident when the arms are outstretched). Tremor is the presenting symptom in the majority of patients with PD. It tends to begin unilaterally and then spreads contralaterally over a course of months to years.

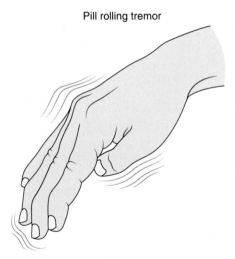

Pill rolling tremor

The resting tremor of PD is most often evident as a pill rolling tremor in the hand, where the fingers and thumb appear to be rolling a pill between them.

Rigidity refers to resistance to passive movement of an extremity. In patients with PD, rigidity is often, but not always, felt on examination as cogwheeling, a jerky stop-and-start (rather than a smooth) resistance to motion. Contralateral activation maneuvers (such as instructing the patient to rapidly open and close their unaffected hand) can help bring out cogwheel rigidity on examination, especially in mild cases.

> ### Box 13.3 Hypertonia
>
> Rigidity is one manifestation of what is termed *hypertonia*. Abnormal muscle tone can be described as low (hypotonic) or high (hypertonic). Hypertonia can further be divided into rigidity and spasticity. Rigidity is velocity independent—in other words, the resistance to passive movement does not change with movement of the limb— and is usually due to extrapyramidal disease, such as is seen with PD. Spasticity is velocity dependent—resistance increases as the limb is accelerated—and is most often due to pyramidal disease. Patients with prior strokes involving the corticospinal tracts (for example, a lacunar stroke involving the corona radiata) often develop spasticity in the affected limb(s). To be clear, though, don't be confused by the seemingly contradictory prefixes: although the rigidity associated with PD is a form of *hypertonia*, PD itself is a *hypokinetic* movement disorder, that is, characterized by the loss of movement.

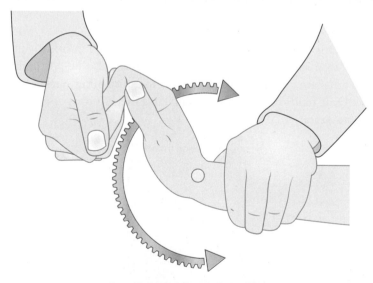

Cogwheel rigidity at the wrist.

Bradykinesia means slowness of movement, but patients often describe this as feeling sluggish or tired. You may notice bradykinesia when you ask your patient to perform a task such as writing or buttoning a shirt, or when your patient enters your office taking short, shuffling steps (arm swing can also be decreased or even absent). Other gait abnormalities may include *freezing* (a sudden, temporary inability to move) and *festination* (a tendency to involuntarily speed up).

The "masked facies" of PD is another example of bradykinesia: spontaneous facial movements are decreased, making the patient appear less emotive. Decreased blink rate gives the patient the appearance of staring. The volume of the patient's voice is also often diminished (referred to as *hypophonia*). *Bradyphrenia*, or mental slowness, is also a common complaint.

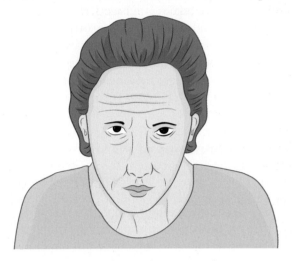

The masked facies of Parkinson disease.

Postural instability manifests itself as difficulty with balance. The "pull test" measures patients' ability to maintain an upright posture when you pull backward on their shoulders (be prepared to catch your patient if they are unable to respond to retropulsion and fall backward).

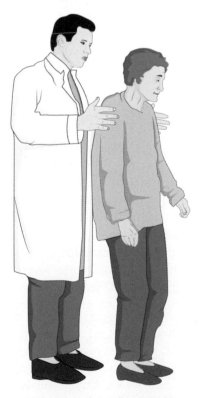

Performing the pull test in PD.

Other clinical symptoms and signs can emerge as the disease progresses. *Neuropsychiatric difficulties* range from issues with impulse control (often worsened by dopamine agonist therapy used to treat PD; see page 339), anxiety, and depression to frank psychosis with hallucinations, memory loss, and dementia. If prominent features of psychosis and dementia appear early on, dementia with Lewy bodies (see page 193) and not PD is the more likely diagnosis. *Autonomic symptoms*, including incontinence, orthostatic hypotension, sexual dysfunction, and constipation are also common. *Insomnia* can be accompanied by or be the result of any of several sleep disorders, notably restless leg syndrome, periodic limb movements of sleep, and especially rapid eye movement (REM) sleep behavior disorder (see page 351).

Box 13.4 Premotor Symptoms of PD

Common premotor symptoms of PD (symptoms appearing before the motor manifestations of the disease) include REM sleep behavior disorder (see page 351), anosmia (lack of smell), constipation, and depression. If you suspect PD in a patient who may not clearly be exhibiting some or all of the classic manifestations of the disease, these are good things to ask about to help guide you in the right direction.

Diagnosis

PD is a clinical diagnosis. *Formal diagnostic criteria include bradykinesia plus at least one other clinical feature of PD.* Routine neuroimaging is not necessary for most patients unless you are concerned about a possible secondary cause of parkinsonism (see page 344). A favorable response to a levodopa challenge will clinch the diagnosis of PD and can often effectively rule out the atypical parkinsonisms (see page 342).

Box 13.5 Advanced Imaging for PD

To reiterate, PD is a *clinical* diagnosis. MRI is not necessary in patients with classic symptoms and a good response to levodopa, but it may be useful to exclude secondary causes (see page 344) in patients with atypical presentations of the disease. More advanced MRI techniques, such as MR spectroscopy and diffusion tensor imaging, may offer higher sensitivity for detecting PD-related neurodegeneration, but their efficacy and diagnostic utility remain unknown. DaTscan, a specific type of single-photon emission computed tomography (SPECT) scan, enables visualization of dopamine transporter levels in the brain and can help distinguish patients with PD or atypical PD syndromes from patients with other diseases such as essential tremor. These scans cannot, however, distinguish between PD and atypical PD syndromes. Thus far, evidence suggests that the diagnostic accuracy of DaTscans is in most cases no better than that of a good clinical history and examination.

Treatment

Because the loss of dopaminergic neurons is responsible for most of the symptoms of PD, it is not surprising that ***levodopa***, the metabolic precursor of dopamine, is the main therapeutic agent. Why not dopamine itself? Because, unlike levodopa, dopamine does not cross the blood-brain barrier. However, levodopa can be converted into dopamine in the periphery, limiting its availability to the brain and causing nausea, vomiting, and orthostatic hypotension. It is therefore combined with ***carbidopa***, a dopa decarboxylase inhibitor that prevents the peripheral conversion of levodopa into dopamine. The combination of these two agents has been the basis of therapy for PD for many years.

Patients typically do well on levodopa for several years, but after a time the beneficial effects wear off. Patients tend to require higher and higher doses of medication and may begin to experience sudden "on-off" fluctuations in their symptoms. The off periods can be severe, resulting in disabling immobility. Medication-induced dyskinesias—involuntary muscle movements—as well as sleep disorders, psychiatric disorders, trouble with speech and swallowing, and dementia can also emerge.

Pharmacologic therapy should be initiated as soon as symptoms become disabling or adversely affect the patient's quality of life. ***Levodopa-carbidopa is the most effective medication and is first-line therapy.*** Other agents can be added as adjunctive treatment for patients who are no longer adequately responding to levodopa-carbidopa alone:

- *Dopamine agonists* (pramipexole, ropinirole, or bromocriptine). These can cause sedation, lower extremity edema, and impulse control issues.
- *MAO-B inhibitors* (selegiline, safinamide, or rasagiline). Insomnia is a common side effect.
- *COMT inhibitors* (entacapone or tolcapone). COMT (Catechol-O-methyl transferase) is an enzyme that breaks down both dopamine and levodopa. COMT inhibitors therefore prolong the half-life of levodopa. They can cause gastrointestinal side effects, sleepiness, and urine discoloration (to dark yellow or orange; this is benign but can be upsetting if patients are not warned beforehand!). Liver function tests must be monitored in patients on tolcapone.
- Anticholinergics (trihexyphenidyl, benztropine). These are used predominantly to treat tremor and drooling. Typical anticholinergic side effects (dry eyes, dry mouth, constipation, urinary retention, *etc.*) are common.
- *Istradefylline.* This adenosine A_{2a} receptor antagonist probably acts by increasing dopaminergic activity and is approved only for use as an adjunct to levodopa-carbidopa therapy in patients with frequent or severe "off" periods.
- *Amantadine.* Its mechanism of action in PD is unknown, although it has been postulated to have both indirect and direct dopaminergic effects. Amantadine can be used as monotherapy in patients with very mild disease. It can also be used as an adjunctive treatment to help reduce levodopa-associated dyskinesias. Side effects are uncommon but can include ankle edema and lace-like skin discoloration referred to as livedo reticularis.

Box 13.6 MAO-B and COMT Inhibitors

The MAO-B inhibitors and COMT inhibitors work by blocking the metabolism of dopamine. These drugs are less potent than levodopa, but they can be dosed less frequently and are less likely to cause dyskinesias. Most often, these drugs are added to levodopa therapy to reduce motor fluctuations in advanced disease and to allow the use of lower doses of levodopa.

Box 13.7 Non-Pharmacologic Therapies

Encouraging physical activity is an important component of improving the quality of life of patients with PD. There is good evidence that starting exercise early, including balance and gait training, resistance and strength exercises, and aerobic exercise, can help patients maintain and often improve their motor function. Physical therapy, occupational therapy, and speech therapy can also be useful when indicated. No complementary or alternative therapies have yet been found to be beneficial. No particular dietary interventions are currently recommended, although ongoing studies are evaluating possible links between altered intestinal microbiota and PD.

No pharmacologic treatment has yet been shown to alter the natural history of the disease.

Neurosurgical therapy is available for patients with advanced disease. The most common technique used is ***deep brain stimulation (DBS),*** in which electrodes are implanted in the brain (typically into the substantia nigra or globus pallidus) where they deliver high-frequency electrical stimulation. DBS has been approved for patients who have had the disease for 4 years or more and are experiencing motor fluctuations. Most patients undergoing DBS experience significantly improved motor function and a lessening of dyskinesia, but other symptoms, including postural instability, cognitive function, speech disorders, and gait freezing, may not improve and can sometimes worsen.

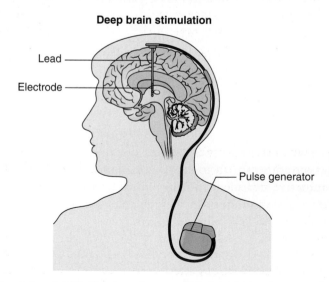

Deep brain stimulation

Lead

Electrode

Pulse generator

Deep brain stimulation for PD. Because the neurons of the brain do not sense pain, the electrode can be left in place without causing any discomfort to the patient.

Prognosis

Despite maximal therapy, most patients will ultimately develop disabling complications. Dementia is common, affecting a significant minority of patients within 5 years. By 10 years, about 25% of patients will require nursing assistance, and average life expectancy from the time of diagnosis is less than 10 years.

Differential Diagnosis: Disorders That Can Mimic Parkinson Disease

Many different disorders, both physiologic and pathologic, can mimic PD. Let's take a few minutes to go through the various types of tremors, as well as the atypical parkinsonian syndromes and secondary causes of parkinsonism that are commonly mistaken for primary or idiopathic PD.

Tremor

Parkinson disease is only one cause of tremor and not the most common one. There are many different types and causes of tremor, but we can sort them into just a few essential varieties.

Parkinson disease. As we already discussed, the tremor of Parkinson disease is usually a resting tremor. It tends to start unilaterally in one hand, but it can also affect the legs, the chin, or the torso. Tremor may persist for years before other symptoms or signs of Parkinson disease develop.

Essential Tremor. Essential tremor (ET) is the most common of all movement disorders. It is primarily an action tremor that is kinetic (brought out by voluntary goal-directed movement such as drinking a cup of coffee) and/or positional (sustaining an anti-gravity posture such as holding the arms outstretched). ET is usually bilateral, although often asymmetric, and can affect the limbs as well as the voice, the neck, and the head. It often improves with alcohol and is worsened by stress and anxiety. Unlike physiologic tremor, it is not typically worsened by caffeine. About half of cases are familial (ET is autosomal dominant), and most begin in adolescence or young adulthood, although onset later in life can occur. It tends to get worse over time. Although traditionally considered a benign condition, it can become quite disabling. Propranolol (a beta blocker) and primidone (an anticonvulsant) are the first-line drugs when medication is required, but they are typically only effective for mild cases. Botox is emerging as a potential alternative option.

> ## Box 13.8
>
> For those of you with a good sense of timing, you may be able to discern that the tremor of ET is faster than the tremor of PD, typically 8 to 10 Hz (*i.e.*, 8 to 10 cycles per second) compared with only 3 to 7 Hz.

Enhanced Physiologic Tremor. We all have this type of tremor to some extent—it is not pathologic—but in some people it can become disabling. It is an action tremor that can be positional or kinetic. It is exacerbated by stress, caffeine, and various medications, including beta-agonists, amphetamines, valproate, lithium, tricyclic antidepressants, selective serotonin reuptake inhibitors, and steroids.

Functional Tremor. This type of tremor is a reaction to stress or trauma or the result of an underlying mood disorder. Unlike the other types of tremor, its onset is often sudden and severe. It tends to improve if the patient is distracted. One common characteristic of functional tremor is entrainment: if you have your patient tap out a rapid rhythm with the unaffected hand, the tremor in the affected hand will change in frequency to match that of the tapping hand.

Other Causes of Tremor. Always consider the possibility of hyperthyroidism (check a thyroid stimulating hormone level!), uremia, and alcoholism (overuse or withdrawal). Other disorders can cause tremor, but they are far less common. One you don't want to miss is Wilson disease, a disorder of copper metabolism (see page 344).

These different types of tremor can usually be sorted out by the nature of the tremor and the clinical context in which they occur. Misdiagnosis, however, is common; patients with early PD are often initially thought to have essential tremor.

Type of Tremor	Description	Example
Resting	Occurs with the relevant body part supported against gravity	Parkinson disease
Action		Essential tremor
Positional or postural	Occurs when trying to hold a position against gravity	
Kinetic	Occurs with voluntary, goal-directed movement	
Functional	Can be anything, typically of sudden onset	Due to stress, trauma, mood disorder

The differential diagnosis of PD can be more challenging when features other than tremor dominate the clinical picture. In some patients with PD, tremor may be minimal or even absent. You then need to consider a group of disorders known collectively as the atypical parkinsonian syndromes, or parkinson-plus syndromes.

The Atypical Parkinsonian Syndromes

All of these disorders are far less common than PD. One key to suspecting these conditions, along with the presence of parkinsonian features and the absence of a predominant resting tremor, is their failure, unlike PD, to respond to therapy with levodopa. There is a lot of clinical overlap among these syndromes, but each has some distinguishing features worth highlighting. The major types of atypical parkinsonian syndromes are:

- Progressive supranuclear palsy
- Corticobasal degeneration
- Dementia with Lewy bodies
- Multiple system atrophy

Progressive Supranuclear Palsy. This disorder is the most common of the atypical parkinsonisms. Rigidity is often prominent, and it tends to impact the axial musculature more than the extremities, resulting in early postural instability and frequent falls. Supranuclear gaze palsy is also characteristic: patients are unable to look up or down when asked to do so, but upgaze occurs involuntarily when the neck is flexed and downgaze occurs when the neck is extended. A resting tremor is usually absent. Magnetic resonance imaging (MRI) classically shows prominent midbrain atrophy resulting in what's known as the "hummingbird sign."

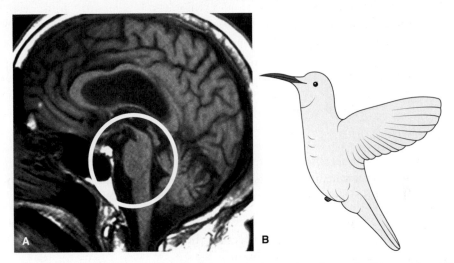

The hummingbird sign, seen in progressive supranuclear palsy. The markedly atrophic midbrain represents the head and the pons represents the body. (*A*, reprinted from Graber JJ, Staudinger R. Teaching NeuroImages: "Penguin" or "hummingbird" sign and midbrain atrophy in progressive supranuclear palsy. *Neurology*. 2009; 72:e81.)

Corticobasal Degeneration. Tremor is not prominent, and patients present instead with predominantly asymmetric rigidity and bradykinesia. Dystonia can lead to painful contractures. Cortical signs, including aphasia, cortical sensory loss (such as agraphesthesia and astereognosis; see page 62), alien limb phenomenon, and dementia, are often prominent and can help distinguish corticobasal degeneration from the other atypical parkinsonian syndromes. Corticobasal degeneration is rare, affecting only about 5 per 100,000 people.

Dementia With Lewy Bodies. We discussed this disorder in detail in Chapter 7. Briefly, the diagnosis requires a combination of dementia with at least one of the key features of PD. Cognitive fluctuations and visual hallucinations are classic features.

Multiple System Atrophy. This disorder should be suspected in patients of middle age who develop features of parkinsonism (again, patients develop rigidity and bradykinesia but not a resting tremor) plus early prominent autonomic dysfunction and/or cerebellar involvement. Autonomic manifestations include orthostatic hypotension and urinary retention or incontinence. The most common cerebellar symptom is ataxia.

Summary of the Atypical Parkinsonian Syndromes. If you remember nothing else, remember that all of the atypical parkinsonian syndromes present with some of the classic features of parkinsonism but (1) tremor is not prominent and (2) response to levodopa is poor.

Disorder	Clinical Characteristics	Pathology
Progressive supranuclear palsy	Early postural instability and frequent falls, supranuclear gaze palsy	Tauopathy
Corticobasal degeneration	Asymmetric dystonia, alien limb, cortical sensory loss	Tauopathy
Dementia with Lewy bodies	Dementia is early and prominent	Alpha synucleinopathy
Multiple system atrophy	Early autonomic dysfunction and/or cerebellar involvement (ataxia)	Alpha synucleinopathy

Secondary Parkinsonism

There are a number of other disease processes, medications and toxins that can cause parkinsonian symptoms; when this occurs, it is referred to as secondary parkinsonism, *i.e.,* parkinsonism caused by something other than primary or atypical PD.

- *Vascular disease.* Multiple small strokes involving the basal ganglia can cause parkinsonian symptoms, typically affecting the lower body and sparing the face and upper body. Tremor is often absent.
- *Normal pressure hydrocephalus* can present with a shuffling gait that can be clinically indistinguishable from that of PD. See page 199.
- *Antidopaminergic medications.* Antipsychotic medications (typical antipsychotics like haloperidol and atypical antipsychotics like risperidone) and antiemetics (metoclopramide and prochlorperazine) can cause features of parkinsonism even months to years after starting the medications.
- *Postencephalitic parkinsonism* can develop after viral infections of the brain parenchyma.
- *Toxins,* such as carbon monoxide, MPTP (an analogue of the opioid meperidine) and manganese, can produce parkinsonian symptoms.
- *Posttraumatic parkinsonism,* a result of repeated head trauma, has been getting a lot of attention lately, but as we mentioned earlier in Chapter 4, the causative relationship is still being investigated.
- *Wilson disease* is one secondary cause of parkinsonism you never want to miss. It typically presents in patients before the age of 40 years and is caused by an autosomal recessive genetic mutation that leads to copper overload (the mutation involves the ATPB7 gene on chromosome 13 that encodes a copper-transporting ATPase). Neurologic symptoms include various movement disorders (including parkinsonism with a resting and/or action tremor, ataxia and chorea) and cognitive decline. Liver disease is often the first sign, but neurologic features can precede evidence of hepatic dysfunction. The diagnosis must be suspected or you will miss it; young patients who present with any features of parkinsonism should always be tested with a serum ceruloplasmin and a 24-hour urine copper measurement. An ophthalmologist may find Kayser-Fleisher rings on slit-lamp examination.

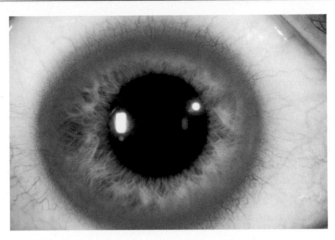

Kayser-Fleisher rings (the dark ring around the iris) are due to copper deposition in Descemet membrane, between the stroma and endothelial layer of the cornea. (Reprinted from Rapuano C. Cornea. 3rd ed. Wolters Kluwer; 2018.)

Box 13.9 Carbon Monoxide Poisoning

Carbon monoxide (CO) is a colorless, odorless gas that is produced any time a fossil fuel is burned. Fires, heaters, and car exhaust are common sources. Acute symptoms of CO poisoning include headache, confusion, and the classic "cherry red" face, which is caused by elevated levels of carboxyhemoglobin in the blood. Parkinsonism can develop days to weeks after acute poisoning. Classic imaging findings include hypodense lesions in the bilateral globus pallidus on CT and hyperintense lesions in the bilateral globus pallidus on MRI (see image below). No parkinsonian drugs have proven effective, but symptoms can spontaneously improve over time.

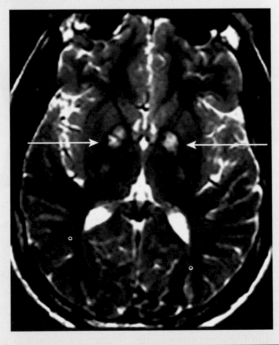

Several months after an episode of acute CO poisoning, hyperintense lesions can be seen in the bilateral globus pallidus on T2-weighted MRI. Modified from Griggs RC, Joynt RJ. *Baker and Joynt's Clinical Neurology on CD-ROM*. Wolters Kluwer; 2004.

Other Movement Disorders

PD is not the only neurologic disease that primarily affects movement. It is by far the most common *hypokinetic* disorder, that is, one that primarily reduces movement, a category that also includes the atypical parkinsonian syndromes and secondary parkinsonism. Tremor is the most common *hyperkinetic* disorder, that is, one that results in excessive involuntary movements. However, there are numerous other abnormal movements and movement disorders in the hyperkinetic category that are important to discuss. Among them are:

- Choreiform disorders and Huntington disease
- Tardive dyskinesia and other drug-induced movement disorders
- Dystonia
- Myoclonus
- Tic disorders
- Sleep-related movement disorders

Choreiform Disorders and Huntington Disease

Chorea, from the Greek word for dance, describes a dyskinesia (defined as any abnormal, involuntary movement) characterized by irregular, relatively rapid movements that can appear to flow smoothly from one part of the body to another, producing a dance-like illusion.

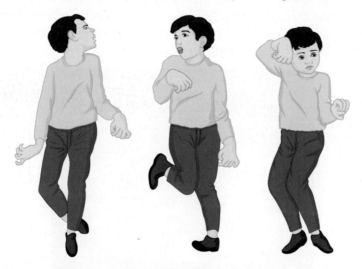

The dance-like movements of chorea.

Chorea was first described as a consequence of beta-hemolytic streptococcal infection, centuries before there were antibiotics to treat the infection. Termed **Sydenham chorea** after Thomas Sydenham who first reported it, it was also referred to as St. Vitus dance (St. Vitus is the patron saint of, among others, dancers). Syndenham chorea occurs months after the infection, is probably autoimmune in origin, and is often preceded by cardiac (rheumatic heart disease) and rheumatologic manifestations. Sydenham chorea is usually self-limited. It is extremely rare today.

Chorea can be acquired or inherited.

Acquired choreiform disorders include chorea associated with *endocrine abnormalities* (such as acute hyperglycemia and thyrotoxicosis), *infections* (HIV and herpes encephalitis), and *autoimmune diseases* (systemic lupus erythematosus and antiphospholipid syndrome).

Chorea gravidarum is the term used to refer to pregnancy-induced chorea. It tends to develop after the first trimester and improve later in the third trimester or after delivery and is more common in women with a history of systemic lupus erythematosus, antiphospholipid syndrome, and other predisposing conditions.

Chorea can occur as a *paraneoplastic* phenomenon. It can also be caused by *medications and drugs of abuse* that share the feature of causing a hyperdopaminergic state (PD, which is a hypokinetic disorder, is caused by the loss of dopaminergic neurons, so it is not surprising that chorea represents the other end of the dopamine spectrum). Among these substances are levodopa, anticonvulsants, lithium, anticholinergic drugs, amphetamines, and cocaine.

Of the *inherited choreiform disorders*, **Huntington disease** is the most common. This progressive neurodegenerative disease is, in its most prevalent form, inherited as an autosomal dominant trait. It is the result of a trinucleotide CAG repeat on chromosome 4 in what is aptly termed the huntingtin (note the spelling) gene, which is involved in multiple intracellular processes including postsynaptic transmission. Expansion of the number of CAG repeats occurs with each successive generation; this phenomenon is known as *anticipation* and results in an increasingly severe and earlier-onset phenotype. The key pathologic finding is the loss of neurons in the caudate and putamen (the caudate and putamen together are known as the striatum; this process is therefore termed *striatal atrophy*). Imaging can show *hydrocephalus ex vacuo* (*i.e.*, expansion of the CSF spaces due to generalized volume loss) and caudate atrophy.

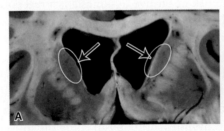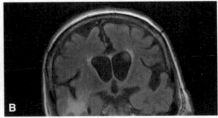

(*A*) Significant caudate atrophy (see arrows) results in enlarged lateral ventricles. (*B*) Enlarged lateral ventricles and cortical atrophy seen on an MRI of a patient with Huntington disease. (Modified from Rubin E, Reisner HM. *Principles of Rubin's Pathology*. Wolters Kluwer; 2018.)

Patients with Huntington disease typically present with chorea but eventually develop aggressive behavior, severe depression, and dementia, as well as profound weight loss. Symptoms usually begin in early adulthood. It is universally fatal. The diagnosis is made by recognizing these clinical features in a patient with a family history of the disease and can be confirmed with genetic testing.

Treatment is supportive. A variety of medications can be used to suppress the movement disorder, among them neuroleptics (*e.g.*, haloperidol), benzodiazepines (*e.g.*, clonazepam), and agents that deplete dopamine (such as reserpine and tetrabenazine; the latter is specifically recommended by the American Academy of Neurology). Deep brain stimulation is also being studied as a therapeutic option.

> ## Box 13.10 Athetosis and Hemiballism
>
> These are two other hyperkinetic movement disorders you should know about that are part of the choreiform spectrum. Compared with chorea, athetosis is characterized by slower, more writhing movements; when the two coexist, the movements are termed "choreoathetoid." Hemiballism is characterized by sudden large-amplitude flinging movements of an extremity and classically localizes to lesions within the subthalamic nucleus.

Benign hereditary chorea is another form of inherited chorea. It presents in infants or young children with hypotonia, generalized chorea, and gait dysfunction. It is inherited as an autosomal dominant disorder most often associated with a thyroid transcription factor gene mutation. Symptoms tend not to progress and may lessen over time, although complete remission is uncommon. It is not always "benign," however, and can be associated with learning disabilities, attention deficit disorder, and a multitude of issues affecting other organ systems (including, not surprisingly, thyroid disease).

Tardive Dyskinesia

Tardive dyskinesia is a complication of long-term use (think *tardy*, or delayed) of dopamine receptor–blocking medications, such as antiemetics and antipsychotics. The risk with the second-generation antipsychotics (such as risperidone, olanzapine, and aripiprazole) is thought to be less than with the first-generation antipsychotics (*e.g.*, chlorpromazine and haloperidol), but this notion has been questioned. The second-generation antipsychotics are increasingly being used to treat depression—approximately one in five nursing home residents is on one of these medications—so the risk of tardive dyskinesia is a real concern.

Patients with tardive dyskinesia experience disabling choreic and choreoathetoid movements of the face as well as the neck and trunk. Why chronic dopaminergic *blockade* should lead to this type of hyperkinetic movement disorder is not well understood; postulated mechanisms include upregulation of dopamine receptors or an imbalance between the stimulation of different classes of dopamine receptors.

The offending medications should be immediately tapered and discontinued when possible. Patients may get better over a period of months, although in some the movement disorder will persist. The same drugs used to treat Huntington disease, as well as deep brain stimulation, can help some patients with tardive dyskinesia. Valbenazine, tetrabenazine, and deutetrabenazine, VMAT inhibitors that limit monamine[1] vesicle packaging and release (known colloquially as monoamine depleters), have been approved for symptomatic relief.

Dystonia

Dystonia is characterized by the sustained or intermittent involuntary contractions of muscle groups resulting in abnormal postures and is often associated with uncontrolled, repetitive twisting movements. The underlying pathophysiology is not well understood. There are multiple types of dystonic disorders that are subdivided based on the part of the body that is affected (generalized vs. focal), etiology (inherited vs. acquired), age of onset,

---

[1]The monoamine neurotransmitters include dopamine, epinephrine, norepinephrine, and serotonin; VMAT stands for vesicular monoamine transporter and is crucial in loading these neurotransmitters into their transport vesicles.

and other associated features. Although the details of these disorders are beyond the scope of this book, there are some essentials you need to know:

Generalized dystonias can affect multiple parts of the body. The most common is the result of a mutation in the dystonia 1 gene. Wilson disease (see page 344) can also cause generalized dystonia.

Focal dystonias affect only a single region of the body. Among these are cervical dystonia (affecting the neck; this is also known as spasmodic torticollis), blepharospasm (the eyelids), vocal cord spasmodic dystonia, and task-specific dystonia (writer's cramp is a common example).

Treatment with anticholinergic agents, muscle relaxers (*e.g.*, baclofen), benzodiazepines, and levodopa can be effective. Botulinum toxin injections are also useful and, unlike the aforementioned options which are all associated with significant side effects, have effectively no side effects.

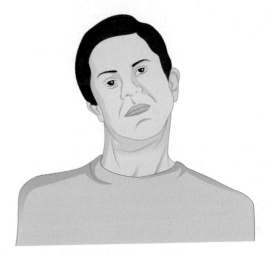

Cervical dystonia. Botox is first-line treatment.

Myoclonus

Myoclonus refers to sudden lightning-like involuntary muscle contractions. It can arise from nearly anywhere in the nervous system and has many different causes. It can be physiologic, secondary to an underlying systemic or neurologic disorder, epileptic, or a primary disease unto itself.

Hiccups (diaphragmatic myoclonus) and *hypnic myoclonus* (the sudden jerk many people get just as they are starting to fall asleep) are examples of physiologic myoclonus.

Causes of secondary myoclonus include *hepatic* and *renal failure. Postanoxic myoclonus*, often seen in post-cardiac arrest patients, is also common. *Asterixis*, a form of "negative" myoclonus, occurs most often in patients with advanced liver disease and is actually the result of a sudden *loss* of muscle tone due to the interruption of ongoing muscle contractions.

When myoclonus arises from abnormal activity in the cerebral cortex, it is considered *epileptic* (see page 163).

Essential myoclonus is the term used when there is no clear cause or if myoclonus is suspected to have a genetic basis. Hereditary essential myoclonus, for example, is an autosomal dominant disorder characterized by upper extremity myoclonus that improves with alcohol ingestion and occurs in the absence of any other neurologic symptoms.

Your evaluation of myoclonus begins with taking a good history and performing a comprehensive examination. If the cause is not obvious, further workup, likely including some combination of laboratory testing (a comprehensive metabolic panel will cover most metabolic possibilities), drug screening, brain imaging, and EEG, should be considered on a case-by-case basis.

Treatment involves correcting any underlying reversible causes, identifying and treating any seizure disorder, and symptomatic therapy with anticonvulsants or benzodiazepines.

Tic Disorders and Tourette Syndrome

Tics are rapid, repetitive involuntary movements or sounds. Motor tics are the most common type of tic (they may be simple, such as single repeated movements resembling myoclonic jerks, or complex, involving a whole sequence of movements). Verbal tics and vocalizations include throat clearing, coughing, and coprolalia (uttering obscenities). Patients typically feel a premonitory urge, often unpleasant, to tic and get relief immediately afterward. Brief, voluntary suppression of the tic is often possible but cannot always be sustained.

Most tics start in childhood and, in a majority of patients, resolve in adulthood. **Tourette syndrome** is characterized by both motor and vocal tics; the diagnosis requires the presence of at least one motor tic and one vocal tic occurring before age 18 years. It is the result of a combination of multiple genetic mutations. The underlying pathophysiology continues to be investigated. Symptoms can be mild or severe. Frequent comorbidities include attention deficit disorder, obsessive compulsive disorder, and mood disorders. Patients may also experience disrupted sleep and difficulties at school.

Treatment depends on the severity of the symptoms. Some patients require little more than reassurance. When tics are disabling, a form of behavioral therapy called *habit reversal training* is first-line management; this technique incorporates awareness training and developing competing responses. If this therapy is not available or if symptoms persist, medications to consider include dopamine depleters (tetrabenazine), antipsychotics (risperidone), and alpha-adrenergic agonists (guanfacine, clonidine). Botulinum toxin, for focal tics, and deep brain stimulation can also be helpful. Symptoms tend to significantly improve if not entirely resolve by adulthood.

Sleep-Related Movement Disorders

We have already mentioned hypnic myoclonus, the myoclonic jerks that accompany falling asleep or transitions from one stage of sleep to another. This condition is benign and requires no further evaluation or treatment.

Restless legs syndrome is characterized by an unpleasant sensation to move one's legs, usually occurring at night in bed. A crawling or itching sensation in the legs is also common. Getting up and moving around relieves the symptoms. Some patients may have a low serum iron level, and all should have their serum iron and ferritin measured. Other causes include uremia, pregnancy, and various medications and other substances (common culprits include antihistamines, nicotine, caffeine, and alcohol). In most patients, no underlying correctable cause will be found. Treatment should focus on stopping any potential offending medications and substances and encouraging regular exercise. If your patient wants to try pharmacologic therapy, gabapentin and dopamine agonists can be helpful. Patients with low ferritin levels often respond to iron replacement therapy.

There are numerous other sleep disorders associated with abnormal movements. Two in particular deserve mention, both of which can be diagnosed with polysomnography:

- *Periodic limb movements of sleep* is a disorder characterized by flexion movements of the legs that repeat in 20-second cycles.

- *REM sleep behavior disorder (RBD)* occurs in patients who lose the normal sleep paralysis that occurs during the REM stage of sleep. They therefore act out their dreams, often in violent fashion with kicking and punching. It appears to respond well to both high-dose melatonin (first-line treatment) and clonazepam. REM sleep behavior disorder is often a prodromal symptom of alpha synuclein neurodegeneration, and thus most patients with RBD will ultimately develop Parkinson disease or one of the other alpha synucleinopathies.

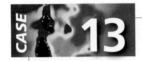

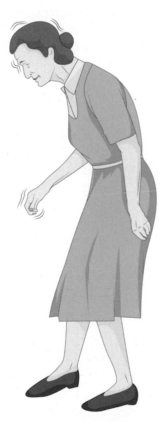

Follow-up on Your Patient: You immediately suspect that Suzanne has Parkinson disease because of her shuffling gait and unilateral resting tremor. Your examination also reveals cogwheel rigidity in her right upper extremity and a positive pull test. Her cognitive testing is normal. You tell her she has Parkinson disease and discuss starting treatment with levodopa-carbidopa. Because her symptoms are interfering with her work in the hospital, she agrees and begins treatment immediately. One month later in follow-up she reports that the medication has helped her immensely and she has been able to continue working much as she has become accustomed to. You arrange to see her on a regular basis to monitor her symptoms and medication.

You now know:

- | How to diagnose and treat patients with Parkinson disease.

- | The mnemonic TRAP (commit this to memory!) that summarizes the basic manifestations of Parkinson disease.

- | How to distinguish between the various types of tremor; in particular, how to differentiate the tremor of Parkinson disease from benign essential tremor.

- | When to suspect the presence of atypical parkinsonian disorders, including progressive supranuclear palsy, corticobasal degeneration, dementia with Lewy bodies, and multiple system atrophy.

- | How to recognize and manage the most common hyperkinetic movement disorders, including choreiform disorders and Huntington disease, tardive dyskinesia, dystonia, myoclonus, tic disorders and Tourette syndrome, and movement disorders of sleep.

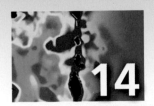

Neurocritical Care

In this chapter, you will learn:

1 | How (and why it matters) to distinguish vasogenic and cytotoxic edema on brain imaging

2 | All about elevated intracranial pressure: what causes it, when to clinically suspect it, and how to emergently treat it

3 | How to clinically and radiographically recognize the major patterns of brain herniation

4 | How to conceptualize and diagnose brain death

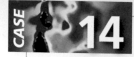

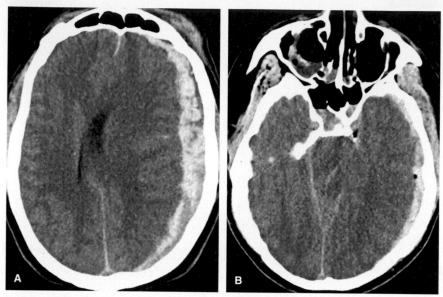

Neha's CT scan. (Modified from Daffner RH, Hartman M. *Clinical Radiology*. 4th ed. Wolters Kluwer; 2013.)

Your Patient: Neha, a 93-year-old mother of four and grandmother of eight, is brought to the hospital by EMS after her daughter found her unconscious on the floor. Her blood pressure is 180/100 mm Hg on arrival. She is largely unresponsive on examination, arousing only briefly to painful stimuli. When you lift her eyelids, you note that her right pupil is 4 mm and reactive, but her left pupil is fixed and dilated. You rush her to CT and obtain the images above. What is the next step in your management?

Neurointensive care encompasses the management of life-threatening neurologic diseases. At this point in the book you are already familiar with the most common neurologic emergencies—acute ischemic and hemorrhagic stroke, subarachnoid hemorrhage, acute spinal cord compression, status epilepticus, myasthenic crisis, uncontrolled cerebral infections, and traumatic brain injury—so we won't spend any more time here on the diagnosis and management of these specific conditions. Instead, we will step back and focus on a few of the worst-case scenarios that unfortunately can be the final common pathways of many of the above presentations. These include:

- Cerebral edema
- Elevated intracranial pressure
- Brain herniation
- Brain death

Dedicated neurological and neurosurgical intensive care units (the first of which opened its doors in 1920) were created with the goals of early identification and—if indicated— aggressive management of these complications. Sometimes, rapid intervention results in remarkable recovery; other times, intervention is unsuccessful, futile, or understandably declined by the patient or patient's family. Compassionate conversation with the patient (and patient's family, particularly if the patient is unable to participate), often involving trained palliative care specialists, can sometimes be the best and most meaningful care a neurological ICU can provide.

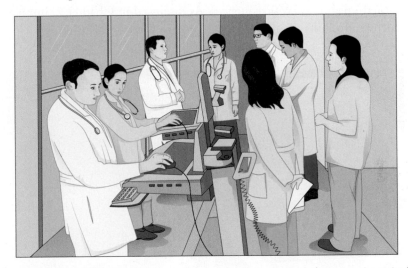

Rounding inside a neurointensive care unit. The team is often a big one and can include an attending, fellow, residents, interns, nurses, physician assistants, pharmacists, and dieticians, all working together to help care for these patients with life-threatening complications.

Cerebral Edema

The term *edema* refers to an excess of fluid within a body compartment or cavity. There are a few types of cerebral edema that you should know, each with specific etiologies and imaging characteristics.

Vasogenic edema is caused by the breakdown of the blood-brain barrier. When intact, the blood-brain barrier prevents many substances that circulate within the blood from entering into the extracellular fluid of the CNS. When the tight junctions of the blood-brain barrier become leaky, fluid accumulates within the extracellular space of the brain. Mass lesions such as brain tumors and abscesses are common causes of vasogenic edema. Acute ischemia causes cytotoxic edema (see page 356) but over time (within hours to days) can cause vasogenic edema as well.

Vasogenic edema has a characteristic finger-like appearance on CT, spreading within the white matter but sparing the gray matter cortex. You can think of it this way: because the white matter is made up of axons and the cortex is made up of tightly packed cell bodies, there is space for extracellular fluid to spread within the white matter but not within the tightly packed cortical regions.

Cytotoxic edema is the result of cell death. It is usually due to the depletion of intracellular adenosine triphosphate (ATP), disrupting the function of the sodium/potassium transporter and causing intracellular osmole accumulation and—because water follows the osmolar gradient—intracellular fluid accumulation. Acute ischemia is the most common cause; other causes include acute liver failure and anoxic injury.

Radiographically, cytotoxic edema is often subtle on CT, appearing as hypoattenuation and blurring of the gray-white junction. On MRI, cytotoxic edema is best identified on diffusion-weighted imaging (DWI) sequences. As discussed in Chapter 2, intracellular fluid shifts and subsequent cellular swelling result in restricted water diffusion, which appears bright white on the MRI.

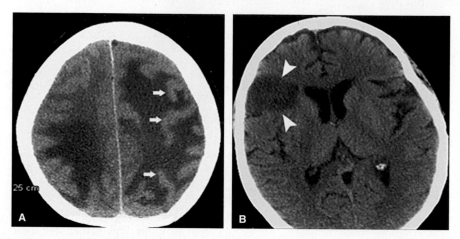

CT scans showing (*A*) vasogenic edema, which has a characteristic finger-like appearance and spares the gray matter cortex (white arrows point to the finger-like extensions of spared cortex that are surrounded by vasogenic edema), and (*B*) cytotoxic edema, which obliterates the gray-white matter junction (white arrows point to the edema). (Reprinted from Weiner WJ, Goetz CG, Shin RK, Lewis SL. Neurology for the Non-Neurologist, 6th Edition. Philadelphia: Wolters Kluwer, 2010.)

These two categories are not exclusive. Various brain lesions and injuries (for example, intracerebral hemorrhage and traumatic brain injury) can cause both cytotoxic and vasogenic edema.

Two other types of cerebral edema to be aware of are *interstitial edema* (also known as transependymal or hydrostatic edema) and *osmotic edema*.

Interstitial edema is the result of obstructive hydrocephalus, when cerebrospinal fluid (CSF) outflow from the ventricles is blocked and CSF is forced into the interstitium of the brain by the high pressure in the ventricular system.

Osmotic edema is due to decreased plasma osmolarity (for example, in the setting of the syndrome of inappropriate ADH secretion [SIADH] or with rapid glucose reduction in patients with hyperosmolar hyperglycemic state). Under normal circumstances, the osmolarity of the CSF and extracellular cerebral fluid is less than that of plasma. If plasma osmolarity falls, fluid shifts into the brain.

Why does cerebral edema matter? Because the skull is a fixed space and any increase in the volume of its contents can result in elevated intracranial pressure, which brings us to our next topic.

 ## *Elevated Intracranial Pressure*

Physiology

Intracranial pressure (ICP) is the pressure within the cranium of the skull.[1] In the eighteenth century, two Scottish surgeons named Alexander Monro and George Kellie came up with a hypothesis that still remains the clearest way to think about ICP. *The Monro-Kellie doctrine*, as it is now known, states that intracranial volume is made up of three components—blood, CSF, and brain tissue—and that this volume must remain constant. Any increase in one component should therefore lead to a decrease in one or both of the other two.

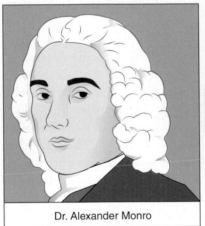
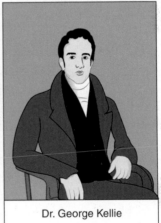

Dr. Alexander Monro   Dr. George Kellie

Let's take an example of a growing brain tumor. As the tumor grows, the tissue component of intracranial volume expands and, because the skull is poorly compliant, even this small increase in volume leads to a relatively large increase in pressure. This increase in pressure, however, will be quickly buffered by displacement of other compartments. In general, the volume of CSF decreases first to compensate. In time, if the tumor continues to expand, blood volume will also decrease (resulting in ischemia) and, ultimately, brain tissue itself will be displaced, forced to herniate outside of the skull.

[1]Normal ICP is approximately 5 to 15 mm Hg in a supine adult.

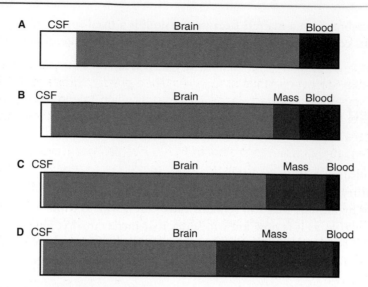

Intracranial volume is made up of three components: CSF, brain tissue, and blood (A). In the setting of a growing mass lesion, CSF tends to decrease first (B), followed by blood volume (C) and ultimately brain tissue (D).

Here is one more way to think about ICP. As we've just discussed, pressure changes within the skull can affect blood flow. In order to adequately perfuse the brain, blood must be pumped against a pressure gradient. If you've ever inflated a basketball, you've experienced this firsthand. At the start, the ball is compliant—not at all like the skull—but as it inflates, the walls become stiff and the pressure inside rises. The higher the pressure rises, the harder it becomes to pump air into the ball. The same effort that, in the beginning, easily pumped air inside the ball becomes less and less effective until it fails: it no longer overcomes the pressure inside the ball, and air entry ceases. The physiologic process that enables brain perfusion is much the same. The heart and arteries generate a blood pressure that forces blood into the blood vessels within the skull. The difference between this pressure (the mean arterial pressure, MAP) and the pressure inside the skull (the ICP) is called the cerebral perfusion pressure (CPP) and is defined as the net pressure gradient that causes blood to flow to the brain.

$$CPP = MAP - ICP$$

When the ICP goes up, the CPP goes down, resulting in a lack of blood flow to the brain and subsequent ischemia.

Box 14.1 Cerebral Autoregulation

How do we maintain stable cerebral blood flow (CBF) and cerebral perfusion pressure (CPP) in the face of drastic fluctuations in systemic blood pressure? Why do we not always immediately pass out or even have a stroke when our systemic blood pressure falls? Conversely, why do we not immediately bleed into our brain when our systemic blood pressure rises?

Box 14.1 Cerebral Autoregulation (Continued)

Cerebral autoregulation is the process by which vasoconstriction and vasodilation maintain stable CBF over a range of CPPs. As blood pressure rises and CPP increases, intracranial vessels vasoconstrict, increasing resistance and thereby maintaining stable CBF and, consequently, ICP. When blood pressure falls and CPP declines, intracranial vessels vasodilate, decreasing resistance to allow the lower CPP to maintain a stable CBF and adequate perfusion to the brain. The precise pathophysiology allowing for appropriate vasodilation and vasoconstriction is unclear (there appear to be metabolic, autonomic, and myogenic factors involved), but the process is an effective one: most people are able to maintain a stable CBF over a range of approximately 50 to 150 mm Hg of CPP. When the limits of autoregulation are exceeded, blood vessels will either collapse (from being underfilled) or be forcibly dilated (from excess pressure). Ischemia and hemorrhage, respectively, can result.

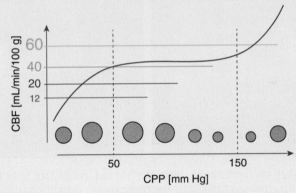

By means of vasoconstriction and vasodilation, cerebral autoregulation allows for a stable CBF over a range of approximately 50 to 150 mm Hg of CPP.

Causes and Presentation of Elevated ICP

Common causes of increased ICP include:

- *Mass lesions* (brain tumors, intracranial abscesses, hematomas)
- *Cerebral edema* (from massive ischemic stroke, severe traumatic brain injury, mass lesions)
- *Obstruction of venous outflow* (venous sinus thrombosis)
- *Obstructive hydrocephalus* (excess accumulation of CSF resulting from mechanical blockage of CSF flow, often caused by tumors or other mass lesions)
- *Communicating hydrocephalus* (excess accumulation of CSF in the absence of mechanical obstruction); there are two major causes:
  - *Decreased CSF absorption* (secondary to intracranial infection, which can clog up the arachnoid granulations with inflammatory exudate and thereby prevent CSF absorption; subarachnoid hemorrhage, which can do the same with blood; and leptomeningeal metastasis, with tumor cells)
  - *Increased CSF production* (secondary to CSF-producing tumors, such as choroid plexus papillomas)

Elevated ICP most often presents with relatively nonspecific symptoms such as headache (thought to be the result of pressure on the pain fibers of CN5 that run in the dura and on blood vessels), nausea, vomiting, and depressed consciousness (presumably a result of distortion of the thalamic and brainstem reticular activating system, which mediates arousal and attention).

Signs on examination can include papilledema (swelling of the optic nerve head due to elevated ICP) and a CN6 palsy (due to pressure on the nerve at the skull base). The development of the so-called *Cushing triad*—bradycardia, hypertension, and respiratory depression—can indicate imminent herniation. See page 363 for a discussion of specific herniation syndromes.

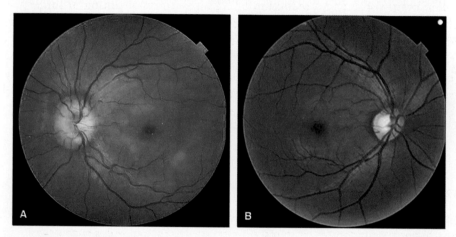

(A) Papilledema seen on funduscopy. Note the blurred margins of the optic nerve head. (B) A normal sharply defined optic disc, for comparison. (Modified from Freddo TF, Chaum E. *Anatomy of the Eye and Orbit*. Wolters Kluwer; 2017.)

Management of Elevated ICP

Patients who are *at risk of elevated ICP*—those with an acutely bleeding tumor, for instance, or with a massive middle cerebral artery (MCA) stroke—should be managed with a guiding set of principles and treatment strategies known as "ICP precautions" that attempt to prevent further elevation in pressure and mitigate its downstream effects. These precautions include maintaining normotension, normothermia, and euglycemia and keeping the head of the bed elevated 30°.

Management of *acutely elevated ICP* involves several steps:

- *Hemodynamic stabilization* (remember your ABCs: airway, blood pressure, and circulation). This prevents the evolution of values lying outside the cerebral autoregulation window and ensures stable cerebral blood flow.
- *Sedation* decreases cerebral metabolic activity, which in turn reduces cerebral blood volume and ICP.

- *Hyperventilation* causes cerebral vasoconstriction, again reducing cerebral blood volume and ICP (in general, this is a temporizing measure and should not be performed for more than 15 minutes or so, as prolonged vasoconstriction can increase the risk of stroke and result in a rebound spike in ICP).

- *Hypertonic osmotic agents* such as mannitol and hypertonic saline can be given to draw fluid out of brain tissue and into the blood vessels, temporarily decreasing both vasogenic and cytotoxic edema. The key word here is *temporarily*: these agents buy you time but will not fix the underlying problem.

- *Surgical decompression* is another option, often performed via hemicraniectomy, whereby a large piece of the skull is removed to allow for the expansion of swollen brain tissue and a reduction of ICP. The optimal timing of surgery, as well as who are the optimal surgical candidates, are still up for debate. In general, hemicraniectomy has been proven to be a *life-saving* procedure, but it is not always a *quality-of-life*-saving procedure, as surgery can leave patients extremely disabled. Whenever possible, it is important to discuss the risks and benefits of surgery in patients at risk of ICP crises early on, to determine if surgical management, should it become a consideration, is within their goals of care.

Box 14.2 Decerebrate and Decorticate Posturing

The term *posturing* refers to abnormal flexion or extension of the extremities that occurs either spontaneously or in response to an external stimulus such as pain, and can indicate severe brain injury.

Decorticate posturing is characterized by arm flexion into the chest and leg extension with feet internally rotated. Decorticate posturing is indicative of damage to the cerebral hemispheres above the level of the red nucleus, a structure located in the midbrain that is involved in motor coordination.

Decerebrate posturing can be clinically differentiated from decorticate posturing by the presence of *both* upper and lower extremity extension. It is caused by brainstem damage *below* the level of the red nucleus. Progression from decorticate to decerebrate posturing can be indicative of uncal or tonsillar herniation (see pages 365–366).

In reality, the clinical distinction between decorticate and decerebrate posturing is often of little localizing value. The takeaway here instead is that abnormal posturing of any sort is an ominous sign and most often indicative of dangerous underlying pathology and a poor prognosis.

Box 14.2 Decerebrate and Decorticate Posturing (Continued)

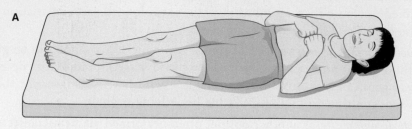

A

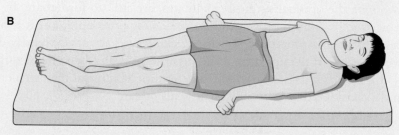

B

Here is a helpful sort of mnemonic: deCORticate posturing (*A*) presents with arms flexed into the CORE of the body, whereas decErebrate posturing (*B*) presents with the arms Extended away.

Box 14.3 ICP Monitoring

Invasive ICP monitoring can be used in neurological or neurosurgical ICUs in patients who are at high risk of developing elevated ICP and for whom monitoring has the potential to significantly guide management and hopefully improve clinical outcome. Intraventricular monitoring, with a catheter surgically placed into the ventricular system, allows for the most precise monitoring and, if indicated, can also treat elevated ICP via CSF drainage. Intraparenchymal devices are also sometimes used.

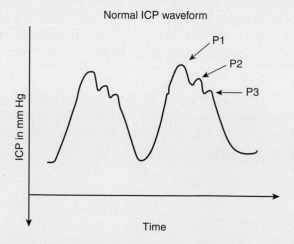

Normal ICP waveform

P1

P2

P3

ICP in mm Hg

Time

A normal ICP waveform as measured by an ICP monitor. P1 correlates with the arterial pulse, P2 with cerebral compliance, and P3 with closure of the aortic valve. Normal ICP is 5 to 15 mm Hg in a supine adult.

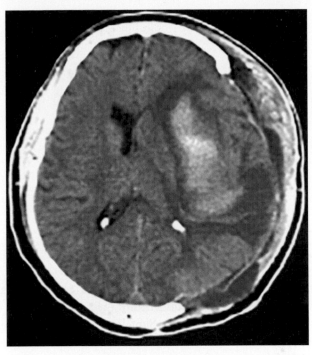

A CT scan several days after decompressive hemicraniectomy, with herniation of edematous brain tissue through the hemicraniectomy skull defect. The hemicraniectomy enables increased skull compliance and expansion of intracranial volume by replacing the hard bone of the skull with more elastic skin. (Reprinted from Louis ED, Mayer SA, Rowland LP. *Merritt's Neurology*, 13th ed. Wolters Kluwer; 2013.)

Herniation Syndromes

For better or worse, there are multiple ways in which brain tissue can be forced into places it shouldn't be. It is important to be able to recognize these different syndromes—both clinically and radiographically—so that you can quickly jump into action.

Herniation here is defined as the displacement of brain tissue from its normal position inside the skull. Before we get into the details, it is important to understand why this can be so devastating. Displacement can result in compression of critical arteries and veins (causing ischemia or hemorrhage) as well as crush injury of brain tissue itself. Because the skull is really just a hard sphere with a single, approximately 3-cm-diameter hole at the bottom (the foramen magnum), the only real way out is down. Consequently, the final common pathway of the herniation patterns listed below is brainstem compression, resulting in damage to pathways controlling respiratory and cardiac function and, eventually, death.

When ICP rises, where can brain tissue go? There are several possibilities:

- From one side of the cranium to the other (subfalcine herniation)
- From the top of the cranium to the bottom (central herniation)
- From the side of the cranium to the bottom (uncal herniation)
- From the bottom of the cranium to outside of the cranium (tonsillar herniation)
- From the inside to the outside of the cranium, through a fracture or surgical site opening in the skull (transcalvarial herniation)

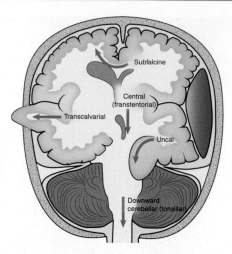

The various herniation patterns.

Subfalcine herniation is the most common herniation pattern. It occurs when the innermost part of the frontal lobe is forced underneath the falx cerebri (the dural sheet that divides the right and left cerebral hemispheres). Subfalcine herniation is often a precursor to other more dangerous types of herniation. The presentation is often nonspecific: headache and increasing somnolence are the most common manifestations. Lower extremity weakness can occur owing to compression of the anterior cerebral artery. The brainstem is generally spared.

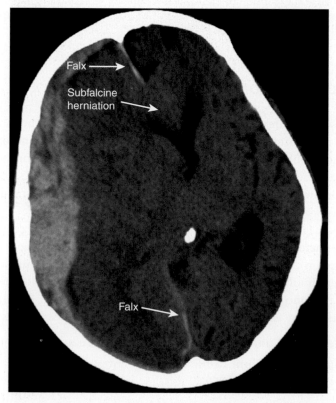

Subfalcine herniation due to an expanding right-sided bleed. (Modified from Daffner RH, Hartman M. *Clinical Radiology*. 4th ed. Wolters Kluwer; 2013.)

Uncal herniation is characterized by the displacement of the medial temporal lobe (*i.e.*, the "uncus") beneath the tentorium cerebelli (the dural sheet that overlies the cerebellum) and into the suprasellar cistern (located above the sella turcica and below the hypothalamus). Ipsilateral CN3 palsy, a result of nerve compression, and contralateral hemiparesis, a result of compression of the corticospinal tract running within the cerebral peduncle of the midbrain, are signs to watch out for.

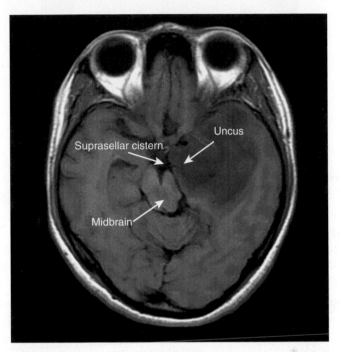

Uncal herniation, characterized by displacement of the uncus resulting in compression of the midbrain. (Modified from Strayer DS, Saffitz JE, Rubin E. *Rubin's Pathology*. 8th ed. Wolters Kluwer; 2019.)

Box 14.4 The Kernohan Phenomenon

Ipsilateral hemiparesis, a so-called false localizing sign, can occur when the brain is compressed against the opposite edge of the tentorium. This is called the Kernohan phenomenon. A right-sided subdural hematoma, for instance, can cause leftward displacement of the brain, resulting in compression of the descending motor fibers located in the left anterior midbrain against the left tentorium cerebelli (at Kernohan notch, hence the name). The result is right-sided weakness caused by a right-sided subdural bleed.

Central tentorial herniation occurs when the cerebral hemispheres are forced downward through the tentorium. This can cause compression of the bilateral third cranial nerves (causing bilateral blown pupils and "down and out" eye deviation), as well as compression of the posterior cerebral and basilar arteries (resulting in posterior circulation ischemia).

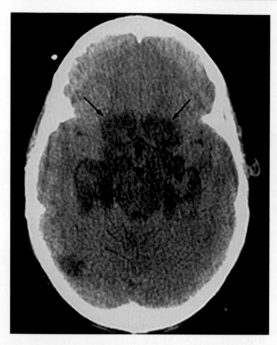

Central tentorial herniation (the arrows point to areas of infarction caused by downward displacement of the cerebral hemispheres). (Reprinted from Shrier DA, Shibata DK, Wang HZ, Numaguchi Y, Powers JM. Central brain herniation secondary to juvenile diabetic ketoacidosis. *Am J Neuroradiol.* 1999;20(10):1885-1888.)

Tonsillar herniation is characterized by the downward displacement of the cerebellar tonsils through the foramen magnum, resulting in brainstem and upper spinal cord compression. The early stages of tonsillar herniation are often missed because there are usually no pupillary changes on examination. Instead, headache, neck stiffness and increasing somnolence are followed by extensor posturing, respiratory failure, and devastating circulatory collapse.

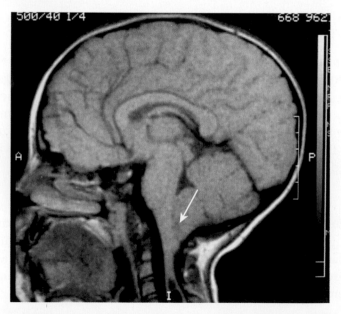

Tonsillar herniation. The arrow points to the downward displacement of the cerebellar tonsils. (Modified from Nelson LB, Olitsky SE. *Harley's Pediatric Ophthalmology.* 6th ed. Wolters Kluwer; 2013.)

Brain Death

Brain death is defined as the complete and irreversible absence of all cerebral and brainstem function. It is nearly universally considered synonymous with death, but the diagnosis can be challenging, as protocols and definitions vary from country to country and even from hospital to hospital. To give you an idea of the requirements needed to declare a patient "brain dead," here is an example of brain death guidelines from a statement issued by a hospital in New York City:

- Clinical requirements:
  - Clinical or radiographic evidence of acute CNS injury that explains the brain dead state
  - The absence of any confounding factors, including medications that depress brain function, neuromuscular blocking agents, hypothermia, hypotension, and other metabolic derangements
- Neurologic examination requirements:
  - The patient is comatose
  - The patient has no brainstem reflexes (see page 427)
  - The patient has no motor response to pain[2]
- A positive apnea test:
  - The apnea test is performed after all of the above criteria have been met. The goal is to prove the absence of the brainstem-mediated respiratory response (*i.e.*, no spontaneous breathing) despite intense stimulation to breathe (Paco$_2$ > 60 mm Hg)

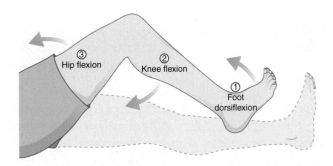

Triple flexion response (see footnote below).

[2]It is important to note that spinal reflexes can persist and appear to be volitional. The *triple flexion* response is a common example, characterized by flexion of the foot, leg, and thigh in response to painful stimuli of the lower extremity. This is a stereotyped spinal reflex, not a voluntary withdrawal response.

If some of the above criteria cannot be adequately performed or assessed, confirmatory tests can help establish the diagnosis. An EEG, for example, will show a complete absence of cerebral electrical activity, including a lack of reactivity to external stimulation. Angiography will usually show absence of blood flow within the intracranial arteries.

There are no known reports of neurologic recovery after a confirmed diagnosis of brain death.

Box 14.5 Coma and Persistent Vegetative State

There is a difference between coma and persistent vegetative state. *Coma* is a state of unarousable unresponsiveness. A comatose patient will not arouse even with strong and continuous stimuli and cannot in any meaningful way interact with the environment.

Persistent vegetative state is a state of wakefulness without awareness. Patients show no awareness of themselves or of their environment. They demonstrate no purposeful movement or any evidence of language comprehension or expression. However, they often maintain normal sleep/wake cycles, and both brainstem and spinal reflexes may be preserved. Guidelines vary, but persistent vegetative state is generally deemed permanent after 3 months to 1 year, depending on the etiology. Meaningful recovery after this point is rare.

Box 14.6 Post-Arrest Prognostication

One of the more difficult jobs of a neurologist is to help establish a patient's prognosis following a cardiac arrest. Various other ICU teams often ask for assistance in determining a patient's chance of neurologic recovery, because having a sense of a patient's prognosis will help guide subsequent management. And families, of course, want answers as soon as possible: Will my mother/father/spouse/partner survive? And if so, what will that survival look like?

Unfortunately, these questions are often hard to answer (the exception is brain death: if confirmed, we know the patient will not recover). The neurologic examination has the best prognostic value. The absence of brainstem reflexes and the lack of any purposeful motor response to painful stimuli portend poorly, suggesting a low likelihood of ever achieving functional independence. EEG and brain imaging are generally less helpful: "malignant" EEG patterns (such as burst-suppression and suppression with continuous periodic discharges) and loss of gray/white differentiation on CT associated with anoxic injury are concerning, but uncommonly patients can still recover. Even in the presence of a poor examination

Box 14.6 Post-Arrest Prognostication   (Continued)

(absent brainstem reflexes except for corneal reflexes, for instance, and no motor response to pain) and burst-suppression EEG, we can offer guidance and help prepare families for what's likely ahead, but we cannot say anything for certain.

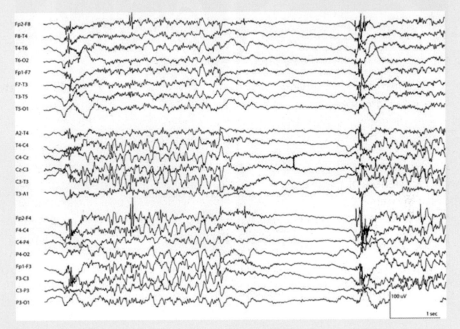

Burst-suppression is characterized by bursts of high-voltage sharp waves superimposed on an otherwise suppressed background and is considered one of the highly malignant EEG patterns associated with a poor prognosis. (Reprinted from Stern JM. *Atlas of EEG Patterns*. 2nd ed. Wolters Kluwer; 2013.)

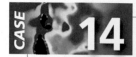

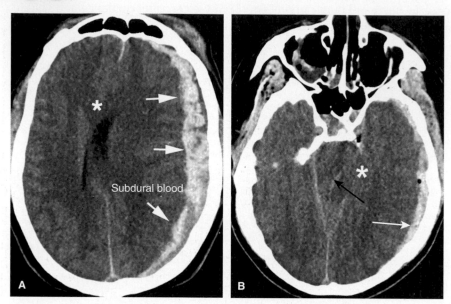

White arrows point to the subdural blood. Asterisks mark examples of herniation (in (A) subfalcine; in (B) uncal). The black arrow points to a Duret hemorrhage. (Modified from Daffner RH, Hartman M. *Clinical Radiology*. 4th ed. Wolters Kluwer; 2013.)

Your Patient's Follow-up: Neha's CT scan shows an acute left-sided subdural hematoma causing significant midline shift to the right and both subfalcine and uncal herniation. Brainstem compression has resulted in what is known as a Duret hemorrhage within the pons—these are small, linear bleeds that are often associated with uncal or downward herniation, likely due to torn arterial branches or ruptured draining veins. The moment you see the scan, you know the bleed is devastating; Neha's chances of meaningful recovery are poor. You step outside the imaging suite to speak to her family, who are waiting for you in the hallway. Her daughter has in hand her mother's do-not-resuscitate/do-not-intubate documentation, and the family is in agreement that Neha—a fiercely independent woman who, over the past few years, had refused to accept help from a home health aide and resisted the use of a walker, despite multiple falls—would want no extraordinary measures taken. She is admitted to the palliative care unit and started on a morphine drip for pain. She passes away peacefully several hours later.

You now know:

- | How to differentiate vasogenic from cytotoxic edema. Vasogenic edema is most often caused by mass lesions and has a characteristic finger-like appearance on CT that preserves the gray-white matter border. Cytotoxic edema is most often caused by acute ischemia and blurs the gray-white border on CT.

- | When to clinically suspect elevated ICP (headache, nausea, vomiting, and worsening somnolence in the appropriate clinical context are the big tip-offs) and the first steps in the management of acutely elevated ICP.

- | How to recognize the major patterns of herniation—subfalcine, uncal, central, and tonsillar herniation—both clinically and radiographically.

- | That decorticate posturing, characterized by upper extremity flexion into the chest and lower extremity extension, is caused by brain damage above the level of the red nucleus. Injury below the red nucleus can result in decerebrate posturing, which is clinically distinguished from decorticate posturing by extension of the upper extremities.

- | How to think about brain death and the potential challenges involved in its diagnosis.

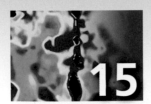

15

Altered Mental Status

In this chapter, you will learn:

1 | What we mean when we talk about altered mental status (AMS)

2 | How to differentiate encephalopathy from aphasia

3 | How to distinguish primary neurologic from secondary causes of altered mental status

4 | The most common—and most dangerous—primary neurologic causes of altered mental status to watch out for; we will also provide you with a quick but comprehensive review of toxic, metabolic, cardiac, and infectious secondary causes of altered mental status, among others

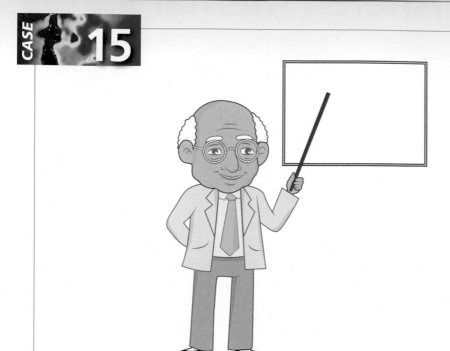

Your Patient: Donald, an 88-year-old retired school teacher, is brought to the emergency department by his wife, who found him slumped over on the toilet seat early this morning. His eyes were closed, and he was unresponsive to vocal or physical stimulation. He has a history of hypertension and diabetes. He was also diagnosed with a urinary tract infection 3 days ago, for which he is now on antibiotics. On arrival at the hospital, he is still unresponsive. He is afebrile, and his blood pressure is 110/75 mm Hg. The emergency department triage nurse calls a stroke code for altered mental status, and you meet the patient and his wife in the hallway outside of the CT scanner. What's the next step in your management?

Altered mental status (AMS) is one of the most common chief complaints encountered by neurologists. But what does it actually mean for a patient to have AMS? AMS is a vague catch-all term that generally describes patients who are somehow, in some way, off their cognitive baseline. It can mean confused, disoriented, delirious, forgetful, somnolent, even comatose.

The first step in identifying the problem is distinguishing primary central nervous system (CNS) causes of AMS—such as seizure, encephalitis, or Alzheimer disease—from secondary causes—such as hypo- or hyperglycemia, systemic infection, or uremia.

We said this in Chapter 1 but it bears repeating: the distinction between neurologic and non-neurologic causes of AMS is difficult, sometimes even impossible, to make. If there is any new focality on examination, assume that the patient's AMS is the result of a primary neurologic cause until proven otherwise (and it *will* sometimes be proven otherwise; for example, in the setting of hypo- and hyperglycemia, see page 377). If, after a comprehensive workup, and even in the absence of focality, there is no alternate explanation for the patient's AMS—no metabolic derangement, no underlying systemic infection—it will likely be up to the neurologist to figure out what's going on.

Before we do a quick dive into the multifactorial causes of AMS, there is one crucial distinction to make.

Encephalopathy Versus Aphasia

Like AMS, *encephalopathy* is a vague term that is often defined as any sort of "brain malfunctioning." Not the most useful definition. Neurologists think of an encephalopathic patient as one who is globally confused (*delirious* is essentially a synonym; see Box 15.1); the term carries connotations of non-neurologic causes of AMS, such as uremia, hepatic failure, hypo- or hyperglycemia, illicit drug or toxin ingestions (in these cases, we refer to it as a *toxic-metabolic encephalopathy*). However, diffuse neurologic problems—such as encephalitis or multifocal scattered cerebral infarcts—can also cause encephalopathy.

Box 15.1 Delirium

The precise difference between *encephalopathy* and *delirium* is hazy, and if you ask 20 neurologists (as we did), you will likely get 20 different answers (as we did!). In general, however, the term *encephalopathy* is used when there is some sort of known or suspected underlying pathology, be it toxic-metabolic or primary neurologic, whereas *delirium* is often used in the setting of no clear-cut cause (*e.g.,* to describe an elderly patient who becomes confused [or "sundowns"] overnight). *Encephalopathy* can also refer to patients who are comatose (*e.g.,* a patient with end-stage liver failure who becomes increasingly somnolent and ultimately unresponsive is diagnosed with *hepatic encephalopathy*), whereas delirious patients are confused but awake.

The hallmark of an encephalopathic patient who is awake is *inattention*: the patient typically requires frequent reorientation and redirection. If, for example, an encephalopathic patient is asked to count backward from 20, he or she may get to 17 and then drift off, start talking about something entirely unrelated or even fall asleep, requiring repeated prompting, vocal and/or physical stimulation to continue to count. Waxing and waning somnolence and disorientation are also common characteristics of encephalopathic patients.

Aphasic patients can appear to be encephalopathic, particularly those with a Wernicke aphasia (see page 59), who cannot follow commands and whose speech often sounds like gibberish. Unlike encephalopathy, however, aphasia is due to *focal* neurologic disease, stroke being the most common cause, not to mention the most urgent to recognize.

So how can you distinguish between aphasia and encephalopathy? Aphasic patients are not usually inattentive. They are typically fully alert and often appear frustrated by their inability to communicate. Depending on the location of the lesion, they may or may not be able to repeat, follow commands, or name objects. They will often have other focal deficits, including weakness and numbness, on exam. The more aphasic patients you encounter, the more easily you will be able to recognize aphasia. The bottom line, however, is that, if you are not sure—and it is ok not to be sure, this stuff is hard!—call for help. If you are in a hospital, that may mean calling a stroke code. If you accidentally mistake encephalopathy for aphasia, the worst thing you have done is taken up a few minutes of a neurology resident's time; if you mistake aphasia for encephalopathy, you may miss an opportunity to treat or abort a stroke.

 ## Neurologic Causes of AMS

The following list is by no means comprehensive, but it includes the most common—and most important to recognize—primary neurologic causes of AMS. Each item below has been or will be discussed in depth elsewhere in this book. The takeaway is that these conditions should be front and center when you see a patient with AMS: these conditions are *why* the patient needs a neurologist, and it is up to you to rule them in or out. How do you do that? Obtain a careful history (this is often reliant on collateral information from family members and caretakers, as patients with AMS rarely will be able to provide the most meticulous of histories), perform a detailed neurologic examination, rule out alternative non-neurologic explanations, and obtain relevant laboratory work and imaging when indicated.

- *Seizure* (see Chapter 6). What we really mean here is the postictal state. Postictal state is most often characterized by lethargy and confusion, but agitation and psychosis can be present as well. Patients can be postictal for minutes to hours following their seizure.
- *Ischemic stroke* (see Chapter 2). Remember, the vast majority of ischemic strokes do not present with AMS. The big do-not-miss exception is a basilar artery occlusion; because of potential involvement of the reticular activating system located in the thalamus and brainstem, basilar artery occlusions can cause somnolence, even coma. Associated oculomotor palsies, visual field deficits, and vertigo are also commonly present.
- *Hemorrhagic stroke* (see Chapter 2). Unlike ischemic strokes, hemorrhagic strokes often present with a decreased level of alertness, likely the result of elevated intracranial pressure and subsequent compression of the reticular activating system.
- *CNS infection* (see Chapter 8). Both encephalitis and meningitis can cause AMS. Because encephalitis affects the brain parenchyma, it can and often does cause both AMS and associated focal deficits. Meningitis affects the pain-sensitive meninges, and AMS in the setting of meningitis is generally attributed to pain and lethargy.
- *CNS malignancy* (see Chapter 16). Big space-occupying tumors can cause AMS because of elevated intracranial pressure in much the same way as an intracerebral hemorrhage. Paraneoplastic encephalitis tends to present with subacute changes in memory, behavior, and/or personality, is often diagnosed prior to cancer diagnosis, and is frequently associated with seizures.

- *Dementia* (see Chapter 7). Whether the result of amyloid accumulation, repeated vascular insult, communicating hydrocephalus, long-standing HIV infection, or a dozen other causes, dementia tends to present with gradual-onset and progressive AMS that can take the form of disorientation and forgetfulness as well as personality and mood changes.

- *Hypertensive encephalopathy.* Sudden and severe rises in blood pressure that exceed the upper limit of cerebral autoregulation can cause cerebral edema and subsequent neurologic deficits. Gradual-onset headache, nausea, vomiting, restlessness, and confusion are common. An MRI can be normal or show posterior bilateral white matter edema (if this sounds familiar, you are right. Posterior reversible encephalopathy syndrome [PRES] and hypertensive encephalopathy exist along the same spectrum; some even argue that the distinction between the two is irrelevant. See page 117 for a discussion of PRES). Symptoms should improve with gradual lowering of the patient's blood pressure.

 ## Non-Neurologic Causes of AMS

This list is a long one but many of these conditions can be easily ruled out with a simple blood test, urine toxicology screen, or electrocardiogram (ECG). All of these disorders can cause some degree of AMS; the key to remembering them lies in their other key distinguishing features (associate pontine demyelination with the rapid development of hypernatremia, for instance, gray lines on the fingernails with arsenic poisoning, etc)

- **Metabolic derangements**
  - *Hypo- and hyperglycemia.* Both hypo- and hyperglycemia can present with confusion, lethargy, and agitation. They can both also present with focal neurologic deficits as well as seizures: hypoglycemic seizures tend to be generalized and are often preceded by diaphoresis and tachycardia; hyperglycemic seizures are most often focal motor seizures.

  - *Hypo- and hypernatremia.* In general, AMS is associated with abnormal sodium levels only in the setting of rapid changes in sodium; patients with chronic hypo- or hypernatremia are often asymptomatic. The rapid development of hyponatremia can cause diffuse cerebral edema, whereas the rapid development of hypernatremia can cause *osmotic demyelination syndrome* (ODS; previously called central pontine myelinolysis). ODS usually presents several days after abrupt correction of hyponatremia and can cause corticospinal dysfunction (including weakness and hyperreflexia), corticobulbar dysfunction (dysarthria, pseudobulbar palsy), generalized confusion and, when severe, seizures and even coma. MRI can show both pontine and extrapontine demyelinating lesions, but these changes may not appear for several weeks.

  - *Hypo- and hypercalcemia.* Tetany, a form of neuromuscular irritability that is characterized by perioral numbness, paresthesias, and muscle spasms, is the hallmark of hypocalcemia, which can also cause nonspecific mental status changes such as lethargy, irritability, anxiety, and depression. Both generalized and focal seizures, as well as QT prolongation on the ECG, can also occur. Hypercalcemia is also associated with anxiety, depression, and generalized cognitive dysfunction, as well as gastrointestinal symptoms (nausea, anorexia, constipation) and renal dysfunction (polyuria, nephrolithiasis).

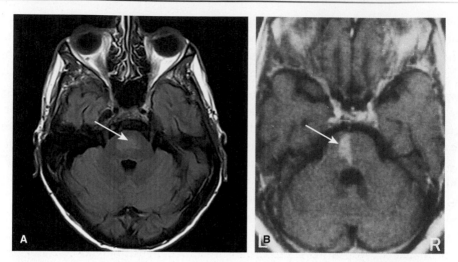

(A) An MRI showing subtle FLAIR hyperintensity in the pons (arrow) consistent with ODS. Note that the lesion is centered in the middle of the pons, helping to distinguish it from (B) stroke (arrow), which is typically unilateral (since the pontine perforating arteries, which come off the basilar, supply either the right or left pons). (A, modified from Klein J, Vinson EN, Brant WE, Helms CA. *Brant and Helms' Fundamentals of Diagnostic Radiology.* 5th ed. Wolters Kluwer; 2018; and B, reprinted from Kataoka S, Hori A, Shirakawa T, Hirose G. Paramedian pontine infarction. Neurological/topographical correlation. *Stroke.* 1997; 28(4):809-815.)

Box 15.2

A helpful mnemonic we learned in medical school and have relied on ever since: from high (sodium) to low (sodium), the brain will blow (*i.e.*, cerebral edema), from low to high, the pons will die (ODS).

Box 15.3 Chvostek and Trousseau Signs

These are classic forms of tetany that you can assess on your examination. Chvostek sign refers to contraction of ipsilateral facial muscles induced by tapping the facial nerve just in front of the ear. Trousseau sign is carpopedal spasm (*i.e.*, involuntary contraction of muscles within the foot or, more commonly, the hand) induced by inflation of a blood pressure cuff.

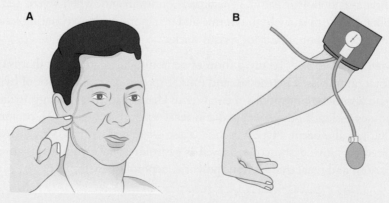

Chvostek (A) and Trousseau (B) signs.

Box 15.4

Did you notice that hypo- and hyperkalemia do not appear on this list of metabolic disorders that can cause AMS? Although certainly dangerous in their own right, changes in potassium concentration do not directly affect the brain.

- *Hypo- and hyperthyroidism.* The manifestations of thyroid disease are highly variable and dependent on the patient's age as well as the acuity and severity of the thyroid disorder. Hypothyroidism is typically associated with fatigue and lethargy (as well as cold intolerance, weight gain, constipation, dry skin, and bradycardia), whereas hyperthyroidism is associated with anxiety and emotional lability (as well as heat intolerance, weight loss, tremor, palpitations, and tachycardia). Both hypo- and hyperthyroidism can cause a non-inflammatory myopathy characterized by the subacute-onset of predominantly proximal weakness. Interestingly, from a neurologic standpoint—if a bit beyond the scope of this book—hyperthyroidism can also cause a form of hypokalemic periodic paralysis in which patients present with sudden attacks of painless muscle weakness, and hypothyroidism can be associated with pseudomyotonia (defined as abnormally slow muscle relaxation following mechanical or electrical muscle stimulation). Hypothyroidism is also a relatively common cause of carpal tunnel syndrome, a result of accumulation of matrix substance on and around the median nerve.

- *Hepatic encephalopathy.* Hepatic encephalopathy can present acutely in the setting of fulminant liver failure (in which case it can be associated with the rapid and dangerous development of cerebral edema), or it can wax and wane, smoldering beneath the surface until triggered by a stress such as dehydration, infection, narcotics, benzodiazepines, or medication noncompliance in patients with underlying chronic liver disease. Early symptoms include irritability, apathy, and altered sleep patterns; AMS, agitation, and coma may develop in more severe cases. *Asterixis*—a form of negative myoclonus characterized by sudden, brief, and involuntary loss of muscle tone in the hand when the wrist is extended—is the characteristic examination finding. The diagnosis is clinical. Although the serum ammonia level can be and often is elevated, the ammonia level does not necessarily correlate with the clinical picture and, in most cases, does not need to be checked. Treatment involves identifying and removing triggers, as well as the use of medications such as lactulose and rifaximin.

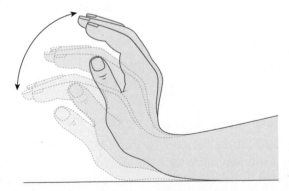

Asterixis is by no means pathognomonic of liver disease; it can also be a sign of renal failure, metabolic derangements, and various medications.

- *Uremic encephalopathy.* Uremic encephalopathy presents similarly to hepatic encephalopathy and can be associated with irritability, disorientation, seizures, tremor, and asterixis. The onset and severity generally parallel the degree of azotemia. Treatment is with hemodialysis, but there is often a lag time of hours to several days post-dialysis before mental status clears.

- **Alcohol Use Disorder**

  Long-standing alcohol abuse can result in *thiamine (B1) deficiency*, which can present acutely as **Wernicke encephalopathy** or chronically as **Korsakoff syndrome.** The classic triad of Wernicke encephalopathy consists of *ophthalmoplegia* (nystagmus, oculomotor cranial nerve palsies), *gait ataxia,* and, yes, *encephalopathy* (often characterized by disorientation, inattentiveness, and apathy) but is actually the exception rather than the rule: only about one-third of patients present with all three findings. The diagnosis is predominantly clinical. Thiamine levels are often low (but they don't have to be), and MRI can show (but doesn't have to show) T2 hyperintensity involving the mammillary bodies and/or bilateral thalami. One quick pearl that comes up often, especially in the emergency department: Wernicke encephalopathy can be precipitated in patients with baseline low levels of thiamine by giving glucose prior to thiamine repletion, so be careful! Treatment is with immediate high-dose intravenous thiamine. Korsakoff syndrome usually occurs as a consequence of untreated Wernicke encephalopathy and presents with deficits in both anterograde and retrograde memory. Confabulation—in which patients unconsciously fill in gaps in memory with distorted or entirely fabricated information—is a classic feature.

Box 15.5 Thiamine Deficiency

Other causes of thiamine (B1) deficiency that can result in Wernicke encephalopathy and Korsakoff syndrome include chronically poor nutrition (*e.g.*, patients with anorexia and patients receiving prolonged intravenous feeding without appropriate supplementation), hemodialysis (due to increased loss of water-soluble vitamins), and hyperemesis of pregnancy. Remember, thiamine deficiency can also cause a length-dependent sensorimotor polyneuropathy (see page 282).

Box 15.6 Alcohol Withdrawal

Seizures associated with alcohol withdrawal tend to occur within the first 12 to 48 hours after the last drink, whereas delirium tremens (or DTs, characterized by tachycardia, hypertension, and hallucinations) presents later, within 48 to 96 hours. Long-acting benzodiazepines, including diazepam and chlordiazepoxide, are standard treatment for mild withdrawal symptoms and are used to help prevent progression to seizures and DTs.

- **Medication overdose and withdrawal**

  - *Benzodiazepines.* Benzodiazepines work by increasing the frequency of GABAa chloride channel opening. Common side effects include sedation, amnesia, and delirium, especially in elderly patients. Benzodiazepine overdose presents with depressed mental status, ataxia, dysarthria, and nystagmus. Unlike opioid intoxication, benzodiazepines do not cause pupillary changes or significant respiratory depression. Treatment is with fluma-zenil (a GABA antagonist), which must be used carefully because it can rapidly lower the threshold for seizure. Benzodiazepine withdrawal—like alcohol withdrawal—can be life-threatening, and—again like alcohol withdrawal—presents with tachycardia, hyper-tension, hyperpyrexia, tremor, and seizures. Treatment is, logically, with benzodiazepines, followed by a slow taper.

Box 15.7

A helpful mnemonic: benZodiazepines increase the frequenZ of GABAa channel opening. Barbiturates, on the other hand, increase the duration of GABAa channel opening.

- *Opioids.* Opioids act on opioid (or mu) receptors. There are several types of opioids: natural opiates (which include morphine and codeine), semisynthetic opioids (*e.g.*, dex-tromethorphan), and fully synthetic opioids (*e.g.*, methadone and fentanyl). Opioid over-dose can be life-threatening and presents with pinpoint pupils, depressed mental status, bradycardia, and respiratory depression. Treatment is with naloxone, an opioid receptor antagonist. Opioid withdrawal—although miserable for the patient—is rarely (but not never) life-threatening; symptoms, which tend to peak within about 72 hours of the last dose, include dilated pupils, fever, yawning, rhinorrhea, lacrimation, nausea, vomiting, and diarrhea. Opioid agonists (such as methadone and buprenorphine) are standard treatment. Clonidine (an alpha-2 adrenergic receptor agonist) can also help mitigate the patient's symptoms.

- **Recreational drugs**
  - *Marijuana.* Marijuana is derived from the *cannabis* plant and contains in varying ratios two natural compounds: tetrahydrocannabinol (THC), which is the pri-mary psychoactive component, and cannabidiol (CBD), which has less psychoac-tive activity and is now sold separately throughout much of the world in the form of supplements, gummies, oils, bubble bath, lotions, and more. Activity is medi-ated via the cannabinoid receptors, CB1 and CB2, in the central and peripheral nervous systems. Conjunctival injection, social withdrawal, paranoia, dry mouth, tachycardia, increased appetite (colloquially known as "the munchies"), and even psychosis can be characteristic of marijuana intoxication. Symptoms of with-drawal can last up to a week and include depressed mood, irritability, anorexia, nausea, and insomnia.

  - *Hallucinogens.* Hallucinogens, including mescaline, psilocybin, and lysergic acid dieth-ylamide (LSD), act as serotonin agonists and can cause altered perception (in the form of visual hallucinations, distortions of time and space, and synesthesias [see Box 15.8]), euphoria, anxiety, panic, and paranoia. Mild dysautonomia—tachycardia, hyperten-sion, and mydriasis—often accompanies these symptoms. There are no withdrawal symptoms (hallucinogens are not addictive drugs) although people can experience "flashbacks" later in life, characterized by a recurrence of symptoms mimicking prior hallucinogen use.

Box 15.8 Synesthesia

Synesthesia is a phenomenon in which stimulation of one sensory pathway results in activation of another. For people with synesthesia, letters or numbers may be perceived as inherently colored: "a" might be red, "2" blue, *etc.* Synesthetes, as people with synesthesia are called, may taste music, hear pain, or visualize specific concepts—like mathematical equations or units of time—as shapes floating around them. The condition is not well understood but more common than previously thought; it has been suggested that up to 1 in every 300 people has some form of it. Vladimir Nabokov[1], author of *Lolita, Ada,* and *Pale Fire*, and physicist Richard Feynman are both believed to have been synesthetes.

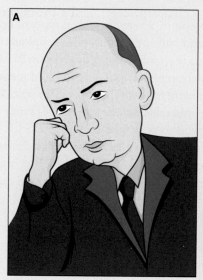 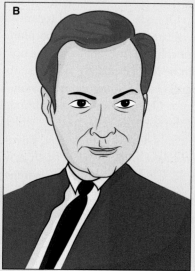

Two synesthetes: (*A*) Vladimir Nabokov and (*B*) Richard Feynman.

[1] His wife and son also were synesthetes!

- *3,4-methylenedioxyamphetamine (MDMA)*. MDMA is a psychostimulant that combines the dopaminergic and adrenergic effects of amphetamines with the serotonergic effects of hallucinogens. Ecstasy and Molly are colloquial terms for MDMA. These are popular recreational drugs—they are used as commonly as amphetamines and cocaine—in part because of the misapprehension that MDMA is relatively safe. Euphoria, empathy toward others, sexual arousal, disinhibition, and psychedelic manifestations are the main effects. However, side effects are common, and the drug accounts for over 20,000 emergency room visits annually. Minor side effects are predictable and include anxiety, insomnia, excessive thirst, loss of appetite, fever, and teeth grinding (bruxism). Overdose can cause dramatic increases in blood pressure (hypertensive crisis) and body temperature (hyperthermia), hyponatremia, cardiac arrhythmias, seizures, psychosis, and death. In addition, because MDMA is currently illegal and unregulated, these popular drugs may be laced with other drugs. It is unclear exactly how addictive MDMA is, but current literature suggests that repeated use can lead to tolerance and dependence, and withdrawal can be associated with fatigue, insomnia, depression, suicidal thoughts, and exacerbation of underlying mood disorders.

- *Phencyclidine.* Phencyclidine (PCP) acts as an NMDA receptor antagonist. PCP intoxication can present with aggressive or belligerent behavior, ataxia, vertical or rotatory nystagmus, mydriasis, tachycardia, and hypertension. There is no specific treatment, but placing patients in a quiet, dark room can help. Benzodiazepines and antipsychotics can be used to help manage behavioral symptoms. PCP, like LSD, is not an addictive drug, so there are no associated withdrawal symptoms. Ketamine is a PCP analogue that is now used as both an anesthetic and a treatment for refractory depression.

Box 15.9 Chasing the Dragon

"Chasing the dragon" is a specific method of heroin use that involves vaporizing and then inhaling the drug. This technique can cause a rare but potentially devastating form of spongiform leukoencephalopathy (*i.e.*, white matter—*leuko*—in the brain—*encephalo*—is damaged—*pathy*). Initial symptoms include confusion and restlessness and can progress to muscle spasms, generalized paresis, central fevers, and even death.

- **Heavy metal poisoning**
  - *Lead.* The effects of acute lead poisoning depend on both the age of the patient and the degree of lead absorption. Sources of lead include old houses (the U.S. banned lead-based paint in 1978) and ceramic dishes with chipped paint, as well as battery and car factories. The mnemonic LEAD is helpful to remember the characteristic features of lead poisoning: **L**ead lines on the gingiva and metaphyses of long bones, **E**ncephalopathy (memory loss, confusion, headaches), **A**bdominal discomfort (as well as **A**nemia and **A**rthralgias), and **D**rops (wrist or foot drops, due to extensor muscle weakness). Children can present with pica behaviors (eating items not normally considered food, such as dirt or grass) and learning delays. Long-term consequences include renal, cardiovascular, and cognitive dysfunction. Treatment includes removal of the source and/or removal of the patient from exposure, as well as chelation therapy (EDTA, DMSA, dimercaprol).

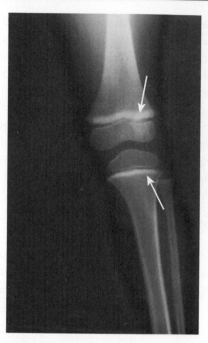

Lead lines (white arrows) visible on x-ray on the bones of the lower extremities. (Modified from Henretig FM. A toddler in status epilepticus. In: Osterhoudt KC, Perrone J, DeRoos F, et al., eds. *Toxicology pearls.* Hanley & Belfus; 2004:S2-S5.)

- *Mercury.* Sources of mercury exposure include metal refineries, gold mining, battery factories, paper manufacturing, and dentistry (amalgam fillings, which are still used worldwide, can release small amounts of elemental mercury, particularly in patients who grind their teeth). Mercury poisoning presents acutely with shortness of breath, cough, chest pain, nausea, vomiting, dyspnea, gum inflammation, dermatitis, and conjunctivitis. Chronic exposure can cause personality changes and memory loss. Treatment consists of supportive care, removal of exposure, and—in certain cases—chelating agents.

- *Arsenic.* Sources include contaminated water (arsenic can seep out of soil and rocks into water and wells) and workplace exposure (primarily inhalation of arsenic dust in refining factories). Acute poisoning can present with abdominal pain, nausea, and diarrhea which can lead to hypovolemia. Cardiac arrhythmias and shock can occur in severe cases. Chronic symptoms include a symmetric sensorimotor polyneuropathy, cognitive dysfunction, and seizures, as well as the appearance of gray lines on the fingernails and pigmentation around the axilla. Arsenic exposure also predisposes to various types of cancer, including skin, bladder, lung, liver, and renal cancer. Acute poisoning often requires advanced life support; chelation with dimercaprol or DMSA can be useful for both acute and chronic exposure.

- **Other Causes**
  - *Hypoxia and hypercapnea.* Both hypoxia and hypercapnea can cause encephalopathy, often in the form of lethargy, confusion, and memory loss that are most likely the result of cerebral vasodilation and increased cerebral blood flow leading to elevated intracranial pressure. The degree of CO_2 retention seems to correlate best with the degree of neurologic dysfunction.

- *Cardiac causes.* Confusion or depressed mental status can be the initial presentation of myocardial infarction or decompensated heart failure, particularly in elderly patients. A careful physical examination and an ECG can quickly assess any underlying cardiac disease.

- *Systemic infection.* Any systemic infection (pneumonia, urinary tract infection, cellulitis, *etc.*) can cause AMS, particularly in the elderly or otherwise fragile patients.

- *Primary psychiatric causes.* In patients with established diagnoses of psychiatric conditions such as bipolar depression or schizophrenia, it can be relatively straightforward to attribute AMS to a primary psychiatric cause. In patients presenting with new psychotic symptoms, however, the differential should remain broad; it is often only after a comprehensive workup (including basic blood tests, urine toxicology screen, lumbar puncture, brain imaging, and so forth, depending on presentation) that a primary psychiatric diagnosis can be convincingly established.

Summary of Non-Neurologic Causes of AMS

Category	Examples
Metabolic derangement	hypo- and hyperglycemia, hypo- and hypernatremia, hypo- and hypercalcemia, hypo- and hyperthyroidism, hepatic and uremic encephalopathy
Alcohol use disorder	
Medication overdose and withdrawal	benzodiazepines, opioids
Recreational drugs	marijuana, hallucinogens, MDMA, PCP
Heavy metal poisoning	lead, mercury, arsenic
Other causes	hypoxia and hypercapnea, cardiac causes, systemic infection, primary psychiatric causes

 ## AMS: Evaluation in a Nutshell

We warned you: it is a long differential. But many of these potential causes can be quickly and easily ruled out. The key is to file this list away and refer to it whenever you are evaluating a patient with AMS. The biggest mistake you can make is to arrive too quickly or carelessly at an answer. Be aware of inherent bias: just because a patient has a history of drug use does not mean that he or she cannot also have an underlying malignancy or a stroke. Approach each case systematically: take a careful history (getting a solid sense of the patient's baseline cognitive function is crucial!), perform a detailed examination and review of pertinent laboratory data, and ask for relevant imaging for patients with new focality on their examination. Involve other services and physicians: the workup of these patients often requires teamwork across subspecialties. Push yourself to think through the full differential. Finally, understand that you do not always need to arrive at an immediate and specific answer. Often the best thing that neurologists can do for patients with AMS is to comprehensively rule out the big do-not-miss neurologic diagnoses.

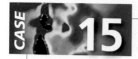

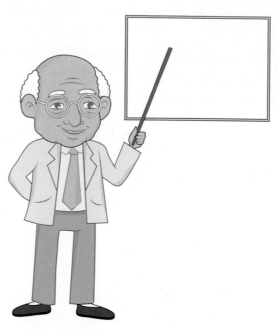

Follow-up on Your Patient: On your way to the emergency department you've quickly thought through the AMS differential, so when you meet Donald and his wife you are ready. You do a quick examination as you wait for the CT scanner— he is, indeed, unresponsive to voice but perks up with strong nail bed pressure. You note that his gaze is midline, he tracks you as you speak, and he is moving all four extremities equally. Within a minute or two, and with repeated prompting, he is able to tell you his name, recognize his wife, and name a few simple objects. He can follow one-step commands but has trouble with two-step commands. As he is positioned in the scanner, you take the opportunity to talk to his wife. She tells you he is "fine" at baseline, although she doesn't like to leave him home alone for extended periods of time because once or twice he has forgotten to turn off the stove. He takes a beta-blocker and antibiotics for his UTI. He was also recently given a "sleeping pill" by his friend and took one or two last night for the first time because he couldn't fall asleep. The CT shows generalized atrophy but is otherwise unremarkable. When you reexamine him, he is even more awake and is now able to tell you where he is and can count backward—slowly but correctly—from 20.

Your assessment at this point is that he is a gradually improving encephalopathic patient: he has nothing focal on examination, and you suspect that the sleeping pill (probably a benzodiazepine or nonbenzodiazepine sedative hypnotic like zolpidem) has triggered this event, its effects superimposed on an already vulnerable cognitive baseline (his age, suspected underlying cognitive impairment, recent infection, and antibiotic treatment all put him at risk). Within a few hours, he has returned fully to his cognitive baseline, and his urine toxicology screen comes back positive for benzodiazepines. You discuss the risks of sleeping medications with him and his wife, and he is discharged home.

You now know:

- | The most common and do-not-miss causes of AMS.
- | That aphasia and encephalopathy are easily confused but critical to distinguish from each other. Encephalopathy generally presents with global confusion and inattention on examination, whereas aphasia is a focal deficit that presents with difficulty understanding, producing, and/or repeating language. Aphasic patients are not typically inattentive and often appear frustrated by their deficits.
- | How to evaluate a patient with AMS. A careful history and examination are crucial, and basic laboratory tests and imaging can help diagnose—or, just as importantly—help cross things off your differential, when indicated.

16 Neuro-Oncology

In this chapter, you will learn:

1 | All about the most common primary brain tumors, including glial tumors (such as glioblastomas), neuronal tumors (such as neuroblastomas), and primary CNS lymphoma

2 | How to differentiate among colloid, dermoid, epidermoid, and arachnoid cysts, and when and how these otherwise benign cysts can cause trouble

3 | About paraneoplastic syndromes, their associated antibodies, and treatments

4 | About immune checkpoint inhibitors: how they work, and how they can cause potentially dangerous neurologic toxicity

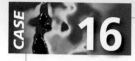

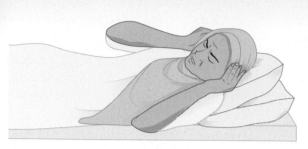

Your Patient: Zhara, a 58-year-old human resources specialist with no past medical history, presents to the emergency department with sudden-onset left arm weakness that began approximately 3 hours ago. She was blow-drying her hair when she noticed that she was having difficulty grasping the brush with her left hand; she says her fingers felt heavy and clumsy, and she had trouble lifting her arm to put the brush away. Her blood pressure is 170/100. Her neurologic examination is notable for 4/5 strength and decreased sensation of her left upper extremity and a subtle left upper motor neuron facial droop. She also reports a headache that began about 2 weeks ago but became much, much worse this morning. What is the next step in your management?

In this chapter, we will focus most of our attention on the brain, for the simple reason that brain tumors are by far the most common of the neurologic malignancies. Many of these tumors can be devastating, but as our understanding of the underlying tumor pathophysiology and genetic make-up has increased, so have our treatment options, and ongoing clinical trials offer more hope each day.

A Quick Word on Mass Lesions

Brain tumors are *mass lesions*: they take up space inside the skull. Abscesses and hemorrhages are other examples of mass lesions. How these lesions present is dependent on only two things:

1. *Their location.* Size matters too, of course—big tumors do tend to be worse than small ones—but location usually matters more. Tiny tumors located in the brainstem, for instance, can present with sudden, dramatic symptoms affecting the cranial nerves, motor pathways, and sensory pathways, whereas tumors located in the right frontal lobe—an area of the brain responsible for (relatively speaking) very little—can remain completely asymptomatic until they grow to become quite large. Cortically based tumors often present with seizures, whereas tumors located deeper in the brain and cerebellum do not.

2. *The rate at which they grow.* Slow-growing tumors typically present insidiously over weeks to months with progressive headache, weight loss, and subtle, progressive neurologic deficits whereas rapidly growing tumors can present with symptoms that develop over days to even hours.

The age of the patient is also something to consider. Because the brain atrophies over time, older patients tend to have more space inside their skull and can therefore "hide" mass lesions for longer than younger patients, who have very little extra space and tend to become symptomatic earlier.

Tumors can cause symptoms by compressing surrounding brain tissue (either directly by the tumor itself or as a result of edema surrounding the tumor) or by obstructing the flow of cerebrospinal fluid (CSF) if the tumor is located within, or compresses against, a ventricle. Tumors can also bleed, and blood can cause compression or obstruction much more rapidly than the tumor itself.

Primary brain tumors can metastasize but rarely do so outside of the central nervous system (CNS). More often, they can cause distant effects—for example, backache, radiculopathies, cranial nerve deficits—as a result of spread into the leptomeninges and CSF (see Box 16.6 on page 402).

For the purposes of this chapter, there are only a handful of things to know about each tumor: its origin (*i.e.*, the cells from which it derives), the population it tends to affect (children, adults or both), where in the brain it likes to grow (this will tell you how it presents), and what it looks like both histologically and on imaging (so you can recognize it when you see it). If we do not mention one or a few of the above categories for a given tumor, it is not because we forgot but because the details are either clinically unimportant or beyond the scope of this book; in either case, nothing for you to worry about. We will also discuss prognosis but will not spend too much time on treatment, since many of the treatment options and algorithms (particularly the newer therapies that are targeted to particular tumor mutations) are constantly changing.

 ## *Primary Brain Tumors*

Primary brain tumors (i.e., tumors that originate in the brain) are actually significantly less common than metastatic brain tumors (i.e., tumors that originate elsewhere in the body). Of the primary brain tumors, meningiomas are the most common, accounting for approximately 35% of all primary intracranial neoplasms. Glioblastomas[1] are the second most common, making up about 15%, followed by schwannomas, which account for approximately 8%.

Glial Tumors

Glial cells are the non-neuronal cells of the CNS. They include *astrocytes* (which form part of the blood-brain barrier and have a role in neurotransmitter metabolism as well as the formation of glial scars), *oligodendrocytes* (which myelinate CNS neurons), and *ependymal*

---

[1]Although glioblastomas are the second most common primary brain tumor, they are the *most* common primary *malignant* brain tumor, accounting for over half of all malignant CNS tumors.

Box 16.1 The World Health Organization Tumor Grading System

Until recently, the WHO graded CNS tumors based largely on their histological features (such as cellularity and mitotic activity) but has now begun to focus on molecular markers as well as a way to improve our understanding of each individual tumor and target potential therapeutic options. The WHO grading scale helps primarily with the diagnosis and prognosis of CNS tumors. The different grades are complicated, but the chart below should help to give a general sense of what they mean. We excluded the newer molecular marker information from this table because it goes beyond the scope of this book.

The WHO Tumor Grading System	
Grade I	Well differentiated cells with low proliferative potential; may be cured with surgery alone
Grade II	Moderately differentiated cells; low recurrence rate but can transform to higher grade tumors
Grade III	Poorly differentiated and infiltrative cells; high recurrence rate following treatment
Grade IV	Poorly differentiated and infiltrative cells with a propensity to spread throughout the CNS and become necrotic; poor prognosis despite treatment

cells (which line the ventricles). *Microglia* (which act as CNS macrophages) are also glia but are not relevant to this chapter for the simple reason that they do not form tumors. All glial cells contain glial fibrillary acidic protein (GFAP), and therefore tumors formed from glial cells will *stain positive for GFAP on histology.*

There are several major types of glial tumors:

- **Ependymomas** are derived from ependymal cells. They are most common in children and young adults and are often located within the fourth ventricle (although they can be supratentorial[2] and cord-based as well). Histology shows perivascular pseudorosettes, which are clusters of tumor cells that surround blood vessels. Depending on their specific molecular make-up, ependymomas can be WHO grade II or III.

- **Oligodendrogliomas** are malignant but slow-growing tumors derived from oligodendrocytes. They are relatively rare, most often diagnosed in young adults, and have a predilection for the frontal lobes. "Fried egg" cells (cells with a dark center surrounded by a pale halo) and "chicken wire" capillaries are the classic findings on histology. These are WHO grade II or III.

---

[2]**Supratentorial** refers to anywhere in the brain above the tentorium cerebelli (i.e., anywhere above the cerebellum). **Infratentorial** refers to anywhere in the brain below the tentorium cerebelli (i.e., in the cerebellum). These terms are often used to describe CNS tumors.

- **Astrocytomas** are derived from astrocytes, and there are multiple types. Discussed below are the two you should know.

  - **Pilocytic astrocytomas** are the most common primary brain tumor in children. They are most often infratentorial (*i.e.*, cerebellar). On histology, they are characterized by Rosenthal fibers (corkscrew-appearing eosinophilic processes of astrocytes). On imaging, they classically appear as cystic lesions with small enhancing nodules inside. They are classified as WHO grade I and, if complete surgical resection is possible, are often completely curable.

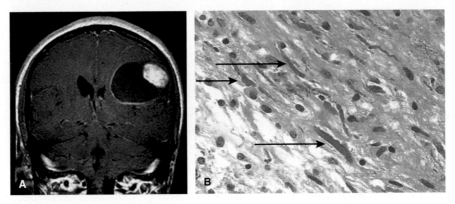

(*A*) The characteristic cystic appearance of an astrocytoma on MRI, with a small enhancing mural nodule (note that, although this astrocytoma is supratentorial, they are most often infratentorial) and (*B*) Rosenthal fibers on histology (black arrows). (*A*, reprinted from Strayer DS, Rubin E. *Rubin's Pathology*, 7th ed. Wolters Kluwer; 2014; and *B*, modified from Schniederjan MJ. *Biopsy Interpretation of the Central Nervous System*, 2nd ed. Wolters Kluwer; 2017.)

- **Glioblastomas** (previously known as glioblastoma multiforme, or GBM) are classified as WHO grade IV. They grow rapidly, are largely resistant to treatment, and have a poor prognosis with an average survival of approximately 15 months. They are typically hemispheric and characteristically cross the corpus callosum to invade the contralateral hemisphere, appearing as big, irregular *butterfly lesions* on imaging with variable enhancement, significant surrounding edema, and often hemorrhagic components. Histology reveals pleomorphic tumor cells with brisk mitotic activity, prominent microvascular proliferation, and areas of necrosis and hemorrhage surrounded by pseudopalisading tumor cells (see image on the next page). Treatment is typically with surgical resection followed by concurrent radiation and chemotherapy (temozolomide, an alkylating agent, is first-line). Ongoing clinical trials are evaluating dozens of other potential therapeutics, including other alkylating agents, anti-angiogenic treatments, targeted mutational drugs, and immunotherapy.

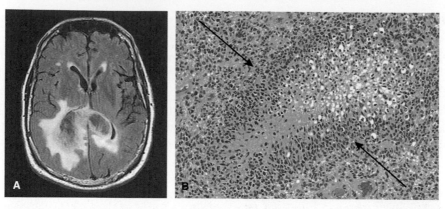

(A) A "butterfly" glioblastoma on MRI and (B) a foci of tumor necrosis surrounded by a hypercellular cuff of tumor cells ("pseudopalisading necrosis;" see black arrows) on histology. (A, reprinted from Griggs RC, Joynt RJ. *Baker and Joynt's Clinical Neurology on CD-ROM*. Wolters Kluwer; 2014; and B, modified from Schniederjan MJ, Brat DJ. *Biopsy Interpretation of the Central Nervous System*. Wolters Kluwer; 2011.)

Neuronal Tumors

Tumors derived from neurons are less common than those derived from glial cells. *Synaptophysin* (a transmembrane glycoprotein involved in synaptic transmission) is a common histological marker for neuronal tumors (just as GFAP is a marker for glial tumors).

- **Neuroepithelial tumors** are derived from neuroepithelial cells, which are undifferentiated cells of the CNS that can ultimately become either neurons or glia.

- **Central neurocytomas** are most common in young adults. They are classified as WHO grade II, are usually located within the ventricles (often involving the septum pellucidum, the thin membrane that separates the anterior horns of the left and right lateral ventricles), and appear as uniform cells with "salt and pepper" chromatin on histology.

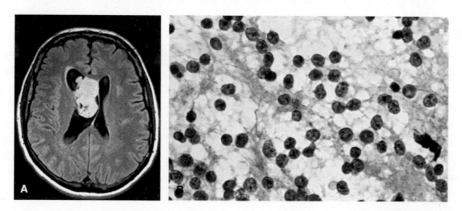

(A) A central neurocytoma on MRI and (B) the salt and pepper appearance on histology. (A, reprinted from Sanelli P, Schaefer P, Loevner L. *Neuroimaging: The Essentials*. Wolters Kluwer; 2015; and B, reprinted from Kini SR. *Cytopathology of Neuroendocrine Neoplasia*. Wolters Kluwer; 2013.)

- **Dysembryonic neuroepithelial tumors** (DNETs) are more common in children. They are rare, benign, and slow-growing, classified as WHO grade I. They have a predilection for the temporal lobe and classically present with intractable focal seizures. On imaging, they have a characteristic "soap bubble" appearance and appear as mucin-rich bubbly nodules on histology.

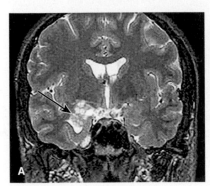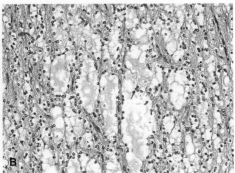

(*A*) A DNET on MRI (black arrow) and (*B*) the soap-bubble appearance on histology. (*A*, modified from Zamora C, Castillo M. *Neuroradiology Companion*, 5th ed. Wolters Kluwer; 2016; and *B*, reprinted from Schniederjan MJ. *Biopsy Interpretation of the Central Nervous System*, 2nd ed. Wolters Kluwer; 2017.)

- **Primitive neuroectodermal tumors** (PNETs) are a subtype of small round blue cell tumors (*i.e.*, they stain blue with standard staining techniques) that tend to be highly aggressive. Both cerebral neuroblastomas and medulloblastomas are WHO grade IV.

  - **Cerebral neuroblastomas** are most common in children and tend to be supratentorial. *Non*cerebral neuroblastomas are most often located in the adrenal medulla but can also grow anywhere along the sympathetic chain. Neuroblastomas appear as clusters of small round blue cells on histology, often in the form of *Homer–Wright rosettes* (dark blue cells surrounding pale fibrils, see image on the next page).

  - **Medulloblastomas** are the most common *malignant* tumor seen in children but can also occur in adults. They tend to be infratentorial, located within the cerebellar vermis or fourth ventricle. They appear similar to cerebral neuroblastomas on histology.

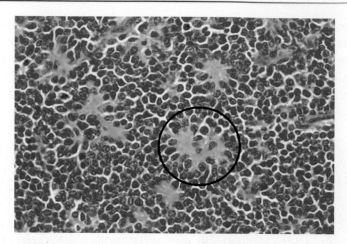

Homer-Wright Rosettes composed of clusters of small round blue cells surrounding pale fibrils (a good example can be seen within the black circle). (Modified from Mulholland MW. *Greenfield's Surgery*, 6th ed. Wolters Kluwer; 2016.)

Other Primary Brain Tumors

- **Meningiomas** are the most common primary brain tumor in adults. They are derived from arachnoid cells and are intradural (most of the time; rarely, they can be extradural) but extra-axial: in other words, they grow beneath the dura but outside of the brain parenchyma, within the concavities of the hemispheres, near bone, and often appear attached to the dura via thickened dural segments known as *dural tails*. The vast majority of meningiomas are WHO grade I (although they can range up to grades II and III), but that does not mean they cannot cause problems: the majority are asymptomatic, but as they grow they can compress and irritate brain tissue, causing focal neurologic deficits and seizures. Characteristic histologic findings include *psammoma bodies* and *whorled cells* (see images below). On imaging, meningiomas are vividly and uniformly enhancing and have a smooth, circular appearance. Treatment is with surgical excision.

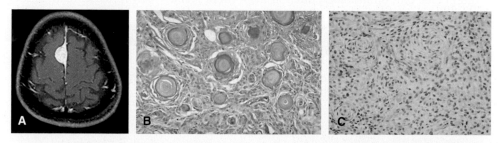

(A) A parasagittal meningioma with dural tails; (B and C) Characteristic psammoma body (B) and whorled cells (C) on histology. (A, reprinted from Tang C, Farooqi A. *Pocket Radiation Oncology*. Wolters Kluwer; 2019; B and C, reprinted from Rubin R, Strayer DS, Rubin E. *Rubin's Pathology*, 6th ed. Wolters Kluwer; 2011.)

- **Schwannomas** are WHO grade I tumors that are derived from schwann cells (the cells that myelinate peripheral nerves) and—logically—grow along peripheral nerves, including the cranial nerves and spinal roots. CN8 schwannomas (*i.e.*, acoustic schwannomas) are the most common and present with progressive hearing loss and tinnitus. Especially when bilateral, acoustic schwannomas are associated with neurofibromatosis type 2 (see Chapter 17). They are characterized by alternating areas of hypercellular "antoni A" tissue (often with *verocay bodies*, see image B below) and hypocellular "antoni B" tissue.

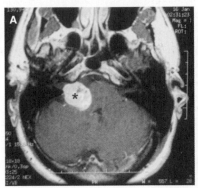
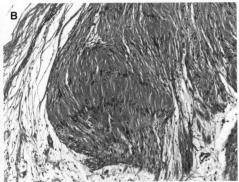

(*A*) An acoustic schwannoma (asterisk) growing along the eighth cranial nerve where it exits the brain at the cerebellopontine angle and (*B*) a close-up of a verocay body, characterized by rows of palisading nuclei (blue dots) separated by areas of acellular pink membrane. (*A*, reprinted from Barker LR, Fiebach NH, Kern DE, Thomas PA, Ziegelstein RC, Zieve PD. *Principles of Ambulatory Medicine*, 7th ed. Wolters Kluwer, 2006; and *B*, modified from Requena L, Requena L, Kutzner H. *Cutaneous Soft Tissue Tumors*. Wolters Kluwer; 2014.)

- **Craniopharyngiomas** are WHO grade I tumors derived from embryonic pituitary tissue (*i.e.*, remnants of Rathke pouch) that grow within the sella turcica and can present with endocrinopathies and bitemporal hemianopia (see Box 16.2 on Sellar and Suprasellar Tumors). There are two common age peaks—young children and adults in their 50s and 60s—and two subtypes—adamantinomatous (which account for approximately 90% of these tumors and appear as cystic and often calcified masses filled with oily fluid) and papillary (masses of metaplastic squamous cells, not calcified).

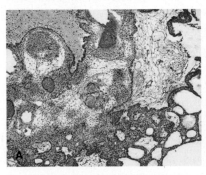
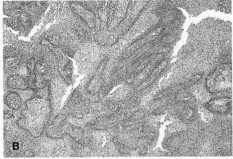

Histology from (*A*) adamantinomatous and (*B*) papillary craniopharyngiomas. (*A*, reprinted from *Biopsy Interpretation: The Frozen Section*, 2nd ed. Wolters Kluwer; 2013; and *B*, reprinted from Mills SE, Greenson JK, Hornick JL, Longacre TA, Reuter VE. *Sternberg's Diagnostic Surgical Pathology*, 6th ed. Wolters Kluwer; 2015.)

Box 16.2 Sellar and Suprasellar Tumors

The sella turcica is a saddle-shaped depression within the sphenoid bone that contains the pituitary gland. Tumors that arise here can cause both bitemporal hemianopia, due to compression of the optic chiasm (remember, light received from the lateral or temporal half of the world falls on the nasal half of each retina and the nasal retinal fibers come together to cross in the chiasm [see page 432]), and endocrinopathies, due to compression of pituitary tissue. In children, the most common sellar and suprasellar tumors include craniopharyngiomas and other gliomas (including hypothalamic and optic nerve gliomas); in adults, pituitary adenomas and meningiomas are more common.

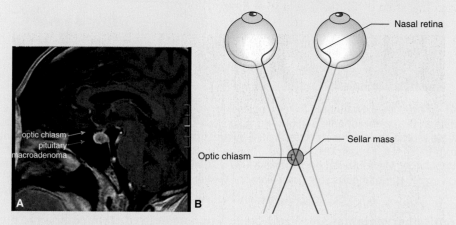

(*A*) A pituitary macroadenoma on sagittal postcontrast MRI. (*B*) A drawing demonstrating how sellar masses can compress the optic chiasm and result in bitemporal hemianopia. (*A*, reprinted from Cheng-Ching E, Baron EP, Chahine L, Rae-Grant A. *Comprehensive Review in Clinical Neurology*, 2nd ed. Wolters Kluwer; 2016.)

- **Hemangioblastomas** are WHO grade I tumors that originate from stromal cells in small blood vessels and are most often located within the cerebellum, brainstem, or spine. About 25% of the time, they are associated with von Hippel–Lindau disease (see Chapter 17); in these cases, the average age of those affected is 20 to 40 years. When hemangioblastomas are sporadic (*i.e.*, not associated with von Hippel–Lindau), the average age is much older, closer to 50 to 70. Histology reveals highly vascularized tissue with foamy cells. Hemangioblastomas can be associated with secondary polycythemia due to erythropoietin production by the tumor cells.

- **Primary CNS lymphoma** is relatively rare, accounting for approximately 5% of all primary CNS tumors. It usually occurs in immunocompromised individuals—HIV and iatrogenic immunosuppression are important risk factors—but can occur sporadically in healthy individuals as well. When it affects immunocompromised patients, primary CNS lymphoma is often associated with an underlying EBV infection, but in the majority of nonimmunocompromised patients no evidence of EBV can be found.

Primary CNS lymphoma can be hemispheric but is often periventricular, located within the deep gray matter. Like glioblastomas, it can also cross the corpus callosum. On MRI, primary CNS lymphoma uniformly enhances and can restrict diffusion on diffusion-weighted imaging (DWI) due to the high cellularity of these tumors. First-line treatment involves steroids, chemotherapy, and—if HIV-related—antiretroviral therapy. Steroids can reduce the diagnostic yield on biopsy and should be delayed if possible until the biopsy is completed. Modern high-dose methotrexate-based chemotherapy regimens have significantly prolonged survival time; however, the relapse rate is high. The survival rate is likely worse in immunocompromised individuals. Surgical resection is not recommended because it has not been shown to increase overall survival. Whole brain radiation is generally used as a salvage therapy; it can be effective but is associated with early relapse and a significant side effect profile including often debilitating cognitive dysfunction.

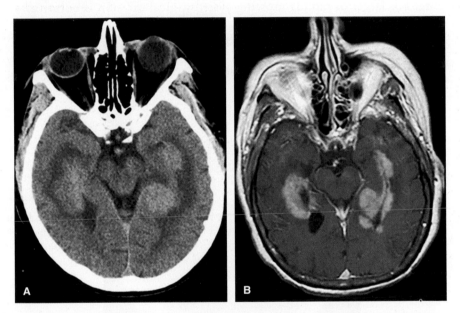

Primary CNS lymphoma. (*A*) Axial CT shows multiple masses along the lateral ventricles. (*B*) These lesions avidly enhance on postcontrast MRI. (Reprinted from Pina Sanelli; Pamela Schaefer; Laurie Loevner. *Neuroimaging: The Essentials*. Wolters Kluwer; 2015.)

Box 16.3 Metastatic Brain Tumors

Metastatic brain tumors are actually more common than primary brain tumors and tend to be located supratentorially along the gray matter/white matter junction. Lung cancer is the most likely to metastasize to the brain, followed by breast cancer and melanoma. All brain metastases can bleed, but lung cancer, melanoma, renal cell cancer, choriocarcinoma, and thyroid cancer metastases are the most likely to do so.

Cysts

A cyst is a membranous pocket that is filled with something—it can be air, CSF, blood, *etc.* They tend to be benign but can occasionally wreak havoc in the brain due to compression of the surrounding tissue or, even more rarely, cyst rupture. Among the most common cysts are:

- **Colloid cysts** are benign mucus-filled masses that are located within the foramen of Monro or third ventricle. They are usually asymptomatic but can occasionally cause sudden headache, drop attacks, rapid neurologic decline, and even herniation and death. These symptoms occur when the cyst shifts so that it obstructs the ventricular system, resulting in acute hydrocephalus and a rapid rise in intracranial pressure. Small, asymptomatic cysts can be monitored with serial imaging. For larger or rapidly growing cysts, surgical excision is curative.

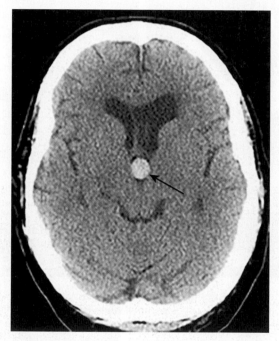

A colloid cyst (arrow) located within the third ventricle on axial CT. (Reprinted from Zamora C, Castillo M. *Neuroradiology Companion*, 5th ed. Wolters Kluwer; 2016.)

- **Dermoid cysts** (also known as teratomas) can occur intracranially (typically in the pons or cerebellum) but can also be found elsewhere in the body, most commonly in the skin or ovaries. They are filled with fully differentiated tissue from just about anywhere in the body, including hair follicles, teeth, and sweat glands. Intracranially, they tend to be entirely asymptomatic until—rarely—they rupture, causing headache, seizure, or potentially life-threatening complications such as vasospasm, ischemia, or chemical meningitis. N-methyl-D-aspartic acid (NMDA) receptor encephalitis (see page 402) is a rare paraneoplastic disease associated with teratomas in the ovaries.

- **Epidermoid cysts** are filled with keratinaceous material and tend to be located intracranially at the cerebellopontine angle. Like dermoid cysts, they are usually asymptomatic unless they rupture.

Box 16.4 Cerebellopontine Angle Tumors

A useful differential to keep in your back pocket: schwannomas account for nearly 75% of all tumors located at the cerebellopontine angle; epidermoid cysts and meningiomas account for the rest.

- **Arachnoid cysts** are filled with CSF and are located near the meninges, typically near the temporal lobe. They are almost always asymptomatic but can grow large enough to compress nearby tissue.

Box 16.5 Epidermoid versus Arachnoid Cysts

On MRI FLAIR sequences, epidermoid cysts appear bright, or hyperintense, whereas CSF-filled arachnoid cysts appear dark. This makes sense: FLAIR sequences are T2-based (in which fat, proteinaceous material, edema, gliosis, and CSF appear bright) but with the CSF signal suppressed. Epidermoid cysts will also typically appear bright on DWI, whereas arachnoid cysts will be dark.

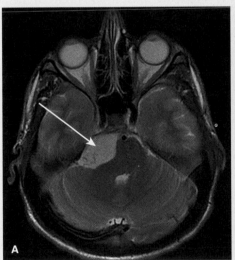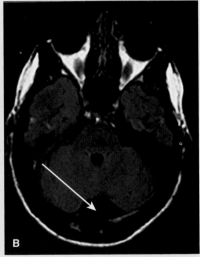

(A) An hyperintense epidermoid cyst (white arrow) located at the cerebellopontine angle and (B) a hypointense posterior fossa arachnoid cyst (white arrow), on FLAIR MRI. (A, modified from Louis ED, Mayer SA, Noble JM. *Merritt's Neurology*, 14th ed. Wolters Kluwer; 2021; and B, modified from Griggs RC, Joynt RJ. *Baker and Joynt's Clinical Neurology on CD-ROM*. Wolters Kluwer; 2004.)

> ## Box 16.6 Leptomeningeal Carcinomatosis
>
> *Leptomeningeal carcinomatosis* is a complication of cancer in which the tumor cells spread to the pia and arachnoid membranes and into the CSF between them. Breast cancer, lung cancer, gastrointestinal cancer, and melanoma are the most common causes. You can remember the symptoms caused by leptomeningeal disease by thinking about where the CSF goes: it bathes the pain-sensitive meninges, causing headache, altered mental status, and multiple cranial nerve palsies (the cranial nerves run through the subarachnoid space and can therefore be "picked off," one by one, as the cancer spreads); and it bathes the cord, resulting in backache and polyradiculopathies due to nerve root involvement. The diagnosis is suggested by leptomeningeal enhancement on brain and/or spine MRI. CSF analysis should reveal a pleocytosis, elevated protein, and positive cytology. However, the cytology test is not sensitive and the lumbar puncture often needs to be repeated several times for a positive result. If the imaging and CSF analysis are nondiagnostic but clinical suspicion remains high, meningeal biopsy is confirmatory. Treatment typically involves whole brain radiation and intrathecal chemotherapy.

 Paraneoplastic Syndromes

Paraneoplastic syndromes are disorders that occur in patients with cancer when antibodies directed against tumor cells are also mistakenly directed against healthy cells of the nervous system. Any part of the CNS, including the brain and spine, and the peripheral nervous system (PNS), including the peripheral nerves, neuromuscular junction, and muscles, can be affected. Paraneoplastic syndromes can—and often do—present before the patient has any awareness of an underlying malignancy.

To be clear, most primary brain tumors do not cause paraneoplastic syndromes. Rather, the brain is more often affected by paraneoplastic syndromes caused by other systemic malignancies: ovarian teratomas and small cell lung cancer are, for example, frequently implicated.

There are dozens of paraneoplastic syndromes that can be caused by an ever-growing list of pathologic antibodies, most of which are associated with particular cancers. However, as we pointed out in Chapter 9, many of these syndromes are not exclusively paraneoplastic; they are, more generally, autoimmune disorders and can be caused by many other types of non-cancer-associated antibodies as well. Important examples include the following:

- **Paraneoplastic encephalitis.** In Chapter 9, we discussed various forms of paraneoplastic encephalitis, including limbic encephalitis, brainstem encephalitis, and encephalomyelitis. Anti-NMDA (most often associated with ovarian teratomas), Anti-Hu (also known as ANNA-1; associated with small cell lung cancer), and Anti-LGI1 (no specific associated tumor) antibodies are commonly implicated.

- **Paraneoplastic cerebellar degeneration.** When antibodies originally directed against tumor cells cross-react with cerebellar cells, the result is relatively rapid cerebellar atrophy that can present with progressive vertigo, dysarthria, dysphagia, diplopia, and gait dysfunction. Anti-Hu (associated with small cell lung cancer, as mentioned above) and Anti-Yo (associated with ovarian cancer) antibodies are common culprits.

- **Opsoclonus myoclonus syndrome.** Characterized by opsoclonus (jerky, uncoordinated and dance-like eye movements) and diffuse myoclonus affecting the limbs and/or trunk, opsoclonus myoclonus syndrome is seen in a small percentage of patients with neuroblastoma.

- **Sensory neuronopathy.** This is a rare condition characterized by patchy asymmetric sensory loss, hypo- or areflexia, and sensory ataxia (a form of ataxia caused by lack of sensory input) due to degeneration of the dorsal root ganglia. Anti-Hu is the most commonly associated paraneoplastic antibody, but sensory neuronopathy can also be associated with Sjogren syndrome, Guillain-Barre syndrome, and various chemotherapy agents, among other causes.

- **Lambert-Eaton myasthenic syndrome.** This is discussed in Chapter 12. About 50% of cases are paraneoplastic, most often associated with small cell lung cancer, and clinical manifestations typically precede the diagnosis of the cancer, often by months to years.

Treatment varies based on the specific syndrome and the underlying malignancy, but there are two general approaches: (1) treat the cancer and (2) suppress the immune response. Intravenous immune globulin (IVIG) and plasmapheresis (PLEX) are the most commonly used immunosuppressants.

Box 16.7 Neurologic Toxicities Associated with Checkpoint Inhibitors

Checkpoint inhibitors are a relatively new form of cancer treatment. They are immunomodulatory antibodies that boost the immune response—essentially blocking the "off signal" that normally prevents the immune response from getting out of hand—by targeting the programmed cell death receptor 1 (PD-1) or cytotoxic T-lymphocyte–associated antigen 4 (CTLA-4), among others. These drugs have significantly improved the prognosis of many late-stage malignancies, most notably metastatic melanoma. However, as their use has become more prevalent, so have their associated toxicities. By boosting the immune system to attack tumor cells, they can also boost production of autoantibodies directed against healthy tissue, resulting in a battery of both systemic and neurologic toxicities. Neurologic complications that can occur include the following:

- encephalitis
- transverse myelitis
- myasthenia gravis
- posterior reversible encephalopathy syndrome (PRES)
- various forms of acute and chronic inflammatory demyelinating polyradiculoneuropathy syndromes (AIDP and CIDP, respectively)

Treatment of these neurologic complications consists of short-term immunosuppression with steroids, IVIG, and/or PLEX. The risks of stopping the checkpoint inhibitor must be weighed against those of the associated toxicity.

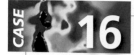

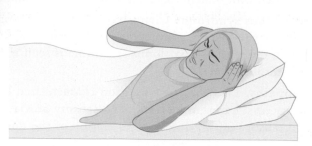

Follow-up on Your Patient: You rush Zhara to CT and simultaneously call the pharmacist to start preparing tPA: remember, acute-onset focal neurologic deficits are stroke until proven otherwise. Her CT, below, shows a hemorrhagic lesion in her right parietal lobe with significant surrounding vasogenic edema, concerning for a mass lesion. You tell the pharmacist to stop preparing tPA (first and most importantly, because she has acute blood on her scan; second, because this right-sided hemorrhagic lesion explains her left-sided symptoms, and you're no longer concerned about an ischemic stroke). You then help move her off the scanner and, as you do, you get a little more history: she has not been feeling well for quite some time, with poor appetite and a nearly 20 lb weight loss over the last few months that she attributed to her stressful job. She has been smoking cigarettes since she was a teenager and, for the past few months, smoking is the only thing that has calmed her down. She has not seen a doctor in over 15 years. You start her on a nicardipine drip to lower her blood pressure and admit her for work-up. Her MRI reveals numerous, rounded lesions (none of which could be clearly seen on CT) located predominantly at the gray/white matter junction in both hemispheres. It is difficult to say for sure because acute blood is obstructing the area, but it looks as though there is a mass underlying the right parietal hemorrhage as well, suggesting that the bleed is due to a bleeding metastasis. Her chest CT reveals a large, spiculated lung mass. She is ultimately diagnosed with metastatic lung adenocarcinoma and is admitted to oncology for further management.

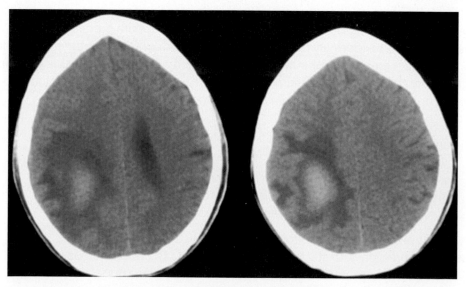

Zhara's CT. (Courtesy of Dr. Bruno Di Muzio, Radiopaedia.org, rID: 25395.)

You now know:

- | The basic epidemiology, histologic, and imaging characteristics of the most common primary brain tumors. Glial tumors, including astrocytomas and glioblastomas, should stain positive for *GFAP*, whereas neuronal tumors should stain positive for *synaptophysin.*
- | How to recognize and treat primary CNS lymphoma
- | How to distinguish between arachnoid and epidermoid cysts on MRI
- | That there is a broad spectrum of paraneoplastic disorders, all of which are associated with specific antibodies that themselves are associated with specific underlying malignancies.
- | The many potential neurologic toxicities associated with the relatively new immune checkpoint inhibitors.

17 Genetic Diseases and Syndromes

In this chapter, you will learn:

1 | How to distinguish among the different lysosomal and glycogen storage diseases

2 | The clinical hallmarks of four important neurocutaneous disorders: *tuberous sclerosis (TS), neurofibromatosis, Sturge-Weber syndrome,* and *von Hippel-Lindau disease*

3 | When to consider the diagnosis of mitochondrial diseases, and how several of these—including *mitochondrial encephalomyopathy with lactic acidosis and stroke-like episodes* (MELAS) and *myoclonic epilepsy with ragged red fibers* (MERRF), among others—present

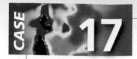

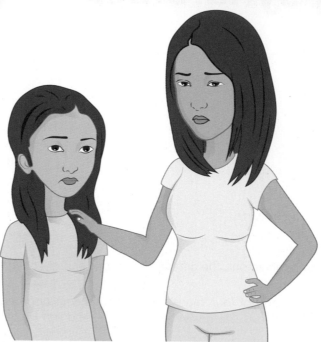

Your Patient: Lila, a 10-year-old girl, comes to your clinic with her mother. She has complained of vision problems for the past 48 hours. Her mother tells you that, starting yesterday, she noticed that Lila was suddenly bumping into things—just this morning, she accidentally walked into a doorway causing a bad bruise on her shoulder. Lila says that she can't see to her right and, indeed, when you examine her, you find a right homonymous hemianopia. Her other medical problems include bilateral hearing loss since she was a baby and recurrent migraine headaches. You also note that she is short for her age. What is the next step in your management?

Many inherited disorders prominently affect the nervous system, some of which we have already encountered in previous chapters. This chapter is by no means an attempt at either an exhaustive list or an in-depth exploration of each disorder, most of which are quite complex and can manifest in many different ways. Rather, we will try to familiarize you with the basic features of the most common among them so that you will know when to suspect their presence.

Because there are so many of these disorders, and because their manifestations are protean, we will be sharing with you some mnemonics along the way that you may find useful for memorizing their principal features. We have found that trying to remember their most distinguishing features—for example, patients with Tay-Sachs disease are typically hyperreflexic, whereas those with Niemann-Pick disease are hyporeflexic—is more useful than attempting to memorize every detail of every disorder.

 ## Lysosomal Storage Diseases

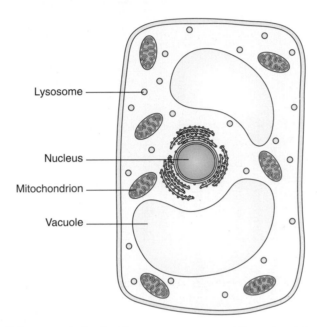

A typical cell; just a reminder that lysosomes are present throughout the cytoplasm.

Lysosomal storage disorders are a group of over 50 inherited diseases characterized by the build-up of abnormal metabolic products within intracellular lysosomes as a result of lysosomal enzyme deficiencies. Many organ systems can be involved, but the neurologic system is often predominantly affected. These disorders are relatively rare, usually inherited in an autosomal recessive fashion (although there are exceptions, which we will point out) and tend to present in infancy or childhood. Prenatal diagnosis is available for most of them. There are two major subsets:

- *Sphingolipidoses* are the result of deficiencies in enzymes that catabolize sphingolipids. The table on the next page (you'll have to turn your head sideways!) contains the basic facts about the most common sphingolipidoses:

Disease	Inheritance	Enzyme Deficiency	Accumulated Substrate	Clinical Manifestations	Histology
Fabry	X-linked recessive	α-Galactosidase A	ceramide trihexoside	Angiokeratomas[a] Acroparesthesias[b] Autonomic dysfunction Cardiomyopathy Nephropathy	Zebra bodies
Krabbe	Autosomal recessive	Galactocerebrosidase	galactocerebroside, psychosine	Excessive irritability Peripheral neuropathy Developmental delay Vision loss	Globoid cells (multinucleated macrophages)
Gaucher	Autosomal recessive	β-Glucocerebrosidase	glucocerebroside	Hepatosplenomegaly Aseptic necrosis of the femur Pancytopenia Developmental delay	Gaucher cells (lipid-laden macrophages with crumpled tissue appearance)
Niemann-Pick	Autosomal recessive	Sphingomyelinase	sphingomyelin	Progressive neurodegeneration Areflexia or hyporeflexia Cherry red spot on macula Hepatosplenomegaly	Foam cells, zebra bodies
Tay-Sachs	Autosomal recessive	Hexosaminidase A	GM$_2$ ganglioside	Progressive neurodegeneration Hyperreflexia Cherry red spot on macula	Lysosomes with an onion skin appearance
Metachromatic Leukodystrophy	Autosomal recessive	Arylsulfatase A	cerebroside sulfate	Progressive demyelination of the central nervous system (CNS) and peripheral nervous system (PNS), resulting in ataxia, vision and hearing loss, developmental delay, behavioral problems	Nonspecific

[a]Angiokeratomas are benign, small, dark capillary lesions that can appear anywhere on the body.
[b]The term "acroparesthesia" refers to burning or tingling pains in the extremities, often exacerbated by very hot or cold weather as well as by exercise; they are thought to be caused by a type of small fiber neuropathy.

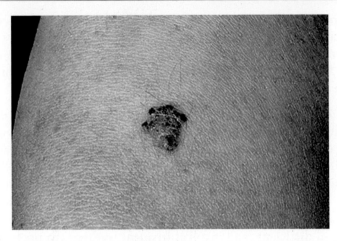

An angiokeratoma in a patient with Fabry disease. (Reprinted from Requena L, Requena L, Kutzner H. *Cutaneous Soft Tissue Tumors.* Wolters Kluwer; 2014.)

• ***Mucopolysaccharidoses*** are the result of deficiencies in enzymes that catabolize glycosaminoglycans (previously known as mucopolysaccharides). There are several, but Hunter and Hurler syndromes are the most common. Again, the nervous system is just one of multiple organ systems that can be affected.

Disease	Inheritance	Enzyme Deficiency	Accumulated Substrate	Common Clinical Manifestations	Distinguishing Feature
Hurler	Autosomal recessive	α-L-iduronidase	heparan sulfate, dermatan sulfate	Developmental delay Macrocephaly Facial dysmorphism (gargoylism) Airway obstruction Hepatosplenomegaly	Corneal clouding
Hunter	X-linked recessive	iduronate-2-sulfatase	heparan sulfate, dermatan sulfate		Aggressive behavior

A mnemonic to help you remember the difference between these two disorders: *the hunter must see clearly to hit the X* (*i.e.*, Hunter syndrome is associated with no corneal clouding and is X-linked recessive).

There are other lysosomal storage diseases, including glycoproteinoses and mucolipidoses, but these are beyond the scope of this book.

For a few of these disorders, new treatments to slow disease progression are currently available or in trials. These include enzyme replacement therapy and gene therapy.

 ## Glycogen Storage Diseases (GSDs)

GSDs are autosomal recessive disorders that result from abnormal glycogen metabolism and subsequent accumulation of glycogen within cells. Prenatal diagnosis is available. Each disorder is associated with a specific deficiency of an enzyme that is crucial to the breakdown of glycogen into glucose. These diseases typically present in infants or young children and characteristically affect the muscles (leading to fatigue, muscle cramps, and often severe exercise intolerance) and the liver (due to glycogen build-up).

There are several GSDs you need to know, and you can remember them by this apt mnemonic: **V**ery **P**oor **CA**rbohydrate Metabolism: **v**on Gierke, **P**ompe, **C**ori, **A**ndersen, and McArdle diseases.

- *Von Gierke Disease (also known as GSD type I)* is the result of a deficiency of glucose-6-phosphatase, an enzyme necessary for glycogen breakdown and the release of glucose from cells. It is the most common form of glycogen storage disease and presents in infants with hypoglycemia, hepato- and renomegaly, doll-like facies and lactic acidosis (the inability to break down glucose-6-phosphate results in shunting of substrates to the glycolytic pathway, resulting in lactate production). There is no specific therapy. Treatment requires a multidisciplinary team that includes doctors, geneticists, and dieticians, and involves frequent feedings (to prevent hypoglycemia) and avoidance of sugars that depend on glucose-6-phosphatase for metabolism (including sucrose, fructose, lactose, and galactose). Patients can live into adulthood, but complications are common, including but not limited to hepatic and renal disease, anemia, hyperlipidemia, and osteopenia.

- *Pompe disease (also known as acid maltase deficiency, or GSD type II)* is the result of a deficiency in acid alpha-glucosidase (also known as acid maltase). It is also classified as a lysosomal storage disorder because it results in the accumulation of glycogen within lysosomes. Pompe disease can present in infants, teenagers, and young adults and is characterized primarily by cardiomyopathy (think *Pompe = Pump*). Generalized muscle weakness, respiratory distress, and feeding difficulties are common in the infantile form. Skeletal myopathy and diaphragmatic weakness are common in older children and adults and typically lead to death from respiratory failure by the third decade of life. Diagnosis is made by muscle biopsy, which reveals periodic acid-Schiff (PAS) positive vacuoles. Treatment involves a combination of enzyme replacement therapy and multidisciplinary support.

- *Cori disease (also known as Forbes disease, or GSD type III)* is the result of a deficiency of a *debranching* enzyme crucial to glycogen breakdown. It typically manifests as a milder form of von Gierke disease, but unlike von Gierke disease, the blood lactate levels are normal. Treatment requires frequent feedings to avoid hypoglycemia and a high-protein diet; avoidance of sugars like fructose and galactose is not necessary.

- *Andersen disease (also known as GSD type IV)*, in contrast to Cori disease, is due to a deficiency of a *branching* enzyme that results in the formation of abnormal glycogen with fewer branch points. Patients typically present in infancy with hepatosplenomegaly and failure to thrive. Liver disease progresses with age and can include cirrhosis, esophageal varices, ascites, and hepatocellular carcinoma. Extra-hepatic disease, affecting predominantly the heart and skeletal muscle, can also occur. There is no specific treatment. Liver transplantation can be considered on a case-by-case basis.

- *McArdle disease (also known as myophosphorylase deficiency, or GSD type V)* is the most common GSD that predominantly affects the muscle. It is the result of a deficiency in myophosphorylase, which causes abnormal glycogen breakdown in muscle cells. Unlike the diseases mentioned above, McArdle disease usually presents in adolescence or young adulthood with exercise intolerance and painful muscle cramps. A "second wind" phenomenon, characterized by gradual improvement in symptoms with sustained exercise, is the classic manifestation. Laboratory work reveals elevated creatine kinase and myoglobinuria. There is no specific treatment. A high carbohydrate diet and regular mild-to-moderate exercise may offer some benefit.

 ## Neurocutaneous Diseases

Neurocutaneous diseases are, as the name suggests, diseases that affect both the brain and the skin. They are present from birth and cause a variety of tumors and lesions to grow within the brain, spinal cord, and skin, as well as other organs and bones. The three most common are Tuberous sclerosis (TS), neurofibromatosis, and Sturge-Weber syndrome; von Hippel-Lindau disease is less common but equally important to recognize, because frequent monitoring of these patients can dramatically improve their outcome.

Tuberous sclerosis (TS) is inherited in an autosomal dominant fashion, but approximately 50% of all cases are due to new sporadic mutations, so that many children are the first cases in their families. Approximately 75% of patients will be found to have a mutation in one of two separate genes: the TSC1 gene (on chromosome 9) and the TSC2 gene (on chromosome 16). There are many associated clinical manifestations; the mnemonic *HAMARTOMAS* below can help you remember them.

- **H**—*Hamartomas in the skin and CNS.* Hamartomas are benign tumors composed of tissue derived from the area in which the hamartoma grows. Glioneuronal hamartomas (also called cortical tubers) and subependymal nodules are two common examples and are present on brain MRI in nearly 90% of affected children.
- **A**—*Autism, behavioral problems* and *other forms of intellectual disability.* Approximately 50% of children with TS have some form of cognitive disability, often with a history of infantile spasms and seizures.
- **M**—*Mitral valve prolapse* and *mitral regurgitation* are potential cardiac complications.
- **A**—*Ash-leaf spots* are hypopigmented skin macules.
- **R**—*Rhabdomyomas* are benign cardiac tumors that are nearly pathognomonic for TS (although not all children with TS have cardiac rhabdomyomas). They are often asymptomatic and can undergo spontaneous regression, but if large enough, can cause heart failure and arrhythmias. *Retinal hamartomas* can also occur.
- **T**—Tuberous sclerosis (yes, the name of the syndrome is in its own mnemonic—this can prove surprisingly helpful if you remember the mnemonic but forget what it is for!).
- **O**—autosomal dOminant.
- **M**—*Myomatosis (more correctly, lymphangioleiomyomatosis, or LAM),* is a diffuse, fibrotic, cystic lung disease that most often presents with progressive shortness of breath or pneumothorax. It is significantly more common in women and can be fatal.

- **A**—*Angiomyolipomas* are benign renal tumors that can bleed and grow sufficiently large to interfere with renal function, occasionally causing secondary hypertension and chronic kidney disease. *Angiofibromas* are another form of benign hamartomatous tumors that often appear on the face.

- **S**—*Seizures* and *infantile spasms* are a common initial presentation of TS. *Shagreen patches* are thick, leathery patches of skin most often seen on the lower back. *Subependymal giant cell astrocytomas* (known as SEGA tumors) are benign slow-growing tumors usually located within the ventricles. These tumors can present with symptoms of obstructive hydrocephalus such as progressive headache, nausea and vomiting, or with other focal neurologic deficits. Treatment is with surgical resection or—for those who are poor surgical candidates (*e.g.*, if they have multiple lesions or difficult-to-access lesions)—the immunosuppressive agent, everolimus, an inhibitor of the protein kinase, mTOR.

The diagnosis of TS can be made based on genetic testing or the fulfillment of several clinical criteria. Management is multidisciplinary and involves seizure control, serial brain imaging, and management of behavioral and neuropsychiatric conditions. The severity of the disease and long-term prognosis vary greatly from person to person.

Neurofibromatosis types 1 (NF1) and 2 (NF2) are both inherited in an autosomal dominant fashion.

- *NF1* is due to a mutation on chromosome 17 involving a tumor suppressor gene called neurofibromin. It is more common than NF2 and is characterized by cafe au lait spots and neurofibromas (benign tumors that can grow along nerves anywhere in the body; they can be small or plexiform, *i.e.*, big and wormy-appearing). Other features may include axillary freckling, lisch nodules (iris hamartomas), optic pathway gliomas (involving the optic nerves, chiasm, and/or optic radiations), pheochromocytomas, and bone abnormalities.

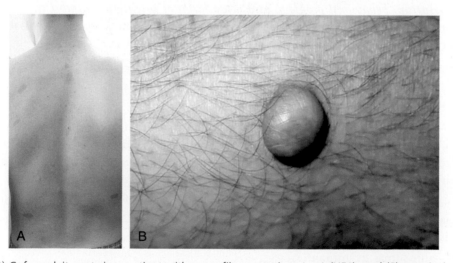

(*A*) Cafe au lait spots in a patient with neurofibromatosis types 1 (NF1), and (*B*) a typical cutaneous neurofibroma. (*A*, Reprinted from Kocher M, Noonan K. *Pediatric Musculoskeletal Physical Diagnosis: A Video-Enhanced Guide.* Wolters Kluwer; 2020. B, Reprinted from Requena L, Kutzner H. *Cutaneous Soft Tissue Tumors.* Wolters Kluwer Health; 2014.)

- *NF2* is due to a mutation on chromosome 22 involving a tumor suppressor gene called merlin. The time-honored NF2 mnemonic is *MISME*: the disease is characterized by **m**ultiple **i**nherited **s**chwannomas (classically bilateral acoustic schwannomas), **m**eningiomas and **e**pendymomas. NF2 can also include neurofibromas (small, not plexiform) and cataracts.

Diagnosis of neurofibromatosis is clinical; it can but does not need to include a positive genetic test. Treatment is multidisciplinary, with frequent tumor screening, surgical tumor resection if indicated, and management of treatable complications.

Sturge-Weber syndrome is congenital, not inherited, and is characterized by a variety of vascular malformations predominantly affecting the face, brain, and eyes. It is the result of an activating mutation of the GNAQ gene, which codes for guanine nucleotide-binding proteins, which in turn affects intracellular signaling and vascular development. We can remember its various clinical manifestations with the mnemonic PIGS (it's a reach, but think of Weber as Wilbur the Pig from E. B. White's novel, *Charlotte's Web*):

- *Port-wine stain* (also known as nevus flammeus) is a common capillary malformation, usually obvious at birth, that appears as a flat pink lesion in the V1-V2 distribution on the face. It is not pathognomonic for Sturge-Weber; most children with a port-wine stain do not have Sturge-Weber. It tends to darken with age and can hypertrophy. Laser treatments are available.

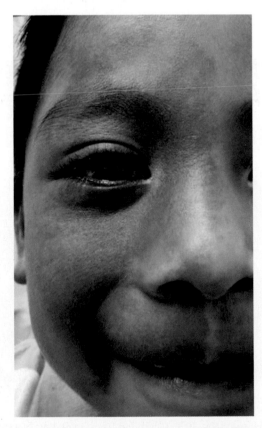

A typical port-wine stain. (Reprinted from *Goodheart's Photoguide to Common Pediatric and Adult Skin Disorders*. 4th ed. Wolters Kluwer; 2015.)

- *Ipsilateral leptomeningeal angiomatosis.* Leptomeningeal capillary-venous malformations usually appear on the same side (*i.e.*, they are ipsilateral) as the port-wine stain; the underlying brain parenchyma is often atrophic and dotted with intraparenchymal dystrophic calcifications. These lesions can cause focal neurologic deficits and seizures.

- *Glaucoma* is the most common ocular abnormality and is the result of the development of episcleral hemangiomas causing elevated intraocular pressure. All patients with Sturge-Weber should see an ophthalmologist regularly for monitoring.

- *Seizures* occur in the majority of patients with Sturge-Weber, usually beginning in childhood, and have a variable response to antiepileptic medications.

The diagnosis of Sturge-Weber syndrome is based on the presence of facial and leptomeningeal capillary malformations, usually best detected with contrast MRI. Treatment requires a multidisciplinary team to manage the cutaneous, neurologic, and ocular manifestations.

Von Hippel-Lindau syndrome is an autosomal dominant condition that results from a mutation in the VHL tumor suppressor gene on chromosome 3. Manifestations are multifocal, and include a variety of benign and malignant tumors, including (but not limited to):

- *Hemangioblastomas:* The most common lesion associated with von Hippel-Lindau; these are benign, highly vascularized tumors that can bleed and are usually located in the cerebellum or spinal cord; for details, see page 398.

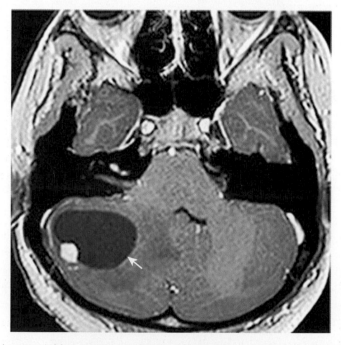

A cerebellar hemangioblastoma in a patient with von Hippel-Lindau syndrome. Note the classic appearance of a cystic lesion with an enhancing mural nodule (similar to the appearance of pilocytic astrocytomas; see page 393). (Modified from Atlas SW. *Magnetic Resonance Imaging of the Brain and Spine.* 5th ed. Wolters Kluwer; 2016.)

- *Cavernomas, also known as cavernous hemangiomas or cavernous malformations:* These are low-flow clusters of abnormal capillaries that can occur throughout the body and are prone to bleeding.

Box 17.1 Cavernous Malformations

Unlike most intracerebral vascular malformations (such as arteriovenous malformations, or AVMs), cavernous malformations are "invisible" on angiography because they have very little blood flow through them. MRI is the gold standard for diagnosis.

- *Clear cell renal carcinoma:* A malignant neoplasm that often requires surgical resection followed by radiation and chemotherapy.
- *Pheochromocytomas:* Benign proliferation of chromaffin cells that characteristically present with the "five Ps": pressure (elevated blood pressure), pain (headache), perspiration, palpitations, and pallor; in von Hippel-Lindau, they tend to occur in younger patients, can be asymptomatic, and can be adrenal or extra-adrenal.
- *Pancreatic tumors:* These include cysts, neuroendocrine tumors, and serous cystadenomas.
- *Retinal capillary hemangioblastomas:* Often multifocal and bilateral; can cause progressive vision loss.
- *Polycystic kidneys and liver.*

The diagnosis of von Hippel-Lindau is typically made by genetic testing. Treatment requires frequent tumor surveillance and management, as indicated.

Box 17.2 Peroxisomal Diseases

Here is one more group of uncommon but important diseases to know about. Peroxisomes are small organelles that, among other things, oxidize very-long-chain fatty acids (VLCFAs). They are most highly concentrated in the liver and kidneys but are found throughout the body. There are three major disorders involving dysfunctional peroxisomes:

1. *Zellweger syndrome* is an autosomal recessive disorder that presents at birth with various craniofacial abnormalities, cataracts, deafness, hepatic and renal dysfunction, severe hypotonia, areflexia, and seizures. Blood work reveals elevated levels of VLCFAs. There is no known treatment and the prognosis is poor.
2. *Refsum disease* is similar, but it can present in infancy or in older children, and tends to be less severe.
3. *Adrenoleukodystrophy* can also present in neonates (an autosomal recessive form known as NALD, or neonatal adrenoleukodystrophy) or in older children or even adults (an x-linked recessive form), and is characterized by both neurologic

Continued

Box 17.2 Peroxisomal Diseases   (Continued)

(seizures, hypotonia, deafness, vision loss) and adrenal (fatigue, vomiting, hyperpigmented skin) dysfunction. The neonatal form tends to be less severe, and less commonly involves the adrenal cortex. As with Zellweger and Refsum diseases, VLCFAs are elevated in the blood. Treatment depends on the precise form of the disease. Routine monitoring is generally recommended for children without evidence of cerebral involvement, whereas hematopoietic stem cell transplant is preferred for children with early cerebral involvement.

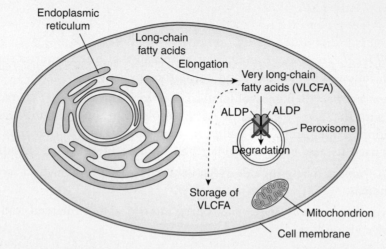

Dysfunction of the adrenoleukodystrophy protein (ALDP)—which transports very-long-chain fatty acids (VLCFA) into the peroxisome to be broken down—results in accumulation of VLCFAs throughout the body.

Mitochondrial Diseases

Genetic mitochondrial diseases are inherited from the mother. They characteristically present with exercise intolerance and unexplained lactic acidosis. Muscle cramps and "second wind" phenomena—as seen in the glycogen storage diseases—are uncommon. There are many mitochondrial diseases; below are several of the most common. There is no proven therapy for these diseases, but there is evidence to suggest that the combination of carnitine, coenzyme Q10, and creatine may provide some benefit.

- *Mitochondrial encephalomyopathy with lactic acidosis and stroke-like episodes (MELAS).* The hallmark of MELAS is recurrent stroke-like episodes that present with acute-onset focal neurologic deficits (the occipital lobe is most often affected, causing visual field cuts and—if bilateral—cortical blindness). We say "stroke-like" because the damage is presumably due to underlying metabolic toxicity and not actual thromboembolic disease; consequently, MELAS-related strokes do not respect vascular territories on MRI, and the diffusion-weighted imaging (DWI) characteristics are variable. Other features of MELAS include short stature, deafness, migraines, cardiomyopathy, and cognitive dysfunction. Symptom onset generally ranges from childhood to young adulthood.

- *Myoclonic epilepsy with ragged red fibers (MERRF)* is characterized by myoclonic seizures and myopathy, with ragged red fibers on biopsy. Other features are similar to those associated with MELAS, including short stature, deafness, cardiomyopathy, and cognitive dysfunction. Lipomatosis (deposits of fat beneath the skin) and optic atrophy may also be seen.

- *Leber hereditary optic neuropathy* presents with painless bilateral vision loss, usually in young men. It often initially affects just one eye but is followed shortly by vision loss in the other. Associated myopathy is uncommon.

- *Leigh syndrome* usually presents within the first year of life with seizures, lactic acidosis, vomiting, generalized weakness, ataxia, and ophthalmoplegia. Developmental delay and psychomotor regression are common, and the prognosis is poor; most children survive only months after the diagnosis is made.

- *Kearns-Sayre syndrome* is characterized by progressive ophthalmoplegia that develops before age 20. Other features can include short stature, pigmentary retinopathy, ataxia, heart block, and cognitive dysfunction. The disease is often fatal by adulthood.

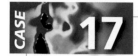

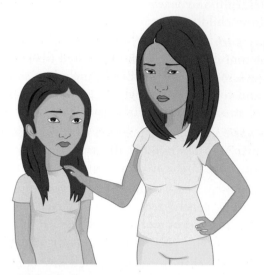

Follow-up on Your Patient: You send Lila to the emergency room for an urgent MRI; the acute-onset of her symptoms is concerning for stroke and—although she is out of the window for any acute intervention—you'd like her to get an expedited work-up. Her MRI shows increased DWI signal predominantly involving the left occipital lobe—the lesion overlaps both middle cerebral artery (MCA) and posterior cerebral artery (PCA) territories and appears swollen on fluid-attenuated inversion recovery (FLAIR). You also can see several other chronic-appearing infarcts. Her laboratory results are unremarkable except for an elevated blood lactate. You suspect MELAS and refer her to a pediatric neurologist and geneticist for further management.

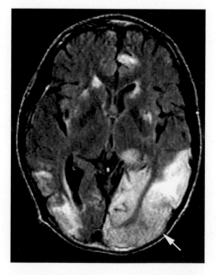

The fluid-attenuated inversion recovery (FLAIR) sequence of Lila's MRI. White arrow points to the large left occipital lesion responsible for Lila's field cut. (Reprinted from Barkovich AJ, Raybaud C. *Pediatric Neuroimaging*. 5th ed. Wolters Kluwer; 2011.)

You now know:

- | The major characteristics of the most common lysosomal and glycogen storage diseases.

- | How to recognize and distinguish among the inherited neurocutaneous diseases that affect the brain and skin: Tuberous sclerosis, neurofibromatosis, Sturge-Weber syndrome, and von Hippel-Lindau disease.

- | To suspect mitochondrial disease when you see a patient with severe exercise intolerance and an otherwise-unexplained elevated blood lactate; glycogen storage diseases can present this way too but are often associated with severe muscle cramps as well.

18 The Cranial Nerves

In this chapter, you will learn:

1 | The basic anatomy and function of each cranial nerve, so that you'll be able to understand where damage to each nerve can occur and what the clinical consequences are

2 | The causes, presentation, and management of oculomotor palsies (*i.e.*, paralysis of one or more of the extraocular muscles due to dysfunction of cranial nerves 3, 4, and/or 6)

3 | Why the seventh cranial nerve can be a bit more complicated than the others, and how to distinguish between lesions of its upper and lower motor neurons

4 | The most common causes of multiple cranial nerve palsies, including cavernous sinus syndrome

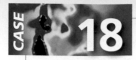

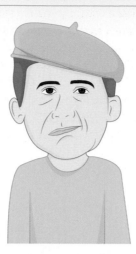

Your Patient: Stanley, a 60-year-old poet, presents to the emergency department with trouble eating for the past 24 hours because of drooling from the right corner of his mouth. You examine him and find that he is unable to fully close his right eye. His face appears symmetric, but when he smiles you note that the right side of his mouth activates less than the left, and when you ask him to raise his eyebrows, you're confident that his right eyebrow doesn't elevate as much as his left. When you rub your fingers together in front of each of his ears, he says he hears better out of his right ear than his left. You look for a ketchup or sugar packet to test Stanley's taste, but can't find anything in the emergency department. His examination is otherwise normal. What's the next step in your management?

The 12 cranial nerves were introduced to you in the first chapter and have continued to pop up throughout this book. This chapter is where we'll condense the most important cranial nerve-related information you need to know. Read it in its entirety, reference it as you go, or use it to solidify what you've already learned; it's up to you. We will be discussing (1) the basic anatomy of the cranial nerves—where they start and where they end—so you will be able to determine where they can run into trouble, (2) what they do, so you can understand what happens when they are damaged, and (3) the most common cranial nerve lesions and pathologies. We will not be discussing pathology involving cranial nerves 8 (discussed in Chapter 5), or 9, 10, 11 and 12 (because disorders involving these nerves rarely come up in practice outside of the brief mentions we've already made of them throughout the text).

Let's start with an overview of cranial nerve anatomy and basic functions.

Cranial Nerve Basics

Except for the olfactory nerve (CN1) and the optic nerve (CN2), all of the cranial nerves are part of the peripheral nervous system. Depending on the particular nerve, they contain motor, sensory, and/or autonomic components and are responsible for most of the non-cognitive things we do with our head: smelling, seeing, tasting, hearing, moving our eyes, chewing, and swallowing. With the exception of the vagus nerve (CN10), which runs from the brainstem down into the thorax and abdomen, they traverse relatively short distances from their nuclei (the collection of cell bodies associated with each nerve) to wherever their functions require them to go.

All of the cranial nerve nuclei are located in the brainstem except for the olfactory (CN1) and optic (CN2) nerves, which originate from the nasal cavity and the retina, respectively. The efferent motor components of the cranial nerves extend from their nuclei to exit the brainstem and ultimately synapse on their motor targets. The afferent sensory components enter the brainstem (or nasal cavity or retina) and terminate on their nuclei, bringing with them sensory information from the face and head. Where the cranial nerves enter and exit the brain is important, because this information will help you localize any lesions. For instance, if you look at the table below, you'll understand why, when a patient presents with acute-onset atraumatic hearing loss, one of the first things to consider is a small pontine stroke.

Exit/Entrance From the Brain	Cranial Nerves
Nasal cavity	1
Retina	2
Midbrain	3, 4[a]
Pons	5, 6, 7, 8
Medulla	9, 10, 12
Superior spinal cord	11

[a]The fourth cranial nerve is the only nerve that exits *dorsally* from the brainstem. It also happens to be the only nerve (besides a branch of the third cranial nerve that you don't need to worry about) that crosses the midline; it decussates to the contralateral side just before it exits the brainstem.

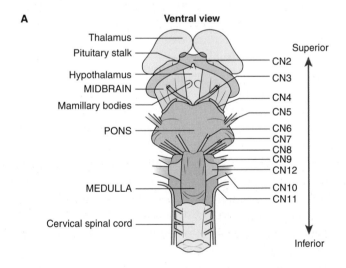

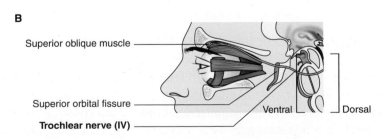

(*A*) A ventral (or anterior) view of the brainstem, showing the entrance and exit of the cranial nerves. (*B*) The fourth cranial nerve exits dorsally (or posteriorly; thus, you can't see its origin on image A), decussates, and then wraps around the pons to head out toward its targets.

CN1, 2, and 8 are pure sensory nerves; CN4, 6, 11, and 12 are pure motor nerves. The rest are some combination of sensory, motor, and autonomic functions. The table below has a lot of important information, so take a minute to look it over. But don't feel like you need to memorize all of this right now. Learn what you need to know at the appropriate time; this table is here to serve as a reference.

Cranial Nerve	Functions
Olfactory (CN1)	Sensory: smell
Optic (CN2)	Sensory: sight
Oculomotor (CN3)	Motor: eyeball movement (superior, inferior, and medial recti and the inferior oblique), eyelid elevation (levator palpebrae)
	Autonomic: pupil constriction (sphincter pupillae), pupil accommodation (ciliary muscle)
Trochlear (CN4)	Motor: eyeball movement (superior oblique)
Trigeminal (CN5)	Sensory: facial sensation (including sensation, but not taste, of the anterior two-thirds of the tongue)
	Motor: jaw movement (muscles of mastication)
Abducens (CN6)	Motor: eyeball movement (lateral rectus)
Facial (CN7)	Motor: facial movement, stapedius (dampens sound)
	Sensory: external ear sensation, taste (anterior two-thirds of tongue)
	Autonomic: lacrimal (tears), submandibular and sublingual (saliva) glands
Vestibulocochlear (CN8)	Sensory: hearing, vestibular function
Glossopharyngeal (CN9)	Motor: stylopharyngeus (pharynx and larynx elevation)
	Sensory: upper pharynx and posterior one-third of tongue sensation, taste (posterior one-third of tongue)
	Autonomic: parotid gland (saliva), chemo- and baroreceptors at the carotid sinus (help to regulate blood pressure and pH)
Vagus (CN10)	Motor: muscles of the palate and pharnyx, cricothyroid (the only laryngeal muscle not innervated by CN11), palatoglossus (the only tongue muscle not innervated by CN12)
	Sensory: pharynx, larynx, and external ear sensation, taste (epiglottis, pharynx)
	Autonomic: thoracoabdominal viscera (heart, lungs, gastrointestinal tract), chemo- and baroreceptors at the aortic arch (help to regulate blood pressure and pH)
Spinal accessory (CN11)	Motor: sternocleidomastoid (turns head to contralateral side), trapezius (scapular stabilization and elevation), intrinsic laryngeal muscles
Hypoglossal (CN12)	Motor: intrinsic tongue muscles

Box 18.1 Tongue Innervation

This can seem complicated and is, for whatever reason, often tested on examinations. So let's make it crystal clear.

- Motor (this is easy): CN12
- Sensory (this isn't as bad as it looks):
  - Sensation: CN5, 9, 10
  - Taste: CN7, 9, 10

	Anterior Two-Thirds	*Posterior One-Third*	*Extreme Posterior, Epiglottis*
Taste	CN7	CN9	CN10
Sensation	CN5	CN9	CN10

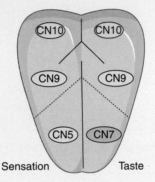

One more way of looking at sensory innervation of the tongue. The posterior one-third is entirely supplied by CN9, and the extreme posterior and epiglottis entirely by CN10.

Brainstem Reflexes

Besides the functions listed above, the cranial nerves also make up several reflexes (aptly known as cranial nerve or brainstem reflexes). These are not routinely tested in awake patients (with the exception of the pupillary reflex) but are a crucial component of examining comatose patients and evaluating patients for possible brain death (see page 367).

The pupillary reflex is worth spending a minute on, because we frequently test it and rely on the information it provides. The pathway below explains why it's a *consensual* reflex: that is, why, if you shine light in one eye, both eyes will constrict.

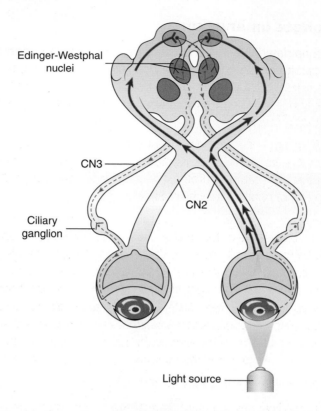

Edinger-Westphal nuclei

CN3

CN2

Ciliary ganglion

Light source

The pupillary reflex pathway, all explained in the text to follow

- **The afferent limb: CN2.** Light strikes the retina, and the information is processed from the outermost layer (which includes the photoreceptors) to the innermost, where the ganglion cell axons travel together in a nerve fiber layer to the optic disc, where they exit the retina as the optic nerve. The optic nerve travels to the optic chiasm (located just below the hypothalamus and above the pituitary gland, the optic chiasm is where the nasal retinal fibers decussate to the contralateral side; see page 432) and then continues as the optic tract. The fibers involved in vision continue on to the thalamus and then the occipital cortex, but those involved in the pupillary reflex separate off to synapse on what are known as the Edinger-Westphal nuclei in the midbrain. The key here is that the optic tract from one eye synapses on BOTH the left and right Edinger-Westphal nuclei, activating both the left and right efferent nerves that will result in bilateral pupillary constriction.

- **The efferent limb: CN3.** Parasympathetic fibers that run within CN3 project from the Edinger-Westphal nuclei to the ciliary ganglion, located just behind the eyeball in the posterior orbit. From here, short ciliary nerves extend to the sphincter pupillae, causing bilateral pupillary constriction.

Box 18.2 A Note on Anisocoria

The term anisocoria describes the condition in which the left and right pupils are of unequal size. It can be physiologic (*i.e.*, entirely normal and benign; the bigger pupil can even switch sides!) or result from a structural or neurologic problem. You also must always ask about the use of medications, in particular eye drops that either constrict or dilate the pupil.

Structural causes are the result of damage within the eye and include trauma, iritis, and angle-closure glaucoma. In these cases, the anisocoria is often also associated with abnormal pupillary shape. Neurologic causes involve damage to or disorders of the nerves that control pupillary reactivity to light.

The first step in evaluating a patient with anisocoria is to determine which pupil is the abnormal pupil, the bigger one or the smaller one. If the smaller pupil is abnormal, the anisocoria should be more prominent in the dark; the normal pupil will dilate appropriately, whereas the affected pupil will remain small. If the larger pupil is abnormal, the anisocoria should be more prominent in bright light; the normal pupil will constrict appropriately, whereas the affected pupil will remain dilated. To help make sense of the various causes of anisocoria, remember that pupillary size is controlled by two opposing muscle groups of the iris: the sphincter pupillae (which constricts the pupil and is parasympathetic mediated) and the dilator pupillae (which dilates the pupil and is sympathetic mediated).

Causes of unilateral miosis (or pupillary constriction) include:

- **Medications:** Medications that stimulate the parasympathetic nervous system (often referred to as "*choline*rgic" medications; acetyl*choline* is the neurotransmitter involved at all parasympathetic targets) will cause miosis. One important example is pilocarpine eye drops. Pilocarpine is a direct acetylcholine receptor agonist that is used to lower intraocular pressure in patients with ocular hypertension or frank glaucoma.
- **Horner syndrome:** This is caused by a lesion along the sympathetic pathway; see page 310 for details. A lesion of the sympathetic pathway results in unopposed parasympathetic activity, hence miosis.
- **Primary ocular pathology:** This can be the result of previous ocular surgery or iritis, among other disorders.

Causes of unilateral mydriasis (or pupillary dilation) include:

- **Medications:** Medications that stimulate the sympathetic nervous system (sympathomimetics) or that block the parasympathetic nervous system (anticholinergics) will cause mydriasis. Among these are anticholinergics such as atropine eye drops and ipratropium nebulizers (sometimes some of the aerosolized medication sneaks into the corner of one eye or the other), as well as sympathomimetics such as topical phenylephrine.
- **Third cranial nerve palsy:** See the discussion coming up on page 434.
- **Adie tonic pupil:** This is a common condition that affects as many as 2 in 1000 in the general population, females more often than males. It is the result of damage to the parasympathetic ciliary ganglion that supplies the eye. Most cases are idiopathic (possibly caused by an undefined viral infection), but the condition

(Continued)

Box 18.2 A Note on Anisocoria (Continued)

can also be the result of an inflammatory, an infectious, or a neoplastic process. The affected pupil is often dramatically larger than the other pupil; it barely constricts to light (if at all) but constricts well to accommodation, after which it remains tonically constricted, remaining small much longer than the unaffected eye. This characteristic—reacting poorly to light but well to accommodation—is known as *light-near dissociation.* Idiopathic Adie pupil is benign and requires no treatment.

- **Ocular trauma:** Injury to the pupillary sphincter muscle can result in abnormal mydriasis.

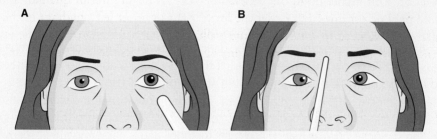

A left-sided Adie pupil. (*A*) The pupil reacts poorly to direct light but (*B*) reacts well to accommodation.

If you remember nothing else from this chapter, however, remember this: *a dilated and unreactive (or so-called blown) pupil in a patient with depressed consciousness should prompt immediate concern for brain herniation* (see page 363). A "blown" pupil in an awake, talking, and otherwise normal patient? Not herniation. Instead, consider the causes in this box for the potential explanation.

Other important cranial nerve reflexes to know include the corneal, lacrimal, jaw jerk, vestibulo-ocular (see page 144), gag, and carotid sinus reflexes.

	Afferent	Efferent	What Actually Happens
Pupillary	CN2	CN3 (to sphincter pupillae)	Bright light causes pupils to constrict
Corneal	CN5	CN7 (to orbicularis oculi)	Touching the cornea causes the eye to blink
Lacrimal	CN5	CN7 (to lacrimal gland)	Touching the cornea causes the eye to tear
Jaw jerk	CN5 (V3; sensory branch from masseter)	CN5 (V3; motor branch to masseter)	Tapping the jaw causes jaw contraction
Vestibulo-ocular	CN8	CN3 (to oculomotor muscles)	Stabilizes vision during head movement
Gag	CN9	CN10 (to pharyngeal muscles)	Irritation in the back of the throat causes pharyngeal muscle contraction
Carotid sinus	CN9	CN10 (to heart)	Pressure on the carotid sinus results in bradycardia

Common Cranial Nerve Pathology

We've discussed a number of these disorders already, but let's take this opportunity to synthesize the information you've already learned and explore a bit deeper into their pathophysiology, presentation, and, when relevant, management.

Visual Field Defects

To understand why a lesion within the thalamus can cause a homonymous hemianopia (*i.e.*, a visual field defect involving either the right or left halves of the visual field of each eye), whereas a lesion a bit higher up in the parietal lobe can cause an inferior quadrantanopia (*i.e.*, a visual field defect involving either the lower right or lower left quadrant of the visual field of each eye), we need to spend a minute walking through the anatomy of the visual pathway (note how these pathways differ from those involved in the pupillary reflex).

How CN2 exits from the eye and orbit:

- As mentioned earlier, when light strikes the retina, information is processed from the outermost layer (where the photoreceptors are located) to the innermost, where the ganglion cell axons travel together in a nerve fiber layer to the optic disc. Here, they exit the retina and the orbit as the optic nerve.

How CN2 enters the CNS:

- As it enters the CNS, CN2 becomes covered in myelin made by oligodendrocytes. It travels to the **optic chiasm**, where the nasal retinal fibers (see diagram on page 432) decussate to the contralateral side. The temporal retinal fibers do not cross and remain on the side of the brain from which they originated. There are therefore two optic tracts that exit the optic chiasm, each containing contralateral nasal fibers and ipsilateral temporal fibers. Thus, each optic tract carries fibers that supply the contralateral visual field of each eye (*i.e.*, the right optic tract supplies the left visual field of both eyes, and the left optic tract supplies the right visual field of both eyes).

- The **optic tracts** synapse at the **lateral geniculate nucleus** of the thalamus.

- From here, the fibers split into the **optic radiations**; those supplying the inferior visual field travel within the parietal lobe, whereas those supplying the superior visual field travel within the temporal lobe.

- The fibers come together again in the occipital lobe, in the **primary visual cortex**. From here, they extend to visual association areas throughout the cortex, where complex visual cues are processed and synthesized.

If your head hurts after reading this, we don't blame you. Take a minute to look at the diagram below, which explains the vision pathway better than words ever could. The most important takeaway lessons here are:

- Lesions of the optic nerve itself (prechiasmal lesions) result in unilateral visual defects (*i.e.*, the entire visual field of one eye is damaged)

- Lesions of the optic tract (postchiasmal lesions) result in bilateral visual field defects (*i.e.*, either the left or right visual field of *both* eyes is damaged)

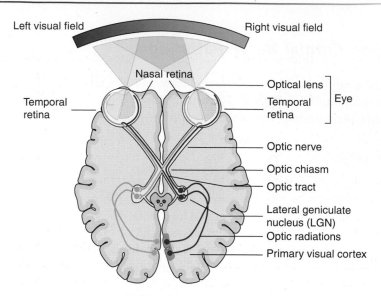

The visual pathway.

You should now be able to work out why the lesions listed below result in the associated visual field defects.

Lesion	Visual Field Defect	
Optic nerve	Unilateral vision loss	A prechiasmal lesion of the optic nerve affects only one eye
Optic chiasm	Bitemporal hemianopia	A lesion at the optic chiasm will catch the bilateral nasal retinal fibers (which supply the bilateral temporal visual fields) as they cross
Optic tract	Homonymous hemianopia	A lesion of the left optic tract will result in loss of the right visual field of both eyes, and vice versa
Temporal radiation	Superior quadrantanopia	The temporal radiations carry inferior retinal fibers, which supply the superior visual field

Lesion	Visual Field Defect	
Parietal radiation	Inferior quadrantanopia	The parietal radiations carry superior retinal fibers, which supply the inferior visual field
Visual cortex	Homonymous hemianopia	The temporal and parietal radiations rejoin in the occipital cortex

One last point: if the lesion of the visual cortex is caused by a posterior cerebral artery (PCA) infarct, it will likely result in ***macular sparing***, because the area of the cortex dedicated to the macula (unlike that dedicated to the rest of the visual field, which is supplied only by the PCA) has a dual blood supply (PCA + middle cerebral artery, or MCA) and is thus spared from ischemia.

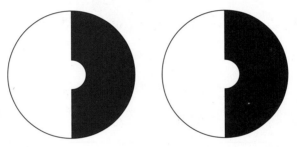

Macular sparing caused by a PCA infarct. The macula is the central area of the retina.

Oculomotor Palsies (Third, Fourth and Sixth Nerve Palsies)

The third, fourth, and sixth cranial nerves are responsible for the extraocular muscles (the muscles that control eye movements). Dysfunction of or damage to these nerves is common and results in various forms of restricted, abnormal eye movements (oculomotor palsies). Here's a summary of the 6 extraocular muscles and what they do:

Extraocular Muscle	Function	Supplied by
Superior rectus	Elevation	CN3
Inferior rectus	Depression	CN3
Medial rectus	Adduction	CN3
Lateral rectus	Abduction	CN6
Superior oblique	Internal rotation, depression	CN4
Inferior oblique	External rotation, elevation	CN3

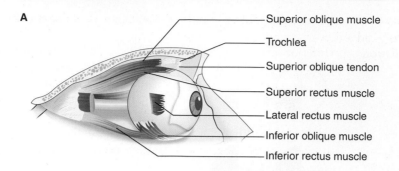

Lateral view of the right eye

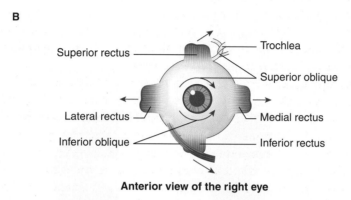

Anterior view of the right eye

Lateral (*A*) and anterior (*B*) views of the 6 extraocular muscles.

Third Nerve Palsy Lesions anywhere along the path of the third cranial nerve, from its nucleus in the midbrain to the extraocular muscles it innervates within the orbit, can result in a third nerve palsy. If you can remember what CN3 does, you already know how a CN3 palsy will present. And remember, besides CN4, no cranial nerves cross the midline; thus, all deficits are ipsilateral to the lesion.

- A "down and out" eye. CN3 supplies the superior, inferior, and medial rectus muscles as well as the inferior oblique, but perhaps more useful is to remember what it *doesn't* supply: the superior oblique (which pulls the eye "down and in") and the lateral rectus (which pulls the eye "out"). When CN3 is damaged, these muscles "take over" and result in an eye that appears "down and out."

- Mydriasis. The parasympathetic fibers of CN3 supply the sphincter pupillae, the muscle that constricts the pupil; damage therefore results in pupillary dilation.

- Ptosis.[1] CN3 supplies the levator palpebrae, which elevates the eyelid; damage results in eyelid drooping, or ptosis.

---

[1]For a review of the causes of ptosis, see page 309.

Patients often won't notice the pupillary abnormalities, but they will complain of diplopia (double vision) and a droopy eyelid.

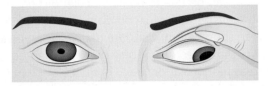

A left third nerve palsy. Notice the down and out position of the eye, the dilated pupil, and the droopy eyelid.

Ischemia (often due to microvascular disease caused by poorly controlled diabetes) is the most common cause of third nerve palsies in adults, but compression of the third nerve by a nearby aneurysm is the most feared. The third nerve runs near the posterior cerebral artery (see diagram on page 49); aneurysmal dilation of the posterior cerebral or posterior communicating arteries can therefore compress the nerve.

Because the parasympathetic fibers of CN3 run on the outside of the nerve, compression of the nerve should always cause pupillary involvement (*i.e.*, mydriasis). Ischemia or infarction of the nerve, on the other hand, often spares the parasympathetic fibers, and pupils can react normally. If you see a complete third nerve palsy with pupil involvement, you are obligated to order vessel imaging (either CT or MR angiogram) to rule out an aneurysm. Most textbooks will tell you that you do not need to order the scan if the third nerve palsy is pupil sparing, but we still often order the scan if possible. Why? Anatomy is variable and examinations are imperfect, and the risk of missing an aneurysm outweighs the risks of a potentially unnecessary scan.

Other causes of third nerve palsies include trauma, neoplasm (pituitary tumor, meningeal carcinomatosis), ophthalmoplegic migraine, cavernous sinus syndrome (see page 441), inflammatory disorders (GBS; see page 284), and uncal herniation (see page 365). It's also worth mentioning that, although most third nerve palsies caused by ischemia are peripheral (*i.e.*, affecting the axons of the nerve itself, due to microvascular disease), they can also be central (due to ischemic strokes affecting the midbrain nucleus of the nerve).

Patching of one eye can be useful for alleviating diplopia, but treatment is otherwise directed at the underlying etiology. In the case of ischemic third nerve palsies, there is no specific treatment besides controlling cardiovascular risk factors (diabetes, hypertension, and hyperlipidemia). Recovery typically takes weeks to months. Deficits that persist at 6 months tend to be permanent.

Fourth Nerve Palsy Fourth nerve palsies are less common than third nerve palsies. Patients will also complain of diplopia, but the eye on examination will be "up and out" owing to dysfunction of the superior oblique muscle (which, to remind you, pulls the eye down and in). A head tilt to the contralateral side will help to correct the diplopia.

Most cases are congenital, even those that present in adulthood. Although patients may insist that the problem is new, more often it is due to a gradually decreasing ability to compensate for the diplopia. Because the fourth nerve has the longest intracranial course

Box 18.3 Diplopia

Diplopia, or double vision, can be due to primary ocular or primary neurologic dysfunction. When you see a patient who complains of diplopia, there is a single question you must ask to sort this out: *does the double vision persist when the patient closes one eye or the other, or is it only present when both eyes are open?* The former (referred to as monocular diplopia) is an ocular problem. Something is wrong in the eye itself. The latter (binocular diplopia) is a neurologic problem. "Neurologic" diplopia is the result of ocular misalignment: one or more of the extraocular muscles is not working properly, and the eyes are not yoked together as they should be. For example, if a patient with a left sixth nerve palsy tries to look to the left, the left eye will be stuck looking straight ahead while the right eye fully adducts to the left. This causes diplopia; the two eyes are unable to focus on the same target. But there is nothing inherently wrong with the left eyeball, and thus, when the right eye is closed, the diplopia disappears.

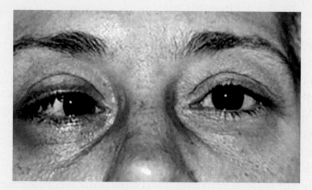

A left sixth nerve palsy. (Reprinted from Nelson L. *Pediatric Ophthalmology*. 2nd ed. Wolters Kluwer; 2018.)

of any cranial nerve, it is also particularly susceptible to compression from trauma, elevated intracranial pressure, and other intracranial lesions. Microvascular disease and ischemia can also cause fourth nerve palsies. As with third nerve palsies, treatment is directed at the underlying etiology.

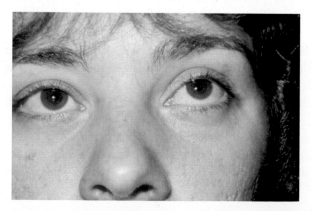

A left fourth nerve palsy. (Courtesy of Leonard B. Nelson, MD.)

Sixth Nerve Palsy Sixth nerve palsies are the most common oculomotor palsy to occur in isolation. Again, patients will present with diplopia but on examination will be unable to fully abduct the affected eye owing to dysfunction of the lateral rectus muscle.

Common causes include ischemia (which, again, can be due to microvascular disease affecting the axons of the nerve itself or stroke affecting its nucleus in the pons), trauma, neoplasm, and elevated intracranial pressure (which can result in bilateral sixth nerve palsies due to traction of the nerves at the skull base). Treatment is directed at the underlying cause.

Box 18.4: What Happened to Fifth Nerve Palsy?

Why have we skipped over the fifth cranial nerve, you may ask? Trigeminal neuralgia is, essentially, the sensory equivalent of a fifth nerve palsy and is discussed in detail in Chapter 3 on headache.

Facial (Seventh) Nerve Palsy

We introduced you to facial nerve palsies in Chapter 11 on peripheral neuropathies. Now it's time to dig a little deeper. When we think about facial nerve palsies, we must distinguish between upper and lower motor neuron lesions. Upper motor neuron (UMN) facial palsies are due to lesions of the nerves that innervate CN7 (*i.e.*, the UMNs that travel between the motor cortex and the facial nerve nucleus in the brainstem). Lower motor neuron (LMN) facial palsies are due to lesions of CN7 itself. We don't make this distinction with other cranial nerve palsies because all other cranial nerves (besides CN12, which has predominantly contralateral innervation) are bilaterally innervated, and thus unilateral upper motor neuron lesions cause no deficits.

The anatomy of the facial nerve motor nucleus is complicated. The part of the nucleus that supplies the upper face receives bilateral UMN innervation; the part that supplies the lower face receives only contralateral UMN innervation. As a result, *a unilateral UMN lesion results in contralateral facial paralysis that spares the forehead, whereas an LMN lesion results in ipsilateral facial paralysis of the entire face.*

Besides making every student's day a little bit worse, what's the point of learning all of this anatomy? As it turns out, the ability to distinguish—and to distinguish quickly—between upper and lower motor neuron lesions of the seventh cranial nerve can be critical for diagnosing the cause of the deficit and determining its subsequent management.

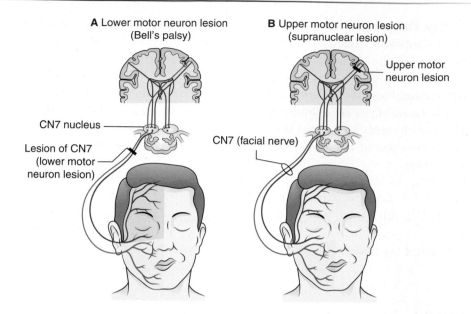

A Lower motor neuron lesion
(Bell's palsy)

B Upper motor neuron lesion
(supranuclear lesion)

Upper motor
neuron lesion

CN7 nucleus

Lesion of CN7
(lower motor
neuron lesion)

CN7 (facial nerve)

Lower versus upper motor neuron facial nerve palsies. Lower motor neuron involvement affects the entire face, whereas upper motor neuron involvement spares the forehead.

Upper Motor Neuron Facial Palsy. Stroke is the most common cause of upper motor neuron facial palsy; other mass lesions affecting the motor fibers that extend to the facial nerve nucleus, such as tumors and abscesses, are less common causes. If a patient presents with a forehead-sparing facial paralysis, assume the patient is experiencing a stroke until proven otherwise and treat the patient as such. If the upper face is involved, however, as is the case with our patient, Stanley, at the beginning of this chapter, who can't fully elevate his eyebrow or shut his eye, you can (most of the time) take a deep breath and relax. Keep in mind, however, that stroke can cause lower motor neuron facial palsy as well. Lateral pontine infarcts, for instance, can involve the nucleus of CN7 and present with a complete ipsilateral facial paralysis. In these cases, however, there are almost always other associated neurologic deficits (in the case of a lateral pontine infarct these can include ipsilateral facial numbness, hearing loss, and Horner syndrome, as well as contralateral body numbness) to tip you off to the correct diagnosis.

Lower Motor Neuron Facial Palsy. This type of facial nerve palsy is far more common than the upper motor neuron variant. Isolated lower motor neuron facial palsies are most often idiopathic; it is then referred to as *Bell palsy.* Herpes simplex virus type 2 (HSV-2) is thought to be responsible for the majority of these "idiopathic" cases, but this can be difficult to confirm. There are also autoimmune causes (especially Sjogren syndrome and sarcoidosis), neoplastic causes, and infectious causes (including HIV, Lyme disease, and shingles [herpes zoster]). When shingles affects the facial nerve, the patient is said to have *Ramsay Hunt syndrome* (aka herpes zoster oticus); you will typically see the characteristic vesicular rash of herpes zoster near the ear. Regardless of etiology, the ipsilateral facial palsy can be accompanied by decreased taste on the anterior two-thirds of the tongue as well as hyperacusis (*i.e.*, normal sounds are perceived as very loud), due to involvement of the stapedius muscle. Vertigo can also be present if the nearby eighth cranial nerve is also affected.

The diagnosis of Bell palsy is clinical. If the presentation is straightforward, that is, if there are no other focal findings on examination in a patient with ipsilateral involvement of the upper and lower facial muscles, imaging is not necessary. Most patients will improve and make a full recovery within weeks to months (but see Box 18.5 for a discussion of some potential long-term complications). A short course of corticosteroids is recommended for patients who present shortly after symptom onset. Although there is no proven benefit, valacyclovir is also often prescribed for patients with severe symptoms; it is well tolerated with few side effects and may offer some additional benefit when combined with corticosteroids in this patient population. The use of eye lubricants or an eye patch can be helpful in preventing dryness, and sunglasses should be worn during the day to protect the eye that cannot fully close.

Box 18.5 Synkinesis

When voluntary muscle activation causes simultaneous, involuntary contraction of other muscles, the phenomenon is called synkinesis, and it is a common long-term sequela of facial nerve palsy. Synkinesis occurs when the axons that regenerate following nerve damage head to the wrong targets and end up innervating incorrect muscles. A common example is involuntary eyelid twitching that occurs with voluntary smiling: misdirected axons that originally supplied the mouth muscles regenerate to supply the orbicularis oculi muscle as well, and thus, when stimulated, cause both smiling and eyelid closure. Another example is known as "crocodile tears," when axons that originally supplied the salivary glands mistakenly innervate the lacrimal glands as well, resulting in tears while eating.

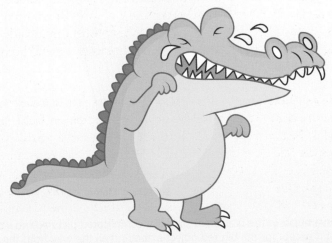

Crocodile tears are a classic example of synkinesis. The term "crocodile tears" has a long history, and goes back to the belief that crocodiles cried - insincerely - before attacking their prey. Alas, this is something our ancestors got completely wrong.

Multiple Cranial Nerve Palsies

There are a handful of diseases that can result in multiple cranial nerve palsies. Some "pick off" cranial nerves gradually and progressively; others damage the nerves simultaneously and all at once. It's good to keep the following differential in the back of your mind, because every single one of these is a "do not miss" diagnosis.

- *CNS infections*, including Lyme disease, listeria, syphilis, and cryptococcus.
- *Autoimmune diseases*, such as Guillain-Barre syndrome and neurosarcoidosis.
- *Malignancy.* Leptomeningeal carcinomatosis (*i.e.*, spread of cancer cells into the cerebrospinal fluid, with involvement of the pia and arachnoid membranes) is discussed further in Chapter 16.
- *Stroke.* Hemorrhagic and ischemic brainstem strokes can and often do involve various combinations of the lower cranial nerves (see page 67). A quick pearl to remember: the nucleus of the fifth cranial nerve is large (the nerve itself exits the brainstem in the pons, but the nucleus extends from the midbrain to the high cervical spinal cord), and thus both lateral pontine and lateral medullary strokes can cause ipsilateral loss of sensation on the face.

Cranial nerve nuclei in brainstem

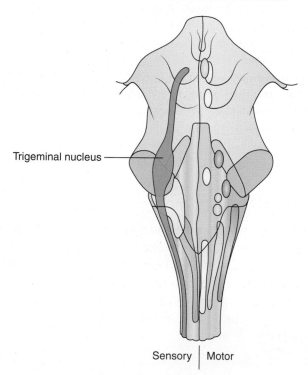

Trigeminal nucleus

Sensory | Motor

The cranial nerve nuclei in the brainstem. This is a complicated picture, and you should feel free to ignore all of it except for the big red object extending all the way from the midbrain into the medulla and high cervical spinal cord: this is the trigeminal nucleus.

- **_Cavernous sinus syndrome._** The cavernous sinus is a collection of dural venous sinuses surrounding the pituitary gland. CN3, CN4, V1 and V2 of CN5, and CN6 pass through it, along with the internal carotid artery (ICA), the sympathetic fibers serving the face and head, and the ophthalmic veins draining blood from the eye. Any pathology within the sinus, most commonly venous sinus thrombosis, mass lesions and fistulas, can result in dysfunction of any of these structures. Classic neurologic symptoms include painful ophthalmoplegia (due to paralysis of one or more of the extraocular muscles; the lateral rectus, supplied by CN6, is the most commonly affected), reduced maxillary and corneal sensation (due to involvement of V1 and V2), Horner syndrome (due to sympathetic damage), and proptosis (due to blocked ophthalmic veins). Visual acuity is preserved, because CN2 does not run through the cavernous sinus.

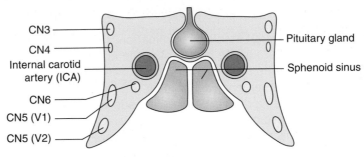

The contents of the cavernous sinus include CN3, CN4, V1 and V2 of CN5, CN6, the internal carotid artery, sympathetic fibers (which run on the surface of the internal carotid artery), and the ophthalmic veins (not pictured here).

Box 18.6 Tolosa-Hunt Syndrome

Tolosa-Hunt syndrome is characterized by idiopathic granulomatous inflammation of the cavernous sinus. It most often presents with severe, unilateral, periorbital headache and painful ophthalmoplegia. Horner syndrome can also occur. Episodes typically resolve spontaneously and then recur every few months to years. MRI with contrast and, if needed, biopsy demonstrating granulomatous inflammation can help make the diagnosis. High-dose steroids are very effective and tend to significantly improve symptoms within a few days.

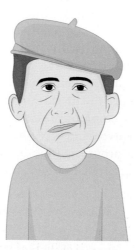

Your Patient's Follow-up: Stanley's examination is consistent with a lower motor neuron facial palsy. Because he has no other neurologic symptoms, you're comfortable telling him that he has a Bell palsy, most likely due to a herpes infection. You reassure the emergency department attending that imaging or any other further neurologic workup is unnecessary and discharge Stanley with a prescription for a short course of corticosteroids and valacyclovir, as well as eye lubricant to help protect his right eye. When you call him 3 weeks later to check in, he tells you that his symptoms, although not fully resolved, have greatly improved and continue to get better each day.

You now know:

- | Where each cranial nerve starts and ends, and what each cranial nerve does
- | The most common causes of third, fourth, and sixth nerve palsies, how they present, and how to treat them
- | How to differentiate between upper and lower motor neuron facial palsies, and why this matters
- | The basic differential diagnosis of multiple cranial nerve palsies

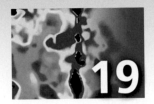

Is That All There Is?

19

Well, no, of course not. There is no limit to the amount of neurology you could stuff into your brain if you chose to, and we certainly don't want to stop you. Hopefully, though, this book has taken you a long way along the path to neurologic nirvana. And for many of you, this really will be *The Only Neurology Book You'll Ever Need*. For others, we hope this is the start of a great adventure in exploring an organ system that is not only an important source of good health (when it works right) and an alarming array of diseases (when it misfires) but one that actually defines who we really are.

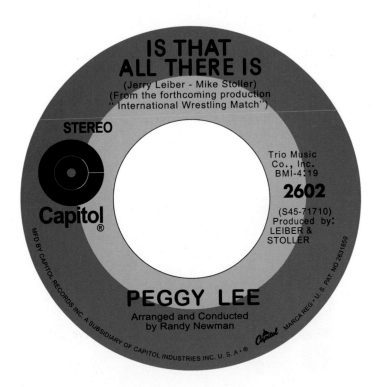

A copy of the 1969 45 rpm recording by Peggy Lee of the Leiber and Stoller classic, "*Is That All There Is.*"

So pat yourself on the back and think about how much you have learned. You are now able to diagnose and manage everything from strokes to multiple sclerosis; seizures to dementia; concussion to neuropathies; dizziness to migraines to confusion. You've also mastered your neurologic toolbox, composed of a careful neurologic history, examination, blood and cerebrospinal fluid (CSF) studies, imaging and electrodiagnostic tools, and can figure out pretty much anything that is going on with your patients, no matter how obscure or complicated.

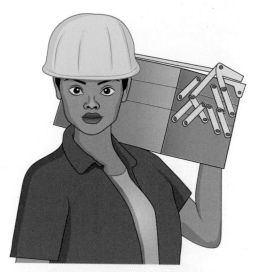

Not a neurologic toolbox, but you get the idea.

It has been a genuine privilege and pleasure to have spent this time with you. We appreciate your patience and your courage. You've worked hard, and it took more than a little *nerve* to follow this journey from beginning to end!

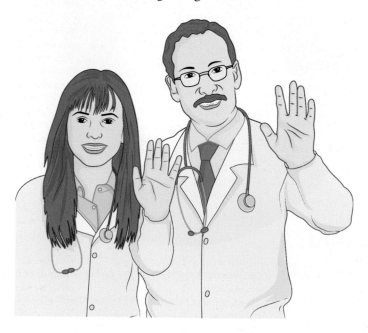

Index

Note: Page numbers followed by "*f*" indicate figures, "*t*" indicate tables and "*b*" indicate boxes.